D0855730

Pediatric
Imaging

A Teaching File

Pediatric
Imaging
A Teaching File

Mahesh Thapa, MD
Associate Professor of Radiology
Director, Pediatric Radiology Fellowship
University of Washington School of Medicine
Seattle Children's Hospital
Seattle, Washington

Edward Weinberger, MD
Professor and Vice Chair of Radiology
Professor of Neurological Surgery
Adjunct Professor of Pediatrics
University of Washington School of Medicine
Director, Department of Radiology
Seattle Children's Hospital
Seattle, Washington

Wolters Kluwer | Lippincott Williams & Wilkins
Health
Philadelphia · Baltimore · New York · London
Buenos Aires · Hong Kong · Sydney · Tokyo

Executive Editor: Jonathan W. Pine, Jr.
Product Manager: Amy G. Dinkel
Vendor Manager: Marian Bellus
Senior Manufacturing Manager: Benjamin Rivera
Senior Marketing Manager: Caroline Foote
Design Coordinator: Holly McLaughlin
Production Service: Aptara, Inc.

© 2013 by LIPPINCOTT WILLIAMS & WILKINS, a Wolters KLUWER business
2001 Market Street
Philadelphia, PA 19103 USA
LWW.com

All rights reserved. This book is protected by copyright. No part of this book may be reproduced in any form by any means, including photocopying, or utilized by any information storage and retrieval system without written permission from the copyright owner, except for brief quotations embodied in critical articles and reviews. Materials appearing in this book prepared by individuals as part of their official duties as U.S. government employees are not covered by the above-mentioned copyright.

Printed in China

Library of Congress Cataloging-in-Publication Data
Pediatric imaging : a teaching file / [edited by] Mahesh Thapa, Edward Weinberger.
   p. ; cm.
 Includes bibliographical references and index.
 ISBN 978-1-60831-856-8 (alk. paper)
 I. Thapa, Mahesh. II. Weinberger, Edward.
 [DNLM: 1. Diagnostic Imaging–methods—Case Reports. 2. Child.
3. Infant. WN 240]
618.92'007575—dc23   2012018450

Care has been taken to confirm the accuracy of the information presented and to describe generally accepted practices. However, the authors, editors, and publisher are not responsible for errors or omissions or for any consequences from application of the information in this book and make no warranty, expressed or implied, with respect to the currency, completeness, or accuracy of the contents of the publication. Application of the information in a particular situation remains the professional responsibility of the practitioner.

The authors, editors, and publisher have exerted every effort to ensure that drug selection and dosage set forth in this text are in accordance with current recommendations and practice at the time of publication. However, in view of ongoing research, changes in government regulations, and the constant flow of information relating to drug therapy and drug reactions, the reader is urged to check the package insert for each drug for any change in indications and dosage and for added warnings and precautions. This is particularly important when the recommended agent is a new or infrequently employed drug.

Some drugs and medical devices presented in the publication have Food and Drug Administration (FDA) clearance for limited use in restricted research settings. It is the responsibility of the health care provider to ascertain the FDA status of each drug or device planned for use in their clinical practice.

To purchase additional copies of this book, call our customer service department at (800) 638-3030 or fax orders to (301) 223-2320. International customers should call (301) 223-2300.

Visit Lippincott Williams & Wilkins on the Internet: at LWW.com. Lippincott Williams & Wilkins customer service representatives are available from 8:30 am to 6 pm, EST.

10 9 8 7 6 5 4 3 2 1

I dedicate this work to my wife, Cindy, and our newborn son, Kishore, who bring joy and balance to my life.

—Mahesh Thapa, MD

I dedicate this work to my mother, Emma Weinberger, my wife, Dr. Sarah Katherine Bloomer, and our two children, Eli and Kate. My life would be empty without them.

—Edward Weinberger, MD

Chaitra Badve, MBBS
Neuroradiology Fellow
Case Western Reserve University School of
    Medicine
Cleveland, Ohio

Puneet Bhargava, MBBS, DNB
Assistant Professor
University of Washington School of Medicine
Staff Radiologist
VA Puget Sound Health Care System
Seattle, Washington

Deepa Reddy Biyyam, MBBS, DMRD
Pediatric Radiology Fellow
University of Washington School of Medicine
Seattle Children's Hospital
Seattle, Washington

Teresa Chapman, MD, MA
Assistant Professor of Radiology
University of Washington School of Medicine
Seattle Children's Hospital
Seattle, Washington

Apeksha Chaturvedi, MBBS
Assistant Professor of Radiology
University of Rochester School of Medicine
Rochester, New York

Deborah Conway, MD
Associate Clinical Professor
Mercer University
Program Director, Radiology Residency
    Program
Director of Pediatric Imaging
Memorial Health University Medical Center
Savannah, Georgia

Megan E. Daigle, MD
Resident, Department of Radiology
Memorial University Medical Center
Savannah, Georgia

Stephen E. Darling, MD
Pediatric Radiology Fellow
University of Washington School of Medicine
Seattle Children's Hospital
Seattle, Washington

Matthew D. Dobbs, MD
Resident, Department of Radiology and
    Radiological Sciences
Vanderbilt University Medical Center
Nashville, Tennessee

Mark R. Ferguson, MD
Assistant Professor of Radiology
University of Washington School of Medicine
Seattle Children's Hospital
Seattle, Washington

Kathleen R. Fink, MD
Assistant Professor
Department of Radiology
University of Washington
Seattle, Washington

Stephen L. Foster, MD
Pediatric Radiologist
Naval Medical Center, Portsmouth
Charette Health Care Center
Portsmouth, Virginia

Gisele E. Ishak MD
Assistant Professor of Radiology
University of Washington School of Medicine
Seattle Children's Hospital
Seattle, Washington

Ramesh S. Iyer, MD
Assistant Professor of Radiology
University of Washington School of Medicine
Seattle Children's Hospital
Seattle, Washington

J. Herman Kan, MD
Assistant Professor
Radiologic Sciences and Pediatrics
Monroe Carell Jr. Children's Hospital at
    Vanderbilt University
Nashville, Tennessee

Paritosh C. Khanna, MD
Assistant Professor of Radiology
University of Washington School of
    Medicine
Seattle Children's Hospital
Seattle, Washington

Anisha Martin, MD
Resident
Department of Radiology
Vanderbilt University Medical Center
Nashville, Tennessee

Prakash Masand, MD
Attending Radiologist
Department of Pediatric Radiology
Texas Children's Hospital
Houston, Texas

Ho Nguyen, MD
PGY-4
Department of Diagnostic Radiology
University of California Davis Medical
    Center
Sacramento, California

Jason N. Nixon, MD
Pediatric Radiology Fellow
University of Washington School of
    Medicine
Seattle Children's Hospital
Seattle, Washington

Randolph K. Otto, MD
Assistant Professor of Radiology
Adjunct Assistant Professor of Cardiology
University of Washington School of
    Medicine
Seattle Children's Hospital
Seattle, Washington

Angelisa M. Paladin, MD
Associate Professor of Radiology
University of Washington School of Medicine
Seattle Children's Hospital
Seattle, Washington

Marguerite T. Parisi, MD, MSEd
Professor of Radiology
Adjunct Professor of Pediatrics
University of Washington School of Medicine
Division Chief, Ultrasound
Seattle Children's Hospital
Seattle, Washington

Grace S. Phillips, MD
Associate Professor of Radiology
University of Washington School of
    Medicine
Division Chief, Computed Tomography
Seattle Children's Hospital
Seattle, Washington

Debra J. Popejoy, MD
Assistant Professor
Pediatric Fellowship Director
Department of Orthopaedic Surgery and
    Pediatric Orthopaedic Surgery
Lawrence J. Ellison Ambulatory Care
    Center
Shriners Hospital for Children
Sacramento, California

Sumit Pruthi, MBBS
Assistant Professor of Radiology
Pediatric Radiology and Neuroradiology
Monroe Carell Jr. Children's Hospital at
    Vanderbilt University
Nashville, Tennessee

Robert P. Raines-Hepple, MD
Pediatric Radiology Fellow
University of Washington School of
    Medicine
Seattle Children's Hospital
Seattle, Washington

Molly E. Raske, MD
Pediatric Radiologist
St. Paul Radiology
Gillette Children's Specialty Healthcare
St. Paul, Minnesota

Marla Sammer, MD
Section Chief
Pediatric Radiology
Children's Hospital at Erlanger
Chatanooga, Tennessee

Sudha P. Singh, MBBS, MD
Assistant Professor
Vanderbilt University
Nashville, Tennessee

Luana Stanescu, MD
Acting Assistant Professor of Radiology
University of Washington School of Medicine
Seattle Children's Hospital
Seattle, Washington

Jonathan O. Swanson, MD
Assistant Professor of Radiology
University of Washington School of Medicine
Seattle Children's Hospital
Seattle, Washington

Kalyan C. Tatineny, MD
Pediatric Radiology Fellow
University of Washington School of Medicine
Seattle Children's Hospital
Seattle, Washington

Jennifer L. Williams, MD
Assistant Professor
Department of Pediatric-Radiology
Baylor College of Medicine
Staff Radiologist
Department of Pediatric Radiology
Texas Children's Hospital
Houston, Texas

Sandra L. Wootton-Gorges, MD
Professor and Director
Pediatric Imaging
University of California, Davis
Medical Director of Imaging
Department of Radiology
Shriner's Hospital of Northern California
Sacramento, California

Teaching Files are one of the hallmarks of education in radiology. There has long been a need for a comprehensive series of books, using the Teaching File format that would provide the kind of personal consultation with the experts normally found only in the setting of a teaching hospital. Lippincott Williams & Wilkins is proud to have created such a series; our goal is to provide residents, fellows and practicing radiologists with a useful resource that answers this need.

Actual cases have been culled from extensive teaching files in major medical centers. The discussions presented mimic those performed on a daily basis between residents and faculty members in all radiology departments.

The format of this series is designed so that each case can be studied as an unknown, if desired. A consistent format is used to present each case. A brief clinical history is given, followed by several images. Relevant findings, differential diagnosis, diagnosis, discussion of the case, questions for further thought, reporting responsibilities and "what the treating physician needs to know" follow. Answers to the questions conclude each case. In this manner, the authors guide the reader through the interpretation of each case, with a strong emphasis on critical thinking.

We hope that this series will become a valuable and trusted teaching tool for radiologists at any stage of training or practice, and that it will also be a benefit to clinicians whose patients undergo these imaging studies.

—*The Publisher*

This book of Pediatric Radiology teaching file cases presents a wide variety of conditions affecting children. Chapters are organized by organ systems, for example, Musculoskeletal Imaging, Neuroimaging, Cardiac Imaging, etc. Multiple scenarios are presented in a chapter. Each scenario begins with a brief clinical history followed by key images and a description of the findings. A differential diagnosis, the actual diagnosis, and relevant discussion then follow. We have also included a few questions for further thought, a radiologist's reporting responsibilities, and what the treating physician needs to know. The case ends with answers to questions and references. Length of the discussion varies from case to case, depending on the complexity of the diagnosis and at the author's/editor's discretion.

The field of Pediatric Radiology is vast, requiring extensive subspecialty knowledge. Therefore, we have carefully chosen a variety of experts to author the individual cases. All modalities, including radiography, fluoroscopy, ultrasound, CT, MRI, and nuclear medicine are presented. This book is not intended to replace a comprehensive textbook. Rather, it has been written to emphasize important concepts and pathologies and to simulate a discussion between a radiologist and a clinician or an expert attending and a trainee in front of a workstation/view box.

The concept for this book began approximately three years ago when Lippincott Williams & Wilkins (LWW) contacted me. I would first like to thank Dr. Felix Chew for recommending me to LWW. I am also indebted to Ed Weinberger, my co-editor and department head, for his expertise, patience, and guidance. I would also like to acknowledge our former directors, Drs. Byron Ward, C. Benjamin Graham, and Eric L. Effmann. I am especially thankful to all the contributing authors from various institutions throughout the country. This project could not have been completed without the support from LWW staff members, including Charlie Mitchell, Ryan Shaw, and Amy Dinkel. Lastly, I want to thank my fellows and residents, who are a constant source of enthusiasm and motivation.

Mahesh Thapa, MD

CHAPTER 2:   **Neuroimaging**

CHAPTER 5:   Airway, Neck, Chest, and Cardiac Imaging

CHAPTER 1

Musculoskeletal Imaging

CASE 1.1

CLINICAL HISTORY *A 13-year-old patient with knee pain*

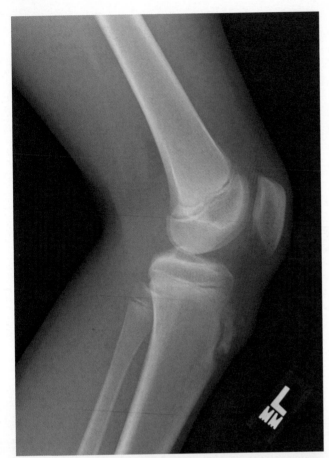

FIGURE **1.1A**

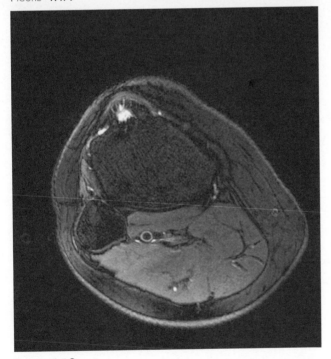

FIGURE **1.1C**

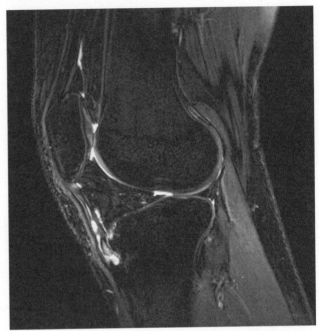

FIGURE **1.1B**

FINDINGS Radiographic findings in **A**: Ill-defined calcification and fragmentation of the tibial tubercle along with a moderate joint effusion and blurring of the patellar ligament.

Magnetic resonance (MR) findings in **B** and **C**: Mild fragmentation at the tibial tubercle, at the attachment site of the patellar ligament. In addition, thickening of the patellar ligament distally with high T2 signal within its substance.

DIFFERENTIAL DIAGNOSIS Osgood–Schlatter disease, normal variant

DIAGNOSIS Osgood–Schlatter disease

DISCUSSION Osgood–Schlatter disease is a chronic avulsion injury thought to result from repetitive microtrauma and traction on the tibial tubercle, or to the patellar tendon at its insertion site. Active adolescents are typically involved, particularly with activities requiring jumping, squatting, and kicking. Boys are more commonly affected with this often unilateral ailment, which can be bilateral in up to 50% of cases. Patients present with localized pain, swelling, and tenderness, oftentimes with a firm palpable mass in the region of the tibial tuberosity.

Most cases will spontaneously resolve. Clinical management of this condition ranges from immobilization and casting to intra-articular steroid injections. Surgical management is only rarely indicated.

Questions for Further Thought
1. Which is the best radiographic view to document Osgood–Schlatter disease?
2. Is plain film radiography diagnostic for this condition?

Reporting Responsibilities
• To rule out neoplasia/infection
• To differentiate from other common patterns of avulsive injury of the pediatric knee in order to facilitate prompt referral and orthopedic management, when indicated

What the Treating Physician Needs to Know
Presence of infection/bone tumor which may closely simulate the above condition.

Answers
1. Lateral radiograph with knee in slight internal rotation.
2. Osgood–Schlatter disease is a clinical diagnosis. Radiography, when used, is mostly to rule out neoplasia or infection. Radiographic findings of a fragmented tibial tubercle closely mimic a normal ossification center.

   Important associated MR findings include soft-tissue swelling and cartilage thickening anterior to tibial tuberosity; indistinctness of sharp inferior angle of infrapatellar fat pad and surrounding tissues, with distension of infrapatellar bursa; enlarged and edematous patellar tendon, with T1 and T2 hyperintensity along its distal aspect, and marrow edema within proximal tibia adjacent to the tuberosity.

REFERENCES
1. Stevens MA, El-Khoury GY, Kathol MH, et al. Imaging features of avulsion injuries. *Radiographics.* 1999;19(3):655–672.
2. Gottsegen CJ, Eyer BA, White EA, et al. Avulsion fractures of the knee: Imaging findings and clinical significance. *Radiographics.* 2008;28:1755–1770.

CASE 1.2

CLINICAL HISTORY *A 13-year-old child with knee swelling*

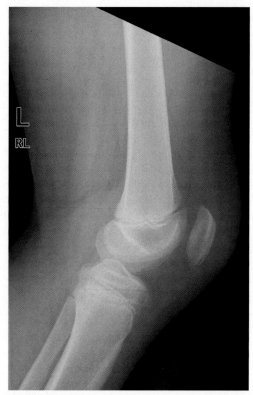

FIGURE **1.2**

FINDINGS Lateral radiograph of the knee demonstrates fragmentation of the apophysis of the inferior pole of the patella, with a small associated knee joint effusion and some superficial soft-tissue swelling.

DIFFERENTIAL DIAGNOSIS Sinding–Larsen–Johansson syndrome, patellar sleeve avulsion, normal variation

DIAGNOSIS Sinding–Larsen–Johansson syndrome

DISCUSSION Sinding–Larsen–Johansson injury results from forceful quadriceps contraction, injuring the inferior aspect of the patella and the proximal patellar tendon. Typically involved are male adolescent athletes.

A spectrum of closely related injuries to the distal aspect of the patella and the proximal patellar tendon consists of "jumper's knee," Sinding–Larsen–Johansson syndrome, and patellar sleeve avulsion. No associated damage to other stabilizing mechanisms of the knee is usually present in these entities.

"Jumper's knee" is a pain syndrome secondary to chronic stress or irritation of the patellar ligament that occurs in young athletes. Radiologically, it manifests only as thickening of the patellar ligament without obvious tear or disruption. The patellar sleeve fracture represents an osteocartilaginous avulsion of the lower pole of the patella, and usually occurs as a result of more violent quadriceps contraction than would precede Sinding–Larsen–Johansson syndrome, which is a pure osseous injury.

Questions for Further Thought

1. Are avulsion injuries to the knee clearly manifest on plain film radiography?
2. When is additional imaging and/or orthopedic referral indicated?

Reporting Responsibilities

- To identify these often subtle injuries on plain films, and to indicate what underlying damage they entail
- To suggest additional imaging, as necessary, to delineate the full extent of damage, and to initiate orthopedic referral, if indicated

What the Treating Physician Needs to Know

Pattern of injury: whether there is involvement of only the osseous or the osteocartilaginous components. This distinction will impact management.

Whether patella alta deformity (abnormally elevated patella in relation to the femur) predisposes to this injury.

Answers

1. These injuries are often quite subtle on plain films and the radiologist needs to maintain a keen eye as well as thorough understanding of the patterns as well as implications of these injuries, to guide appropriate work-up and management.

2. On plain films, the extent of some avulsion injuries is underestimated, and a precise estimate of associated chondral injury can be obtained by MR. Ultrasound can aid in identification of periosteal avulsion. The assessment is important because minimally displaced fractures such as those seen with Sinding–Larsen–Johansson syndrome will respond to conservative management, whereas displaced patellar sleeve avulsion fractures will require open reduction and possible internal fixation, as well as extensor mechanism reconstruction.

REFERENCES

1. Gottsegen CJ, Eyer BA, White EA, et al. Avulsion fractures of the knee: Imaging findings and clinical significance. *Radiographics.* 2008;28:1755–1770.

2. Peace KA, Lee JC, Healy J. Imaging the infrapatellar tendon in the elite athlete. *Clin Radiol.* 2006;61(7):570–578.

Apeksha Chaturvedi and Mahesh Thapa

CASE 1.3

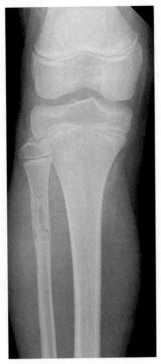

FIGURE **1.3A**

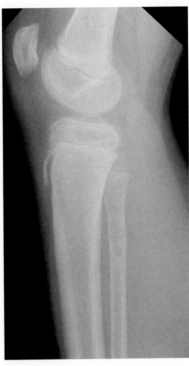

FIGURE **1.3B**

FINDINGS Anteroposterior (AP) (**A**) and lateral (**B**) radiographs of the knee demonstrate a multiloculated osteolytic corticomedullary defect in the proximal fibular metaphysis/diaphysis. The lesion has a sclerotic rim and clearly defined, geographic margins. No matrix calcification or pathologic fractures are visible.

DIFFERENTIAL DIAGNOSIS Nonossifying fibroma (NOF), benign fibrous histiocytoma, fibrous dysplasia (FD)

DIAGNOSIS NOF

DISCUSSION On the basis of their location, benign osseous lesions may be categorized into fibrous cortical defects (intracortical), fibrous endosteal defect, and NOF (corticomedullary or entirely medullary). NOFs are believed to arise from medullary extension of a fibrous cortical defect, and represent part of an identical spectrum.

Most frequently discovered incidentally in an adolescent male, these lesions are occasionally complicated by fracture and may then present with pain. Usually, they heal spontaneously.

Imaging findings are characteristic, comprising a multilocular expansile lytic lucency causing overlying cortical expansion. A sharp zone of transition is between the lesion and surrounding bone, and a thin rim of sclerosis (<1 mm) around its periphery. No periosteal reaction, cortical destruction, or accompanying soft-tissue masses are seen with the uncomplicated lesion.

Questions for Further Thought

1. Which metabolic disturbances or additional processes can accompany an NOF?
2. When is further imaging (beyond plain film radiography) indicated?

What the Treating Physician Needs to Know

Benign fibrous lesions of the bone are innocuous and resolve spontaneously. Radiographic findings are classical. Follow-up is not typically necessary unless they are complicated by pain, in which case a pathologic fracture needs to be looked for. A study reported an increased risk of pathologic fracture if an NOF involves more than 50% of the transverse diameter of the bone or measures more than 33 mm in length. Also, cortical destruction and accompanying soft-tissue masses, which may signify a potentially malignant process, should be carefully excluded.

Reporting Responsibilities

- Is there a fracture?
- Can we definitely exclude a malignant process?

Answers

1. NOFs are believed to secrete a substance that increases tubular reabsorption of phosphorus, and may be associated with vitamin D-resistant hypophosphatemic rickets and osteomalacia. Another possible association is with extraskeletal manifestations of mental retardation, ocular, cardiovascular, and dermal lesions (Jaffe–Campanacci syndrome).

2. Stress fractures sometimes complicate these fibro-osseous lesions, in which case a lamellated solid periosteal reaction is seen, sometimes mistaken for sarcoma. Cross-sectional imaging may then be indicated to determine the true nature and extent of the process.

REFERENCES

1. Eisenberg RL. Bubbly lesions of bone. *AJR Am J Roentgenol.* 2009;193(2):W79–W94.

2. Kumar R, Madewell JE, Lindell MM, et al. Fibrous lesions of bones. *Radiographics.* 1990;10:237–256.

3. Shimal A, Davies AM, James SL, et al. Fatigue-type stress fractures of the lower limb associated with fibrous cortical defects/non-ossifying fibromas in the skeletally immature. *Clin Radiol.* 2010;65:382–386.

4. Arata MA, Peterson HA, Dahlin DC. Pathological fractures through nonossifying fibromas. *J Bone Joint Surg Am.* 1981; 63A:980–988.

CASE 1.4

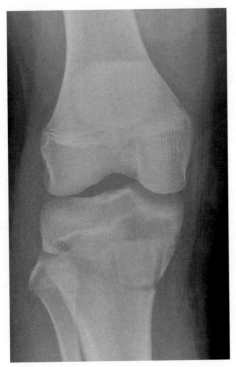

FIGURE **1.4A**

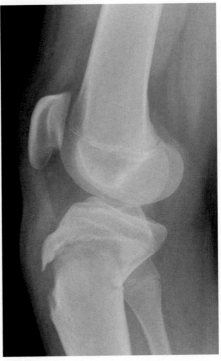

FIGURE **1.4B**

FINDINGS AP (**A**) and lateral (**B**) radiographs of the knee demonstrate a mildly displaced, triangular tibial metaphyseal fracture, extending to the growth plate.

DIFFERENTIAL DIAGNOSIS Salter–Harris injury, appearance of normal apophysis at the knee

DIAGNOSIS Salter–Harris type II fracture

DISCUSSION The Salter–Harris classification consists of five types of injury:

(a) Type I: exclusively physeal injury.
(b) Type II: most common. The line of fracture extends through the physis and then through a margin of the metaphysis.
(c) Type III: epiphyseal fracture, extending horizontally to the periphery of the physis.
(d) Type IV: extends across the epiphysis, physis, and adjacent metaphysis.
(e) Type V: crush injury of the epiphysis or physis.

The higher the Salter–Harris classification, the more serious the injury is with greater potential for complications such as growth retardation. Plain film radiography is the initial imaging modality. This includes the standard AP and lateral projections, to which oblique and cross-table lateral views may be added if findings are equivocal. X-rays generally allow depiction of the fracture itself, together with the periarticular soft-tissue planes and assessment of joint effusions.

Questions for Further Thought

1. What is the most important complication of Salter–Harris fractures?
2. When is further evaluation indicated in Salter–Harris injury?

Reporting Responsibilities

• Is there a fracture; if so, does it extend to involve the growth plate?
• Is there bone bridging as a consequence of physeal injury?

What the Treating Physician Needs to Know

Involvement of the physis distinguishes the Salter–Harris spectrum from other pediatric fractures. Classifying injuries based on the Salter–Harris system has predictive and prognostic value, and should be an integral component of radiographic interpretation.

Answers

1. Bone bridging across the growth plate is a feared complication of Salter–Harris injuries. Eccentric tethering of the growth plate causes angular deformity. Central involvement causes shortening of the bone. Complications are more severe in the younger child. Indications for resection of bridges include bridging of less than 50% with more than 2 years of growth remaining. Surgery is contraindicated if there is more extensive bridging.

2. MR is indicated only with subtle or nondisplaced physeal fractures. MR images should be assessed for widened physis, fracture lines through the epiphysis or metaphysis, marrow edema, and periosteal elevation.

REFERENCES

1. Salter RB, Harris WR. Injuries involving the epiphyseal plate. *J Bone and Joint Surg.* 1963;45-A:587–622.
2. Close BJ, Strouse PJ. MR of physeal fractures of the adolescent knee. *Pediatr Radiol.* 2000;30:756–762.
3. Basener CJ, Mehlman CT, DiPasquale TG. Growth disturbance after distal femoral growth plate fractures in children: A meta-analysis. *J Ortho Trauma.* 2009;23(9):663–667.

CLINICAL HISTORY *A 6-year-old child with right hip swelling and painful limp*

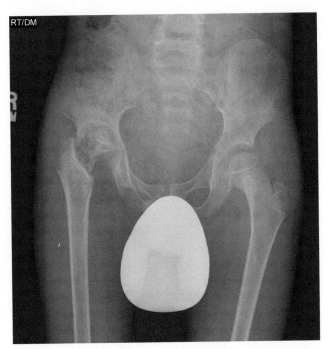

FIGURE **1.5A**

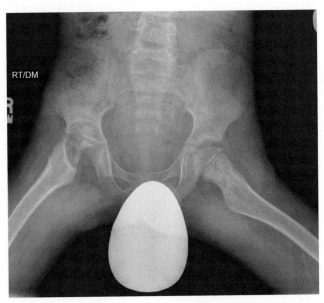

FIGURE **1.5B**

FINDINGS AP (**A**) and frog-leg lateral (**B**) views of the pelvis demonstrate marked destruction of the right femoral head and neck, with narrowed hip joint space. Also, the femur is displaced proximally with a lucency through the femoral neck, indicating a pathologic fracture.

DIFFERENTIAL DIAGNOSIS Septic arthritis, osteomyelitis, toxic synovitis, slipped capital femoral epiphysis (SCFE)

DIAGNOSIS Septic arthritis with osteomyelitis

DISCUSSION Septic arthritis is a severely disabling, and, potentially life-threatening disease. Most common implicated pathogen in septic arthritis is *Staphylococcus aureus.* *Escherichia coli,* group B *Streptococcus,* other gram-negative rods, and *Candida albicans* are also frequently implicated in the neonate. Fungal, parasitic, and mycobacterial infections occur in the immunocompromised and in endemic regions.

Three main routes of spread of infection to the bone/joint are hematogenous or via direct or indirect contamination.

Before secondary ossification centers appear, the cartilaginous epiphyses derive their blood supply directly from the metaphyseal blood vessels. This accounts for the increased susceptibility of the neonatal joint to septic arthritis arising as a sequelae to osteomyelitis. Later in life, the blood supply of the epiphysis and metaphysis becomes separate, and secondary involvement of the joint from an infective process in the metaphysis becomes less common.

Avascular necrosis (AVN) of the femoral head due to compression and vascular compromise as a result of inflammatory swelling can occur as a sequelae to septic arthritis. Prompt diagnosis and management are thus critical. Subluxation and dislocations can also occur. Imaging confirms presence and site of infection, aids in differentiating unifocal from multifocal disease, locates and guides aspiration of collections, and identifies present or impending complications such as joint involvement.

Questions for Further Thought

1. What is the most common cause of acute hip pain in a limping child?
2. What is the role of plain hip radiography in evaluation of patients with suspected septic arthritis/osteomyelitis?

Reporting Responsibilities

- Describe the extent and location of abnormality.
- Describe presence of associated complications, such as abscesses and dislocation/subluxation.

What the Treating Physician Needs to Know

On plain films, the presence of joint effusion manifested as joint widening or displaced fat planes, and the presence of epiphyseal lucency must be actively sought and reported. Ultrasound is frequently used to detect effusions and guide emergency joint aspirations. Synovial enhancement on MR, altered marrow signal, and decreased first-pass perfusion are also characteristic. As with any illness with potentially devastating complications, the threshold for ordering additional imaging is low.

Answers

1. Transient synovitis is the most common cause of acute hip pain. It is a self-limited illness with no adverse residual sequelae. Nevertheless, differentiating this entity from septic arthritis is potentially challenging, especially in the setting of a negative radiograph.

2. Plain film radiography is frequently normal, or reveals subtle findings of joint effusion or widening, especially in early stages of the disease. Findings of osteomyelitis often develop after destruction of at least one-third of the bone matrix. Plain radiographs can document hip dislocation/subluxations and establish a baseline for further follow-up.

REFERENCES

1. Pruthi S, Thapa MM. Infectious and inflammatory disorders. *Magn Reson Imaging Clin N Am.* 2009;17(3):429–438.

2. Caird MS, Flynn JM, Leung YL, et al. Factors distinguishing septic arthritis from transient synovitis of the hip in children. A prospective study. *J Bone Joint Surg Am.* 2006;88(6):1251–1257.

3. Lin HM, Learch TJ, White EA, et al. Emergency joint aspiration: A guide for radiologists on call. *Radiographics.* 2009;29(4):1139–1158.

4. Yang WJ, Im SA, Lim GY, et al. MR imaging of transient synovitis: Differentiation from septic arthritis. *Pediatr Radiol.* 2006;36(11):1154–1158.

CASE 1.6

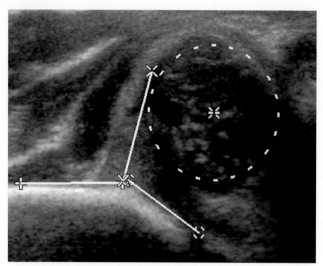

FIGURE **1.6A**

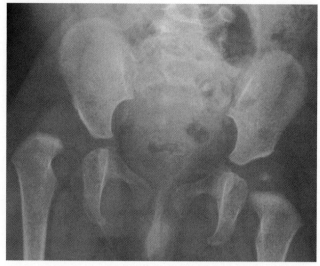

FIGURE **1.6B**

FINDINGS Neonatal hip ultrasound (**A**) and plain film radiographs (**B**) of an older infant document a severely subluxed/dislocated hip, with associated acetabular dysplasia. In **A**, the alpha angle was measured at 36°, and femoral head coverage was estimated at 37%. In **B**, the right femur is superolaterally displaced and the corresponding acetabulum is shallow. There is also asymmetric appearance of bilateral femoral head ossific nuclei.

DIFFERENTIAL DIAGNOSIS Developmental dysplasia of the hip (DDH); AVN

DIAGNOSIS DDH

DISCUSSION The spectrum of DDH ranges from a very mild acetabular dysplasia with a stable hip to severe acetabular and femoral head dysmorphism associated with a dislocatable, subluxed, or frankly dislocated hip. The incidence is 1.5 to 20 cases per 1000 births, is bilateral in 20% cases, and has a female to male ratio of approximately 4:1.

Clinically, it is most sensitively diagnosed by limited hip abduction (<60°) in 90° of hip flexion. Barlow and Ortolani maneuvers are alternatively described.

Risk factors include connective tissue laxity, shallow acetabulum, breech delivery, a large-for-gestational-age baby, oligohydramnios, multiple gestation, and a positive family history of a sibling with this condition.

At <4.5 months of age, ultrasound is helpful to assess the hip using both static and dynamic assessment. Ultrasound uses a modified Graf (Rosendahl) technique, using standard coronal sections and the alpha angle, which is a measure of acetabular depth. Radiographically, it is diagnosed by drawing a horizontal line along the triradiate cartilage (Hilgenreiner line) and dropping a perpendicular (Perkin line) through the most superolateral portion of the ossified acetabulum. The ossified femoral head, when present, should localize to the inferomedial aspect of this quadrant.

Most affected hips will respond to a Pavlik harness, if treatment is initiated before 6 to 8 weeks. If this fails or initial presentation is delayed, surgery may be necessary.

Questions for Further Thought

1. How should a slightly abnormal hip ultrasound (alpha angle 55°) be interpreted?
2. Should ultrasound screening of the hip be universally implemented?

Reporting Responsibilities

On initial screening ultrasound, the alpha angles should be carefully reported and interpreted in accordance with suggested guidelines (see later).

What the Treating Physician Needs to Know

An assessment of severity of involvement of the affected hip, based on which the plan for further management can be formulated, is important from the treatment standpoint. Also, imaging is useful for excluding hip dysplasia and alleviating parent anxiety, especially in context of an affected sibling.

Answers

1. Results are interpreted as follows:

   Alpha angle >60°: Normal.

   Alpha angle between 50° and 60°: Immature.

   Alpha angle from 43° to 50°: Mild dysplasia.

   Alpha angle <43° with or without changes in the acetabular labrum: Severe dysplasia.

   Given the above, an alpha angle of 55° should be interpreted as functional immaturity of the hip.

2. According to current guidelines, the screening algorithm is as under:

   Newborn with normal hip examination and no risk factors: Clinical examination at 6 weeks.

   Newborn with normal hip examination but with risk factors: Ultrasonogram at 6 weeks if immediate treatment necessary. If not, ultrasound at 4 weeks to allow time for results and referral.

   Newborn with abnormal hip examination: Ultrasound at 2 to 3 weeks, referral to specialist (may repeat scan). Initiate treatment.

REFERENCES

1. Sewell MD, Rosendahl K, Eastwood DM. Developmental dysplasia of the hip. *BMJ.* 2009;339:b4454.
2. Gelfer P, Kennedy KA. Developmental dysplasia of the hip. *J Pediatr Health Care.* 2008;22(5):318–322.

CASE 1.7

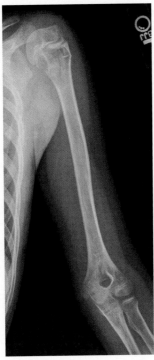

FIGURE **1.7A**

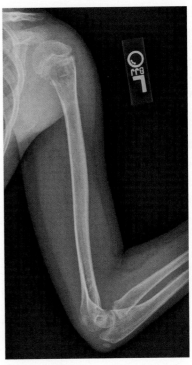

FIGURE **1.7B**

FINDINGS AP (**A**) and lateral (**B**) views of the left humerus demonstrate an oval lytic bone lesion with well-defined margins in the proximal metaphysis. There is an associated pathologic fracture with a sliver of bone lying at the bottom of the cyst cavity. No associated soft-tissue or periosteal reaction is seen.

DIFFERENTIAL DIAGNOSIS Simple bone cyst (SBC), aneurysmal bone cyst (ABC), monostotic FD

DIAGNOSIS SBC

DISCUSSION SBC (also known as unicameral bone cyst) is of uncertain etiology. Though radiographically these cysts are most often solitary, they are seldom unilocular. Common age of presentation is 5 to 15 years with male to female ratio of 2.5 : 1.[1] Classical presentation is with pathologic fracture

after sports trauma. Commonest site is proximal humerus followed by proximal femur.[1] The lesion starts in the proximal metaphysis and extends into the diaphysis with skeletal growth. By the time they heal, the lesions are usually located at the junction of middle and distal thirds of the shaft. SBCs in the calcaneum have a characteristic triangular appearance.[2]

Questions for Further Thought

1. What is the "fallen fragment" sign?
2. What are the magnetic resonance imaging (MRI) features of an SBC?

Reporting Responsibilities
Identify the benign nonaggressive appearance of the lesion and detect pathologic fractures.

What the Treating Physician Needs to Know
Presence of a pathologic fracture. Identify lesion as benign.

Answers

1. It is a radiographic sign seen in about 20% of SBCs and refers to a fragment of cortical bone lying dependently within the cyst in the setting of a pathologic fracture. Sometimes the fragment of cortical bone may project into the lumen of the SBC in a hinge-like fashion, also known as the "hinged fragment" sign.

2. MRI demonstrates the fluid content of the lesion. The appearance may be altered by presence of fracture, in which case fluid–fluid levels are seen due to hemorrhage.

REFERENCES

1. Adam A, Dixon AK, Grainger RG, et al., eds. *Diagnostic Radiology*. 5th ed. Churchill Livingstone: Elsevier; 2008.
2. Helms CA. *Fundamentals of Skeletal Radiology*. 3rd ed. Philadelphia, PA: Elsevier/Saunders; 2005.

CASE 1.8

CLINICAL HISTORY *Left elbow pain and swelling*

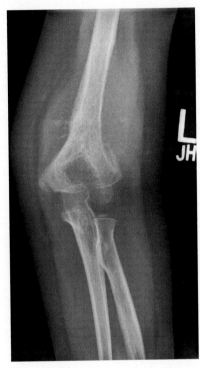

FIGURE **1.8A**

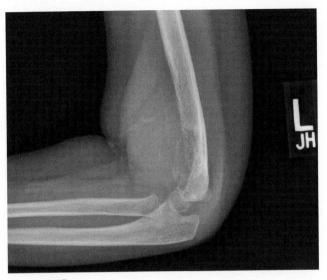

FIGURE **1.8B**

FINDINGS AP (**A**) and lateral (**B**) views of the left elbow show a predominantly sclerotic lesion of the distal humeral metadiaphysis with a wide distal zone of transition and associated cortical destruction. There is a sunburst type of periosteal reaction with spiculations and Codman triangle formation. Associated soft-tissue mass with calcification is noted. There is no pathologic fracture.

DIFFERENTIAL DIAGNOSIS Osteosarcoma, Ewing sarcoma

DIAGNOSIS Osteosarcoma

DISCUSSION Osteosarcoma is the most common primary bone tumor in adolescents and young adults.[1] Usual presentation is bone pain or swelling after a sports-related injury. Predisposing conditions include exposure to ionizing radiation, Paget disease of bone, enchondromatosis, hereditary multiple exostosis, FD, and genetic conditions such as hereditary retinoblastoma and Li–Fraumeni syndrome.[1] It commonly affects the metaphysis of long tubular bones such as femur, tibia, and humerus.[1] Epiphysis can be infiltrated even with open physis. Radiologically, conventional central osteosarcoma shows fluffy cloud-like areas of increased bone density with permeative lytic areas of bone destruction.[2] The classical type of periosteal reaction is sunburst appearance with spiculations and formation of Codman triangle.[2] Associated soft-tissue mass with variable matrix mineralization is common. MRI is the technique of choice for presurgical staging and demonstrating the extent of marrow infiltration.[3] Computed tomography (CT) chest and bone scan are useful in metastatic work-up. Pathologically, osteosarcoma is characterized by formation of immature bone and malignant osteoid matrix.[2] Metastasis is common to the lungs and sometimes to bones. Treatment is by limb salvage surgery with or without chemotherapy and radiation.

Questions for Further Thought

1. What are some other tumors that can show fluid levels on MRI?
2. How does one differentiate myositis ossificans from parosteal osteosarcoma?

Reporting Responsibilities

The lesion should be recognized as aggressive. MRI report should identify extent of marrow infiltration, presence or absence of skip lesions, involvement of epiphysis, joint space infiltration, presence of pathologic fracture, soft-tissue infiltration, and involvement of the neurovascular structures.

What the Treating Physician Needs to Know

Site, extent, pathologic fracture, soft-tissue mass, skip lesions, involvement of epiphysis, joint space and neurovascular structures, and lung and bone metastasis.

Answers

1. ABC, simple/unicameral bone cyst, and giant cell tumor (GCT).

2. In myositis ossificans, the ossification tends to be more marked at the periphery than at the center.

REFERENCES

1. Arndt CAS, Crist WM. Common musculoskeletal tumors of childhood and adolescence. *N Engl J Med.* 1999;341:342–352.
2. Suresh S, Saifuddin A. Radiological appearances of appendicular osteosarcoma: A comprehensive pictorial review. *Clin Radiol.* 2007;62:314–323.
3. Saifuddin A. The accuracy of imaging in the local staging of appendicular osteosarcoma. *Skeletal Radiol.* 2002;31: 191–201.

CASE 1.9

CLINICAL HISTORY *Short stature*

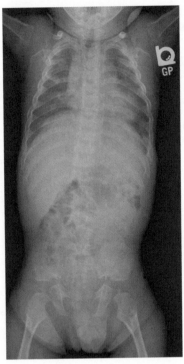

FIGURE **1.9A**

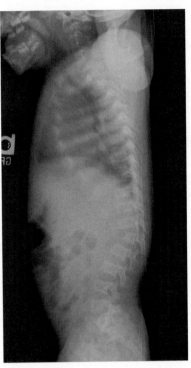

FIGURE **1.9B**

FINDINGS AP view (**A**) of the thoracolumbar spine reveals marked narrowing of the interpediculate distance of the lumbar vertebrae. The acetabular roof is horizontal, the iliac wings are small and squared, and the sacroiliac notches are short. On the lateral radiograph (**B**), there is AP shortening of the L1 vertebra causing a gibbus deformity. There is also posterior vertebral scalloping.

DIFFERENTIAL DIAGNOSIS Achondroplasia, achondrogenesis, campomelic dysplasia

DIAGNOSIS Achondroplasia

DISCUSSION Achondroplasia is the most common skeletal dysplasia caused by a mutation of fibroblast growth factor receptor-3 and inherited in autosomal dominant fashion.[1]

The key radiologic feature is narrowing of interpediculate distance from L1 to L5 in an AP radiograph of the spine. The other associated anomalies include frontal bossing, midface hypoplasia, rhizomelic short stature, radial head dislocation, genu varum, thoracolumbar kyphosis, and lumbar hyperlordosis. The neurologic complications include foramen magnum stenosis that may result in brain stem compression with apnea and sudden death and spinal canal stenosis. Medical and surgical options are available to increase patient height, corrective osteotomy for genu varum.[1]

Questions for Further Thought

1. What are the extraskeletal manifestations of achondroplasia?
2. What is the role of MRI in achondroplasia?

Reporting Responsibilities

The potential complications of achondroplasia must be kept in mind while reviewing any imaging on these patients.

What the Treating Physician Needs to Know

Foramen magnum stenosis, especially if there is brain stem compression.

Answers

1. Hydrocephalus requiring ventricular shunts, otolaryngeal problems, obesity. Cognitive development is typically normal.

2. MRI plays a role in evaluating complications such as foramen magnum and spinal canal stenosis.

REFERENCE

1. Shirley E, Ain M. Achondroplasia: Manifestations and treatment. *J Am Acad Orthop Surg.* 2009;17:231–241.

CASE 1.10

CLINICAL HISTORY *Painless bump over the right knee*

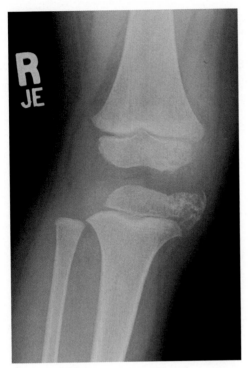

FIGURE **1.10A**

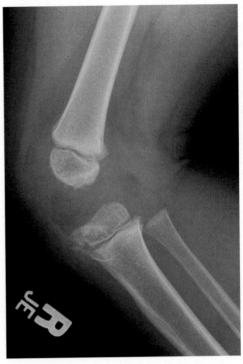

FIGURE **1.10B**

FINDINGS AP (**A**) and lateral (**B**) views of the right knee show a well-defined bony process on the medial aspect of the proximal tibial metaphysis fused with the epiphysis, suggesting an epiphyseal outgrowth. It shows symmetric calcification. The adjacent bone appears otherwise normal. There is no fracture or periosteal reaction. The knee joint is normal.

DIFFERENTIAL DIAGNOSIS Dysplasia epiphysealis hemimelica (DEH)

DIAGNOSIS DEH or Trevor disease.

DISCUSSION DEH (Trevor disease) is a rare skeletal dysplasia characterized by cartilage proliferation in the epiphyses, usually of the lower extremity bones. Age at onset is usually between 2 and 14 years. Boys are affected three times as often as girls. The most common presentation is that of a painless mass; other reported manifestations include pain, swelling, restricted range of motion of the affected joint, and occasionally axial deformity or limb length discrepancy.

Azouz et al.[1] have classified DEH as follows:

1. Localized: involving only one epiphysis.
2. Classic: affects more than one area in a single limb, most common form. Most common sites are distal medial epiphyses of distal femur, talus, proximal and distal tibia, and the tarsal bones. Upper limb involvement is rare.[2]
3. Generalized: affecting the whole lower limb from pelvis to foot.

CT and MRI are helpful in planning surgical resection and deformity correction. Anatomic relationship between the mass and the underlying bone is well seen on cross-sectional imaging. MRI also demonstrates the extent of the mass and joint deformity and the status of the articular cartilage. A plane of cleavage between the lesion and the normal epiphyseal ossification center can be demonstrated.[2]

Questions for Further Thought

1. What is the role of biopsy in Trevor disease?
2. How is Trevor disease treated?

Reporting Responsibilities

The radiologist must be aware of this entity and its benign nature to avoid unnecessary and aggressive work-up.

What the Treating Physician Needs to Know

Describe the lesion and stress the concept that the lesion is benign and aggressive work-up such as biopsy is not necessary.

Answers

1. The radiographic appearance is usually characteristic and diagnosis can be reached on imaging features alone.

Biopsy might be useful in cases with atypical radiographic appearance and location.[1]

2. No treatment is required in asymptomatic patients with incidentally detected lesions. In patients with pain or growth deformity, surgical correction is required.

REFERENCES

1. Azouz EM, Slomic AM, Marton D, et al. The variable manifestations of dysplasia epiphysealis hemimelica. *Pediatr Radiol.* 1985;15:44–49.

2. Lang IM, Azouz EM. MRI appearances of dysplasia epiphysealis hemimelica of the knee. *Skeletal Radiol.* 1997;26:226–229.

Deepa Reddy Biyyam and Mahesh Thapa

CASE 1.11

CLINICAL HISTORY *Child presenting with facial asymmetry and deformity*

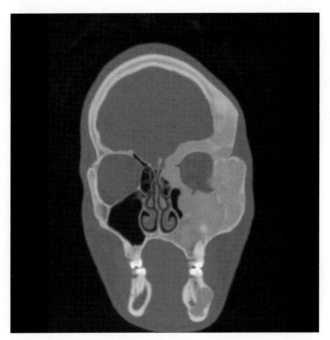

FIGURE **1.11**

FINDINGS Coronal CT image of the skull and facial bones demonstrates marked expansion of the diploic spaces of the left-sided craniofacial bones, with a "ground glass" appearance.

DIFFERENTIAL DIAGNOSIS None

DIAGNOSIS Polyostotic FD

DISCUSSION FD is a benign developmental abnormality in which the normal marrow and cancellous bone are replaced by immature woven bone and dense fibrotic stroma. It can involve any bone. Most patients present with a painless swelling or deformity. Ground glass appearance on plain radiographs and CT is characteristic. Seventy to eighty per cent are monostotic and 20% to 30% are polyostotic. Craniofacial involvement is seen in 50% of patients with polyostotic disease. Other signs and symptoms include sinus or nasal obstruction, malocclusion of teeth, proptosis, and cranial neuropathy (diplopia, hearing loss, and blindness).[1]

Question for Further Thought

1. What is the most common extraskeletal manifestation of FD?

Reporting Responsibilities

- Describe the location and extent of abnormality
- Describe any associated pathologic fracture, particularly with the monostotic variety

What the Treating Physician Needs to Know

Bone scan can help identify additional lesions, particularly in polyostotic FD.

Answer

1. Abnormal cutaneous pigmentation (café au lait spots). Polyostotic FD, café au lait spots, and precocious puberty constitute McCune–Albright syndrome.

REFERENCE

1. Resnick D. *Bone and Joint Disorders.* 4th ed. Philadelphia, PA: Elsevier; 2004.

Deepa Reddy Biyyam and Mahesh Thapa

CASE 1.12

CLINICAL HISTORY *A 16-month-old child refusing to bear weight*

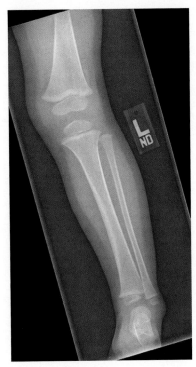

FIGURE **1.12A**

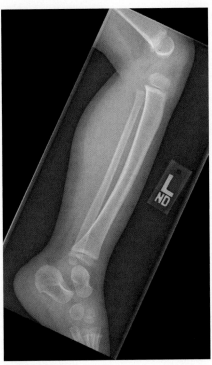

FIGURE **1.12B**

FINDINGS There is a curved nondisplaced fracture in the distal tibial shaft, seen on the AP (**A**) radiograph. The fracture is not clearly seen on the lateral (**B**) radiograph.

DIFFERENTIAL DIAGNOSIS Accidental fracture, nonaccidental injury

DIAGNOSIS Accidental fracture (toddler's fracture)

DISCUSSION Toddler's fractures are subtle lower extremity fractures and should always be suspected in a toddler or young child refusing to bear weight.

The classic "toddler's fracture," often called toddler's fracture type I originally referred to a nondisplaced oblique fracture of the distal tibial diaphysis, which usually results from a twisting or rotational force applied to the foot or lower extremity. A hairline fracture is often visible, although rarely the fracture is occult. In these cases, a radionuclide bone scan may be helpful, although is not specific. Alternatively, the limb is immobilized and a repeat radiograph is obtained in 10 to 14 days, which may demonstrate periosteal new bone formation indicating healing. Toddler's fracture type II consists of a knee hyperextension injury leading to posterior cortex, distracting fracture of the upper tibial metadiaphysis. There is associated compression and buckling of the anterior cortex and deepening of the notch for tibial tubercle.[1]

Question for Further Thought

1. What are the other common sites of occult fractures in toddlers?

Reporting Responsibilities

- Describe site and extent of fracture.
- Describe whether displaced or nondisplaced.

What the Treating Physician Needs to Know

A similar fracture in a nonambulatory child should raise the suspicion of nonaccidental injury.

Answer

1. Occult fractures commonly occur in the bones of the foot, particularly the calcaneus, cuboid, and the meta-tarsals. These fractures may be very subtle and comparison views or bone scans may be needed to detect these fractures.[2]

REFERENCES

1. Jadhav SP, Swischuk LE. Commonly missed subtle skeletal injuries in children: A pictorial review. *Emerg Radiol.* 2008;15:391–398.
2. John SD, Moorthy CS, Swischuk LE. Expanding the concept of the toddler's fracture. *Radiographics.* 1997;17:367–376.

CLINICAL HISTORY *A 10-year-old boy presenting with knee pain*

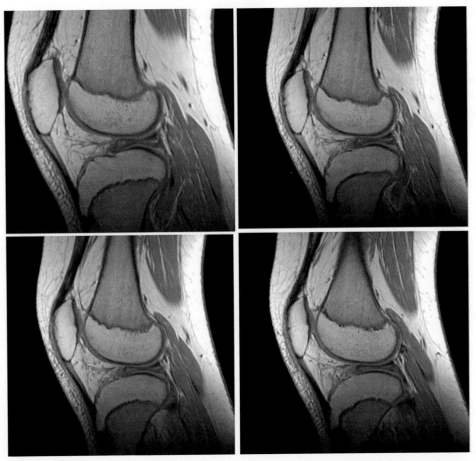

FIGURE **1.13A**

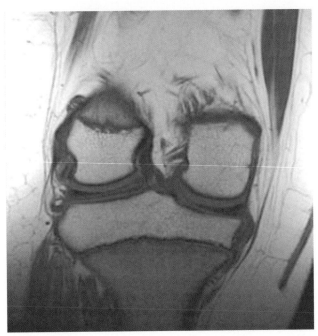

FIGURE **1.13B**

FINDINGS Sagittal proton density (PD) images (**A**) of the lateral meniscus demonstrate continuity of the anterior and posterior horns of the lateral meniscus on four consecutive images. On the coronal image (**B**), the lateral meniscus does not taper into the intercondylar notch. There is abnormal intermediate signal within the lateral meniscus.

DIFFERENTIAL DIAGNOSIS Discoid meniscus, disc degeneration

DIAGNOSIS Discoid meniscus with disc degeneration

DISCUSSION Discoid meniscus is a developmental abnormality in which the meniscus is shaped like a disc, instead of the normal C shape. Possible etiologies include abnormal development secondary to deficiency in the normal meniscal attachments and failure of fetal discoid form to involute. The lateral meniscus is more commonly involved, compared to the medial. Most children with discoid meniscus are asymptomatic, although they may present with pain, locking, snapping, or "giving away."

Plain radiograph findings include widening of the lateral tibiofemoral joint space, cupping of the lateral tibial plateau, hypoplastic lateral tibial spine, and hypoplastic femoral condyle. MRI is the imaging modality of choice. The normal meniscus is hypointense on both T1- and T2-weighted MR images, and the meniscal size varies from 5 to 13 mm from the capsular margin to free edge on a central coronal image. Continuity of the anterior and posterior horns of the meniscus (meniscal bowties) in three or more consecutive sagittal MR images at 4 to 5 mm slice thickness and meniscal size more than 13 mm in cross section are diagnostic of discoid meniscus.[1] Increased intrameniscal T2 signal indicates a tear or mucoid degeneration.

Question for Further Thought

1. What are the types of discoid meniscus?

Reporting Responsibilities

- Describe any abnormal signal in the meniscus if present.
- Describe location, type, and extent of meniscal tear when present.

What the Treating Physician Needs to Know

MR arthrogram can be helpful in distinguishing a tear from degeneration. If contrast enters into the meniscus, it indicates a tear.

Answer

1. Type I (complete) extends into the intercondylar notch; type II (incomplete) partially extends into the intercondylar notch; and type III (Wrisberg ligament type) lacks the normal posterior meniscotibial attachment, thus allowing increased mobility and producing the classic "snapping knee" syndrome.[2]

REFERENCES

1. Silverman JM, Mink JH, Deutsch AL. Discoid menisci of the knee: MR imaging appearance. *Radiology*. 1989;173(2):351–354.
2. Yaniv M, Blumberg N. The discoid meniscus. *J Child Orthop*. 2007;1:89–96.

CLINICAL HISTORY *An 11-year-old boy presenting with left groin pain*

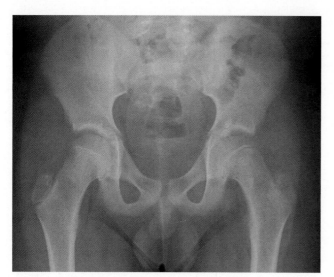

FIGURE **1.14A**

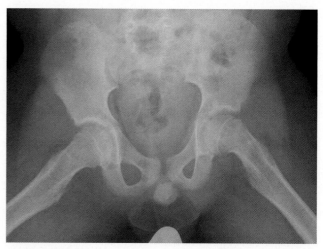

FIGURE **1.14B**

FINDINGS AP radiograph of the hips (**A**), demonstrating subtle widening of the femoral physis on the left. An imaginary tangential line drawn along the lateral border of the femoral neck (line of Klein) should normally intersect a part of the physis. In this case, it fails to intersect any part of the physis on the left, indicating medial displacement of the capital epiphysis in relation to the metaphysis. Frog lateral view of the hips (**B**) of the same patient shows posterior displacement of the left capital femoral physis.

DIFFERENTIAL DIAGNOSIS SCFE, traumatic Salter–Harris type I fracture

DIAGNOSIS SCFE

DISCUSSION SCFE is displacement of the femoral head relative to the femoral neck through the open growth plate due to repetitive stress of weight bearing, typically occurring in adolescents. Contributing factors include adolescent growth spurt, hormonal influences (decreased sex hormones), obesity, and increased physical activity. Most of the patients present with hip pain, although about one-fourth of the patients complain of knee pain. Bilateral involvement is noted in 20% to 35% cases.[1]

Except for the adductor group, most muscles about the hip joint insert laterally, just below the greater trochanter and thereby pull the femoral shaft laterally and anteriorly. The femoral head seated in the acetabulum is located posteriorly and medially with respect to the femoral shaft. Conventionally, in SCFE, reference is made to the movement of the femoral head with respect to the shaft, when in actuality the opposite is occurring.[2]

Plain radiographs remain the imaging modality of choice. Both the AP and lateral/frog-leg lateral views should be obtained.[2] MRI appears to be more sensitive to early diagnosis of this condition, when the plain radiographs appear normal. MRI findings include physeal widening, marrow edema in the periphyseal bones, and synovitis.

Questions for Further Thought

1. How is SCFE treated?
2. What are complications of SCFE?

Reporting Responsibilities

• Describe the severity of slippage: mild, moderate, or severe depending on the displacement of the capital femoral physis by <1/3, 1/3 to 2/3, or >2/3 of its diameter on the femoral metaphysis.

- On follow-up radiographs, it is important to document physeal fusion when it occurs. Document complications such as progression of slip, hardware failure, chondrolysis, AVN, and secondary osteoarthritis, if evident.

What the Treating Physician Needs to Know

1. Both AP and lateral or frog-leg lateral views are mandatory. The hip is abducted and externally rotated in the frog-leg lateral view. Do not apply force to secure frog-leg lateral position as there is a possibility of increasing the slip due to increased pressure.

2. Both hips should be imaged as there is a possibility that the asymptomatic contralateral side may also be affected.

Answers

1. Treatment of SCFE consists of stabilization across the physis with pins or screws. Attempted reduction is associated with a greater risk of AVN, hence avoided.

2. The early complications include slip progression, hardware failure, chondrolysis, and AVN, whereas the late complications include pistol grip deformity of the femoral neck, secondary osteoarthritis, and limb length discrepancy due to premature physeal fusion.

REFERENCES

1. Boles CA, El-Khoury GY. Slipped capital femoral epiphysis. *Radiographics.* 1997;17:809–823.

2. Resnick D. *Diagnosis of Bone and Joint Disorders.* 3rd ed. Philadelphia, PA: WB Saunders; 1995.

CASE 1.15

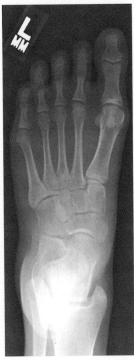

FIGURE **1.15A**

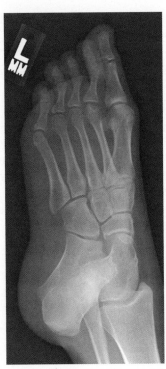

FIGURE **1.15B**

FINDINGS AP (**A**) and oblique (**B**) radiographs of the foot demonstrate flattening of the second metatarsal head with sclerosis and irregularity.

DIFFERENTIAL DIAGNOSIS Secondary osteoarthritis, Freiberg infraction

DIAGNOSIS Freiberg infraction

DISCUSSION Location and appearance are classic for Freiberg infraction, an osteochondrosis of the second metatarsal head that typically affects skeletally immature teens.[1] Etiology is not completely understood, but is thought secondary to osteonecrosis.[2] Repetitive stress has also been postulated as etiology when the disease process occurs in middle-aged females. Differentiation from secondary osteoarthritis is primarily made on classic imaging appearance. However,

osteoarthritis related to prior trauma or inflammation could result in similar dysplasia within the metatarsal head though one may expect to see more arthritic change in the adjacent proximal phalanx.

Questions for Further Thought

1. What is the underlying mechanism for osteochondroses?
2. What are the other common articular osteochondroses?

Reporting Responsibilities

- An attempt to differentiate from secondary osteoarthritis should be made, with signs of a primary etiology if present, reported.
- An associated fracture or malalignment should be reported (though these are not expected).

What the Treating Physician Needs to Know

1. Further progression may be halted by treatment (initially mobilization).

2. Anatomy may predispose to injury (long second metatarsal may increase its susceptibility to this stress-related injury).

Answers

1. Abnormality in epiphyseal blood supply (which may be idiopathic or secondary to insult such as trauma, low-grade infection, or endocrinopathy).

2. Legg–Calve–Perthes disease (LCPD; femoral head), Kohler disease (tarsal navicular), Panner disease (capitellum)

REFERENCES

1. Scartozzi G, Schram A, Janigian J. Freiberg's infraction of the second metatarsal head with formation of multiple loose bodies. *J Foot Surg.* 1989;28(3):195–199.

2. Doyle SM, Monahan A. Osteochondroses: A clinical review for the pediatrician. *Curr Opin Pediatr.* 2010;22(1): 41–46.

CASE 1.16

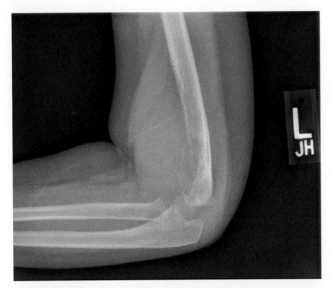

FIGURE **1.16A**

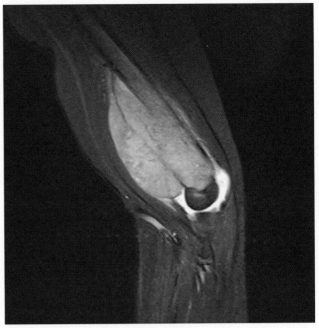

FIGURE **1.16B**

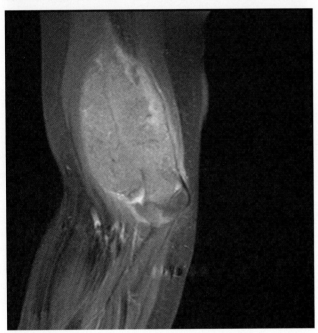

FIGURE **1.16C**

FINDINGS Lateral radiograph of the left elbow (**A**) demonstrates a destructive lesion of the distal humerus with a large soft-tissue component and aggressive periosteal reaction. Sagittal short Tau inversion recovery (STIR) MR image (**B**) of the humerus demonstrates a large soft-tissue mass arising from the distal humeral metadiaphysis, with enhancement following Gadolinium administration (**C**).

DIFFERENTIAL DIAGNOSIS Osteosarcoma, Langerhans cell histiocytosis (LCH), osteomyelitis, Ewing sarcoma

DIAGNOSIS Ewing sarcoma

DISCUSSION Ewing sarcoma is an aggressive small round blue cell tumor arising from bone, closely related to primitive neuroectodermal tumors that arise in other tissues. The tumor results from a translocation of chromosomes 11 and 22, resulting in the fusion gene EWS/FL11. The disease most often presents in the second decade of life, with a male to female ratio of 1.6:1. Of those affected, 95% are Caucasian. It is the second most common primary bone malignancy after osteosarcoma.

Of all the lesions, 75% will be either in the flat bones of the pelvis or the long tubular bones of the extremities.

Patients most often present with bone pain and a palpable mass. Systemic signs are less common, presenting in about one-third. Approximately 30% have overt metastatic disease at presentation, most frequently to the lung.

The classic imaging description is of a large soft-tissue mass arising from the diaphysis or metadiaphysis of a long bone, with "sunburst" or "onion skin" periosteal reaction, a Codman triangle, and a permeative or "moth-eaten" appearance of the bone. CT will demonstrate the extent of bony destruction and periosteal reaction. It is also useful to look for lung metastases. MR will show a large soft-tissue component and better delineate the extent of disease for treatment planning. Positron emission tomography (PET) imaging is used to assess response to therapy.

Neoadjuvant chemotherapy is typical utilized, followed by local radiation therapy and surgical resection. Limb salvage surgery is often attempted.

Questions for Further Thought

1. Should a patient with no overt lung metastases proceed directly to surgical excision?
2. Are Ewing sarcoma and osteosarcoma easily distinguished by their imaging and clinical characteristics?

Reporting Responsibilities

- This is a high-grade, highly malignant lesion, and should generate an immediate call to the referring provider to initiate further management.
- The radiologist should recommend additional imaging with MR for tumor delineation, and likely CT of the chest for exclusion of pulmonary metastases.

What the Treating Physician Needs to Know

1. That imaging favors Ewing sarcoma, and additional imaging may be needed as described above.
2. Prompt evaluation by orthopedic oncology is required.
3. Biopsy should only be performed by or in conjunction with the orthopedic surgeon who will do the limb salvage surgery. The biopsy tract generally also must be excised, and thus the approach is crucial in determining later reconstructability.

Answers

1. No. Most patients are felt to have occult metastases at the time of diagnosis. Neoadjuvant chemotherapy is therefore utilized, which may also help with local control and limb sparing surgery.
2. No. There is great overlap in the two entities. Both affect similar patient populations, males in the second decade of life. Both are common in long bones, with aggressive bone changes. The presence of dense ossification will point toward osteosarcoma, but this is not universally present. Biopsy may be required to differentiate these entities.

REFERENCES

1. Stoller DW. *Magnetic Resonance Imaging in Orthopaedics and Sports Medicine.* 3rd ed. Baltimore, MD: Lippincott; 2007.
2. Slovis TL, ed. *Caffey's Pediatric Diagnostic Imaging.* Philadelphia, PA: Mosby/Elsevier; 2008.
3. Donelly L. *Diagnostic Imaging: Pediatrics.* Salt Lake City, UT: Amirys; 2005.

CASE 1.17

CLINICAL HISTORY *Child with multiple "lumps and bumps"*

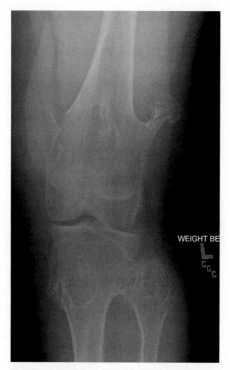

FIGURE **1.17A**

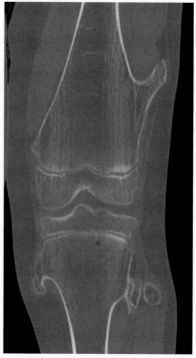

FIGURE **1.17B**

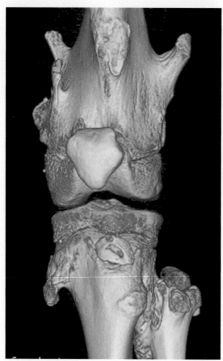

FIGURE **1.17C**

FINDINGS The key finding in this condition is the presence of innumerable osteochondromas, located at multiple places on the body. These are bony excrescences primarily seen on the long bones at the metaphyses. These classically are pedunculated, and point away from the joint space, as seen in these images of the knee: radiograph (**A**), coronal CT reconstruction (**B**), and 3D CT reconstruction (**C**). There is continuity of the normal cortical and medullary bone with that of the lesion.

Undertubulation of the long bones is also encountered, as seen in the knee images as widening of the proximal tibial and distal femoral metaphyses.

DIFFERENTIAL DIAGNOSIS Clinically, the lumps and bumps could represent subcutaneous nodules such as neurofibromas in neurofibromatosis. From an imaging standpoint, the multiplicity and appearance of the lesions are classic for this entity.

DIAGNOSIS Multiple hereditary exostoses (MHE). This is also known as multiple osteochondromatosis.

DISCUSSION MHE is an autosomal dominant hereditary disorder with 96% penetrance. Most cases are familial, though 10% to 20% of patients are a new spontaneous mutation. The incidence is approximately 1:52,000, males are more commonly involved, and have increased severity.

The exostoses are not present at birth, but develop during childhood. The patients will present with multiple palpable masses about the joints. Symptoms are most often attributable to mass effect from the exostoses themselves, causing limitation of joint range of motion, or direct inflammation or impingement on local muscles or nerves. The lesions can fracture, with subsequent pain. Undertubulation of the long bones can also lead to short stature and bowing deformities of the lower extremities.

Treatment is palliative, with many patients undergoing numerous surgeries for local management. The lesions tend to grow until adulthood before stabilizing.

The feared complication of any osteochondroma is degeneration of the cartilaginous end-cap into a chondrosarcoma. This is very uncommon in solitary lesions, <1%, but has been reported to be as high as 8.3% in MHE. In an adult, enlargement of the cartilaginous cap >1 cm, renewed growth, or pain is concerning for malignant change. In children, the cap may be as large as 3 cm, and enlargement is normal until puberty. MR is often performed to evaluate these lesions for aggressive features, and differentiate other potential sources of pain such as muscle inflammation, bursa formation, or nerve impingement.

Questions for Further Thought

1. Are there any subpopulations with a higher incidence of MHE?
2. When is advanced imaging of lesions required?

Reporting Responsibilities

- Initial findings of multiple exostoses should prompt investigation of other family members due to the autosomal dominant inheritance pattern.

- Any aggressive features should prompt orthopedics referral and a recommendation of advanced imaging to evaluate for malignant degeneration.

What the Treating Physician Needs to Know

1. Multiple and multifocal lesions are expected, and new lesions will arise. Cataloging of asymptomatic lesions with imaging is not necessarily required.
2. Growth of exostoses is expected in the growing child. Growth or new pain in a postpubertal patient is more concerning and should be addressed.

Answers

1. Yes. Natives of the island of Guam, known as Chamorros, have an incidence of approximately 1:1000. In the Ojibway natives of Canada, the incidence is 13%.
2. Advanced imaging should be performed in consistently painful lesions in children, or those that limit joint movement. Growth is expected and does not necessarily require advanced imaging. New pain or renewed growth postpuberty is cause for advanced imaging to evaluate the cartilaginous cap for malignant degeneration.

REFERENCES

1. Lachman R. *Taybi and Lachman's Radiology of Syndromes, Metabolic Disorders and Skeletal Dysplasias.* 5th ed. Philadelphia, PA: Mosby/Elsevier; 2007.
2. Stoller DW. *Magnetic Resonance Imaging in Orthopaedics and Sports Medicine.* 3rd ed. Baltimore, MD: Lippincott; 2007.
3. Kivioja A, Ervasti H, Kinnunen J, et al. Chondrosarcoma in a family with multiple hereditary exostoses. *J Bone Joint Surg Br.* 2000;82(2):261–266.

CLINICAL HISTORY *A 14-year-old male athlete with chronic knee pain, worse with exercise*

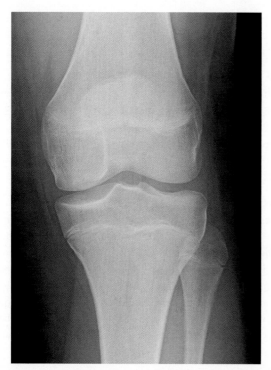

FIGURE **1.18A**

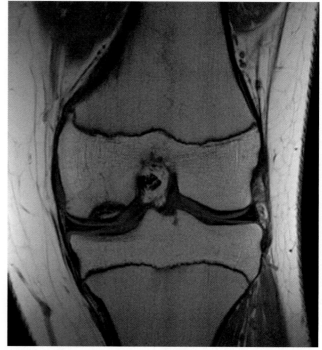

FIGURE **1.18B**

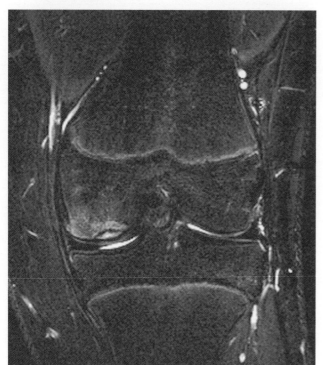

FIGURE **1.18C**

FINDINGS There is a lucent lesion on plain radiographs located at the medial femoral condyle (**A**). Subsequent coronal T1W (**B**) and STIR (**C**) MR images demonstrate a 1-cm lesion surrounded by a rim of high T2 signal. No definite irregularity of the overlying articular cartilage is seen.

DIFFERENTIAL DIAGNOSIS Normal irregular distal femoral epiphyseal ossification, AVN of the femoral condyle, osteochondral fracture from direct impact, stress fracture, osteochondritis dissecans (OCD)

DIAGNOSIS OCD of the knee

DISCUSSION OCD of the knee is a relatively frequent cause of knee pain in athletic children, with a male to female ratio of 3:1. It is most commonly seen at the lateral aspect (primary weight-bearing surface) of the medial femoral condyle, extending toward the intercondylar notch. Talar dome and capitellum are other common sites.

This lesion is felt to be the sequela of repetitive microtrauma of the weight-bearing surfaces. It is frequently diagnosed on plain radiographs as a circumscribed lucency of the condyle. MRI is often helpful in determining the stability of the lesion. The grading system typically used in adults may not be as applicable in children or teenagers, as the latter group tends to be more resilient. For example, in adults, the presence of high T2 signal around an OCD lesion is often described as "unstable." However, in children, instability requires the surrounding bright T2 signal to be as bright as fluid, not just hyperintense with respect to the surrounding marrow.

In a child, it is important to differentiate OCD from normal, irregular ossification of the femoral condyles. Normal developmental irregularity will typically be located more posteriorly in the condyle and away from the articular surface. Multiple accessory ossification centers are often seen, and the centers will have a more spiculated margin than the OCD lesions. MR will also fail to show the marrow edema seen with osteochondral lesions.

Questions for Further Thought

1. Are AVN and OCD the same entity?
2. Should MR arthrography be performed routinely?

Reporting Responsibilities

- Presence of loose bodies within the joint space on plain radiographs must be documented, as this means an unstable and fragmented lesion.
- Components of the MR classification system must be commented upon to determine an unstable and thus surgical lesion.

What the Treating Physician Needs to Know

1. Orthopedics referral and MRI of the knee should be done in a patient with knee pain and an OCD demonstrated on plain radiographs.
2. MR findings of an unstable fragment require orthopedic evaluation, and this should be relayed to the referring primary care physician.

Answers

1. AVN and OCD are not the same entity. OCD is a result of osteonecrosis from repetitive microtrauma, not a lack of vascularity. The joint with the most overlap of these entities is the elbow. Panner disease or "little league elbow" is AVN of the capitellum. This will show sclerosis and fragmentation rather than a focal, single defect. The condition is typically seen in boys under 10.
2. MR classification of instability is based on findings from conventional MR, and arthrography is not routinely performed. In equivocal cases where treatment will be altered based on the presence of subtle articular defects, gadolinium arthrography may then be helpful in determining the patient's course.

REFERENCES

1. Stoller DW. *Magnetic Resonance Imaging in Orthopaedics and Sports Medicine.* 3rd ed. Baltimore, MD: Lippincott; 2007.
2. Slovis TL, ed. *Caffey's Pediatric Diagnostic Imaging.* Philadelphia, PA: Mosby/Elsevier; 2008.
3. Donelly L. *Diagnostic Imaging: Pediatrics.* Salt Lake City, UT: Amirys; 2005.

CLINICAL HISTORY *Otherwise healthy child with asymmetric lower extremities*

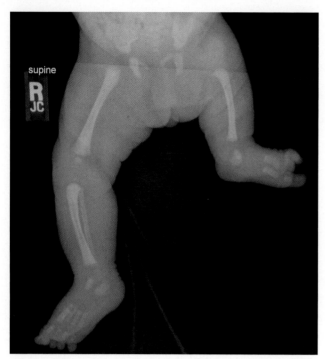

FIGURE **1.19A**

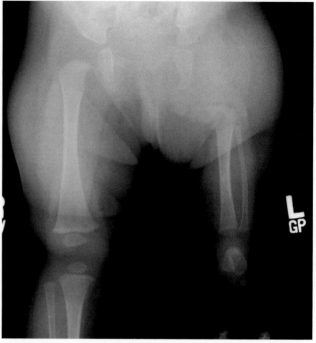

FIGURE **1.19B**

(**A**) Newborn. (**B**) Later with early femoral ossification. Different child, same syndrome with a milder presentation.

FINDINGS Early imaging (**A**) fails to demonstrate any component of the left femur. The limb is foreshortened, and there is a flat and insufficient acetabulum. While femoral head ossification is not expected at this age, the acetabular abnormality is consistent with a poorly formed or absent femoral epiphysis. Later imaging (**B**) shows a minimally formed and ossified left femur, with no evident femoral head. The contralateral limb is normally formed, and the remaining bones are normal in appearance.

DIFFERENTIAL DIAGNOSIS Congenitally short femur, proximal focal femoral deficiency (PFFD), congenital coxa vara, DDH

DIAGNOSIS PFFD

DISCUSSION PFFD is a spectrum of abnormal development of the femur and acetabulum. This is a sporadic condition occurring in approximately 1:52,000 births, about twice as frequently in males. It is a developmental insult occurring around 4 to 6 weeks. It is bilateral in10% to 15% of cases, and usually quite severe when it does affect both sides. There is a high association with ipsilateral fibular hemimelia. Other findings include tibial shortening, and an unstable knee secondary to insufficient cruciate ligaments. Abductor musculature about the hip may also be poorly developed.

Classification is based on the degree of femoral and acetabular insufficiency. Several classification systems have been developed, but the most commonly used is the Aitken system. This was developed in 1968, and is based upon plain radiographs.

Aitken A: Femoral head is present and there is a normal acetabulum. Early, there may be a defect separating the femoral head from the shaft, but this eventually ossifies with no defect. Subtrochanteric varus angulation is seen.

Aitken B: Femoral head is present with a formed acetabulum, though both are mild to moderately dysplastic. There is a non-ossified gap between the femoral head and shaft.

Aitken C: Femoral head is completely absent or merely a small ossicle. Subsequently, the acetabulum is extremely dysplastic.

Aitken D: Femoral head and acetabulum both absent, severely diminished femoral segment, obturator foramen of pelvis is enlarged.

Ultrasound or MRI can allow better classification early on in infancy, before ossification of the femoral segments. MRI can also evaluate for ligamentous insufficiency in the knee. This can help treatment planning. Treatment is aimed at leg lengthening for function in less severe cases. In the higher grades, hip and knee reconstruction, rotationplasty of the tibia, foot amputation, and other procedures can be performed to maximize mobility.

Question for Further Thought

1. What percentage of patients with PFFD will have associated ipsilateral fibular hemimelia?

Reporting Responsibilities

• The key to the Aitken classification is the degree of acetabular dysmorphology, so this must be stressed in the report.
• The other lower extremity must be imaged, as bilaterality is common and will impact management.

What the Treating Physician Needs to Know

1. Bilaterality and associated abnormalities of the fibula
2. MRI may be indicated to determine non-osseous connection between the femoral components in mild cases, and may be necessary to evaluate ligamentous integrity of the knee to guide later management.

Answer

1. Of all patients with PFFD, 50% will have ipsilateral fibular hemimelia.

REFERENCES

1. Slovis TL, ed. *Caffey's Pediatric Diagnostic Imaging.* Philadelphia, PA: Mosby/Elsevier; 2008.
2. Donelly L. *Diagnostic Imaging: Pediatrics.* Salt Lake City, UT: Amirys; 2005.

Stephen L. Foster, Luana Stanescu, and Mahesh Thapa

CASE 1.20

CLINICAL HISTORY *Short stature, evaluate for syndrome/dysplasia*

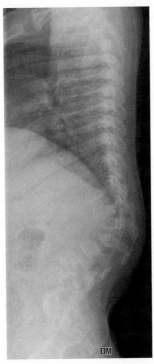

FIGURE **1.20A**

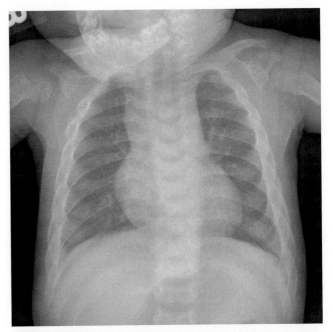

FIGURE **1.20B**

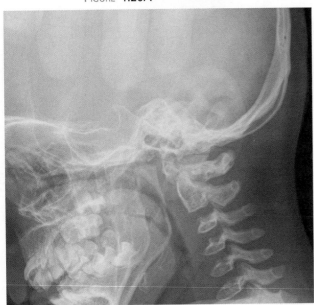

FIGURE **1.20C**

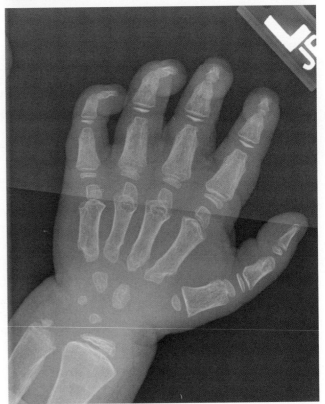

FIGURE **1.20D**

FINDINGS A skeletal survey is performed on any child suspected of a skeletal dysplasia. At our institution (Seattle Children's Hospital), this consists of frontal and lateral views of the skull, chest, spine, frontal pelvis, long bones, feet, and hands. Classic features known as dysostosis multiplex are demonstrated.

Spine (**A**): Dorsolumbar gibbus deformity with characteristic "beaking" of the anterior vertebral bodies (beaking along the inferior margin in this case). This beaking can help differentiate the mucopolysaccharidosis (MPS) types by radiographs. Hurler and Hunter syndrome (MPS 1 and 2) tend to have beaking at the inferior margin of the vertebral body. Morquio syndrome (MPS 4) tends to be in the middle, and Sanfilippo syndrome (MPS 3) tends to be along the superior margin.

Chest (**B**): Wide, "paddle"- or "oar-" shaped ribs. Short, thickened clavicles.

Skull (**C**): J-shaped sella turcica and hypoplastic dens.

Hands (**D**): Broad diaphyses of the metacarpals, proximal, and middle phalanges; proximal pointing of the second to fifth metacarpals.

Pelvis: Narrowed/tapered iliac bones, flat acetabula.

DIFFERENTIAL DIAGNOSIS Dysostosis multiplex (DM) is seen to a varying extent in the various storage diseases that cause dysplasia; primarily MPS including Hunter, Hurler, Morquio, and Sanfilippo syndromes among others. Other dysplasias such as spondyloepiphyseal dysplasia (SED) or spondylometaphyseal dysplasia (SMD) could share some similar findings.

DIAGNOSIS Hurler syndrome, MPS I-H

DISCUSSION Hurler syndrome is the most severe type of the lysosomal storage disorders known as MPS. This is an autosomal recessive deficiency of the enzyme α-L-iduronidase, which is responsible for the breakdown of glycosaminoglycans, aka mucopolysaccharides. This results in accumulation of these substances within developing bones, giving rise to the classic radiographic appearance.

A rare condition, it is present in approximately 1:100,000 live births. The children will usually present between 1 and 2 years of age due to a change in the child's appearance secondary to glycosaminoglycan deposition. Subsequently, the patients will experience developmental delay and loss of milestones due to central nervous system (CNS) involvement. Hirsutism, hepatosplenomegaly, frequent respiratory tract infections and airway narrowing, deafness, corneal clouding and glaucoma, and cardiac valve insufficiency are other associated findings.

Life expectancy without treatment for these children is generally less than 10 years. Bone marrow transplant (BMT) therapy has been shown to be of some benefit, with decreased hepatosplenomegaly, better cardiac function, and improved airway patency. Neurologic deficiency is also lessened with early BMT. Dysplastic bone changes are unaffected by BMT. Recombinant α-L-iduronidase supplementation is also used, though the lack of blood–brain barrier passage means the severe mental retardation will persist.

Questions for Further Thought

1. Do all MPS carry a poor prognosis?
2. Do these patients have a tendency toward more fractures?

Reporting Responsibilities

- Isolated imaging findings of DM should prompt a full skeletal survey and consideration of laboratory or genetic testing.
- The craniocervical junction should be imaged, as there is a strong association with odontoid hypoplasia and C1/C2 instability.

What the Treating Physician Needs to Know

1. DM is seen with a number of dysplasias related to lysosomal storage diseases. Further genetic testing is indicated to fully classify the patient and help determine prognosis. If MPS testing is negative but imaging findings are classic, mucolipidoses should also be considered.
2. C1/C2 instability secondary to odontoid hypoplasia is common and should be evaluated with imaging. Clinical concern for hydrocephalus may require cross-sectional evaluation.

Answers

1. The degree of severity of the skeletal dysplasia does not necessarily correlate with the degree of clinical severity. While Hurler syndrome has both severe DM and severe mental retardation, Sanfilippo syndrome has mild DM with severe mental retardation and Morquio syndrome has severe DM but often normal metal function.
2. While the bones do have abnormal deposition of glycosaminoglycans, mineralization is normal and the bones do not have an excessive tendency toward fracture.

REFERENCES

1. Lachman R. *Taybi and Lachman's Radiology of Syndromes, Metabolic Disorders and Skeletal Dysplasias.* 5th ed. Philadelphia, PA: Mosby/Elsevier; 2007.
2. Jones KL. *Smith's Recognizable Patterns of Human Malformation.* 6th ed. Philadelphia, PA: Elsevier/Saunders; 2006.

Debra J. Popejoy and Sandra L. Wootton-Gorges

CLINICAL HISTORY *A 14-year-old girl with knee pain after twisting injury*

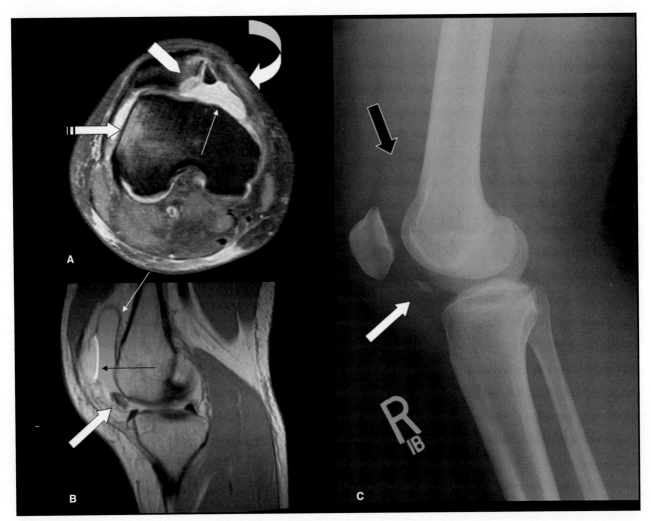

FIGURE 1.21A–C

FINDINGS (**A**) PD fat-saturated (FS) axial MRI image shows marrow edema and an osteochondral fracture of the medial patella (*arrowhead*). There is edema and stranding in the medial patellar retinaculum and medial patellofemoral ligament (*curved arrow*). Marrow edema is seen at the lateral distal femur as well (*dashed arrow*). (**B**) Sagittal PD MRI image shows a large knee joint effusion with hemarthrosis (*thin white and black arrows*). The osteochondral fragment is seen inferior to the patella (*white arrow*). (**C**) Lateral radiograph of the knee shows a large joint effusion (*black arrow*) and a loose body inferior to the patella (*white arrow*)

DIFFERENTIAL DIAGNOSIS Transient acute patellar dislocation, OCD of the patella, osteochondral injury of the patella

DIAGNOSIS Transient acute patellar dislocation with associated osteochondral injury

DISCUSSION Transient patellar dislocation occurs most commonly in the 14- to 20-year-old age range.[1] It almost always occurs laterally and results from twisting injury or direct trauma. Most frequently, the dislocation spontaneously reduces and the only plain radiographic abnormality may be a joint effusion.[2] Because of concern for internal derangement, almost all of these adolescents undergo MRI of their knee, where the injury pattern of (1) bone contusion involving the inferomedial patella and lateral distal femoral condyle; (2) concave impaction deformity or cartilage injury of the inferomedial patella;[3] (3) strain, partial, or complete tear of the patellar retinaculum and MPFL; and (4) patellar tilting and a shallow trochlear notch[1-3] is seen. In addition, joint effusion and edema in Hoffa's fat pad may be present. The patella, as in this case, may undergo osteochondral fracture as it collides with the lateral distal femoral condyle during relocation, resulting in an intra-articular loose body.

Questions for Further Thought

1. What is the main soft-tissue restraint to lateral movement of the patella?
2. What fractures are specific for transient patellar dislocation?

Reporting Responsibilities

- Describe the bony and soft-tissue injuries seen, and recognize the pattern of transient acute patellar dislocation.
- Identify a dysplastic or shallow trochlear groove.
- Identify and report any osteochondral injuries to the patella.

What the Treating Physician Needs to know

1. The only plain film abnormality seen after injury may be a joint effusion; however, one should search for evidence of osteochondral fracture with a loose body.
2. MRI is excellent in detection of this injury, and in defining osteochondral injury of the patella.

Answers

1. The MPFL is the primary soft-tissue restraint to lateral movement of the patella, and accounting for 50% to 80% of the medial restraint. It extends from the medial femur between the adductor tubercle and the medial epicondyle to the upper half of the medial patella. Since the MPFL is often difficult to identify, secondary signs such as edema at its origin and elevation of the vastus medialis obliquus by edema can be used to infer its disruption.[1]
2. Impacted fractures of the inferior medial border of the patella are specific for transient patellar dislocation.[3]

REFERENCES

1. Davis KW. Imaging pediatric sports injuries: Lower extremity. *Radiol Clin North Am.* 2010;48:1213–1235.
2. Sanchez TRS, Jadhav SP, Swischuk LE. MR imaging of pediatric trauma. *Radiol Clin North Am.* 2009;47:927–938.
3. Elias DA, White LM, Fithian DC. Acute lateral patellar dislocation at MR imaging: Injury patterns of medial patellar soft-tissue restraints and osteochondral injuries of the inferomedial patella. *Radiology.* 2002;225:736.

Debra J. Popejoy and Sandra L. Wootton-Gorges

CLINICAL HISTORY *A 14-year-old female who presents with a rib deformity*

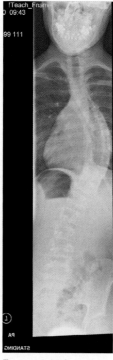

FIGURE **1.22A**

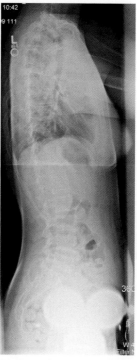

FIGURE **1.22B**

FINDINGS (**A**) This posteroanterior (PA) view of the spine shows a rightward thoracic spinal curve measured as 60°. The thorax is centered to the right of the pelvis. No underlying segmentation anomalies, paraspinal masses, or other lesions are identified. The visualized lungs and heart appear normal.

(**B**) On the lateral view, the normal thoracic kyphosis is decreased.

DIFFERENTIAL DIAGNOSIS Adolescent idiopathic scoliosis (AIS), neuromuscular scoliosis, congenital scoliosis, developmental scoliosis, tumor-associated scoliosis

DIAGNOSIS AIS

DISCUSSION Scoliosis is one of the most common deformities of the pediatric spine. Primary idiopathic scoliosis accounts for 80% of all cases of scoliosis. AIS is more common in girls, and usually includes a rightward thoracic curve.[1] The underlying cause of AIS is unknown. AIS is a diagnosis of exclusion and can only be made after excluding a neuromuscular (such as cerebral palsy or muscular dystrophy), congenital (such as segmentation anomalies),

developmental (such as skeletal dysplasia or neurofibromatosis), or tumor-associated (such as osteoblastoma or spinal cord tumor) cause for the curvature. This is done by careful clinical and radiographic examination, as well as by an MRI in certain instances. MRI is reserved for those patients who have an atypical presentation of presumed idiopathic scoliosis, including patients with complaints of neck pain and headaches, abnormal neurologic findings, a leftward thoracic curve, and those with absence of apical segment lordosis on the lateral projection.[2] MRI findings of syrinx, Arnold–Chiari malformations, diastematomyelia, spinal cord tumors, and tethered spinal cord have all been reported in patients with presumed idiopathic scoliosis.

Treatment is based on the severity of curvature, the likelihood of progression, and symptoms. Treatment options include observation, bracing, and surgical correction with instrumentation and fusion.

Questions for Further Thought

1. Should a PA or an AP image be used for imaging scoliosis?
2. In reviewing a spine MRI image of a child with congenital scoliosis, what other organ system should be closely scrutinized?

Reporting Responsibilities

• Describe the location, degree, and direction of the curvature. Most current PACS systems have a Cobb angle measuring tool. If not, the reader is referred to Ref. 1 for the description of Cobb angle measurement.
• Describe any bony or soft-tissue lesions (such as segmentation anomalies and paraspinal masses) that may be the underlying etiology for the scoliosis.

What the Treating Physician Needs to Know

1. The severity of the curve.
2. Is the scoliosis idiopathic, or is there an underlying etiology for the curve?

Answers

1. The PA radiograph is recommended, as this significantly decreases the amount of radiation to breast and thyroid tissues. Studies have shown that patients undergoing multiple scoliosis studies have a slightly increased risk of these cancers.[3]
2. The genitourinary (GU) system develops at the same time as the spine, and 20% of children with congenital scoliosis have a GU abnormality.[4]

REFERENCES

1. Kim H, Kim HS, Moon ES, et al. Scoliosis imaging: What radiologists should know. *Radiographics*. 2010;30:1823–1842.
2. Davids JR, Chamberlin E, Blackhurst DW. Indications for magnetic resonance imaging in presumed adolescent idiopathic scoliosis. *J Bone Joint Surg Am*. 2004;86:2187–2195.
3. Levy AR, Goldberg MS, Mayo NE, et al. Reducing the lifetime risk of cancer from spinal radiographs among people with adolescent idiopathic scoliosis. *Spine*. 1996;21:1540.
4. Riccio AI, Guille JT, Grissom L, et al. Magnetic resonance imaging of renal abnormalities in patients with congenital osseous anomalies of the spine. *J Bone Joint Surg Am*. 2007;89:2456–2459.

CASE 1.23

CLINICAL HISTORY *A 15-year-old female with multiple sites of bone pain*

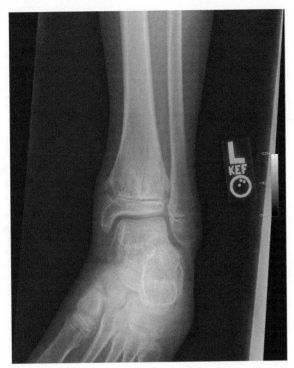

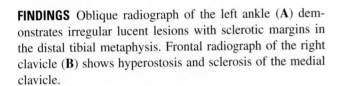

FIGURE **1.23A**

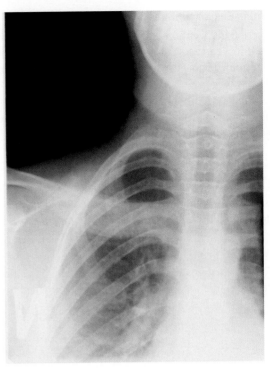

FIGURE **1.23B**

FINDINGS Oblique radiograph of the left ankle (**A**) demonstrates irregular lucent lesions with sclerotic margins in the distal tibial metaphysis. Frontal radiograph of the right clavicle (**B**) shows hyperostosis and sclerosis of the medial clavicle.

DIFFERENTIAL DIAGNOSIS Chronic recurrent multifocal osteomyelitis (CRMO), multifocal pyogenic osteomyelitis, metastases

DIAGNOSIS CRMO

DISCUSSION CRMO is most likely a noninfectious inflammatory disorder. The prolonged clinical course is punctuated by episodic multifocal bone pain. The vast majority of cases (up to 85%) occur in females, with a median age of onset of 10 years. The lesions are predomi-nantly situated in the metaphyses of tubular bones, followed by the clavicle and spine.[1] Among tubular bones, there is a predilection for the lower extremities. CRMO has a variable imaging presentation depending on active versus reparative phases. In its active phase, there is lytic destruction centered in the metaphyses with sclerotic margins. In its reparative phase, hyperostosis and sclerosis are typically present. Abscess or sequestra formation are typically absent, distinguishing CRMO from pyogenic osteomyelitis. MR during active disease demonstrates T2/STIR hyperintense marrow edema and ill-defined enhancement within the affected bone.[2]

Questions for Further Thought

1. How does spinal CRMO present on imaging?
2. What are long-term sequelae of CRMO?

Reporting Responsibilities

- Identify and describe the locations and extent of abnormalities.
- Identify disease phase—active, reparative, or mixed—if possible.

What the Treating Physician Needs to Know

CRMO is often a diagnosis of exclusion. Offer the most likely alternative diagnoses, particularly pyogenic osteomyelitis and tumor.

Answers

1. Spinal CRMO typically mimics spondylodiscitis. There is irregularity and edema involving a single vertebral end plate, without crossing the intervertebral space. CRMO can also manifest as vertebra plana.

2. Most cases are self-limited and resolve without major sequelae. However, some patients do suffer from premature closure of epiphyses, bony deformity, and kyphosis.

REFERENCES

1. Jurik AG. Chronic regional multifocal osteomyelitis. *Semin Musculoskel Radiol.* 2004;8(3):243–253.
2. Jurik AG, Egund N. MRI in chronic recurrent multifocal osteomyelitis. *Skeletal Radiol.* 1997;26:230–238.

Ramesh Iyer and Mahesh Thapa

CLINICAL HISTORY *A 12-year-old girl with back pain.*

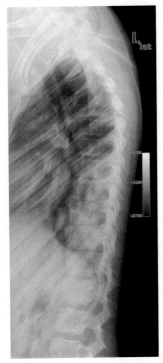

FIGURE **1.24A**

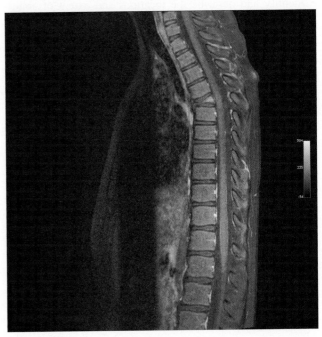

FIGURE **1.24B**

FINDINGS Lateral radiograph (**A**) and sagittal T1-weighted, post-contrast MR image of the thoracic spine (**B**) demonstrate complete collapse of a single upper thoracic vertebral body. There is no involvement of the adjacent disks, central canal, or posterior elements.

DIFFERENTIAL DIAGNOSIS Vertebra plana (multiple etiologies, see later)

DIAGNOSIS Vertebra plana from eosinophilic granuloma (EG)

DISCUSSION Vertebra plana is an imaging diagnosis of complete vertebral body collapse. Criteria for this diagnosis include the following: (1) collapse of one vertebral body only, (2) normal adjacent intervertebral disks, (3) height of the intervertebral space increased by at least one-third compared to normal, and (4) increased density of the collapsed vertebra.[1]

Vertebra plana is a manifestation of numerous diseases, often indistinguishable on imaging. The most common etiology is EG. The differential diagnosis also includes malignant tumors (Ewing sarcoma, osteosarcoma, lymphoma, leukemia, metastasis), benign tumors (GCT, ABC), trauma, and infection.[1,2]

Questions for Further Thought

1. What are indications for biopsy in cases of vertebra plana?
2. How can one distinguish between EG and osteomyelitis as a cause for vertebra plana?

Reporting Responsibilities

- Identify the spinal level affected.
- Identify any associated central canal or neural foraminal compromise.
- Identify and describe any soft-tissue lesion components.

What the Treating Physician Needs to Know

1. If there is central canal stenosis, MR signal changes within or compression of the spinal cord, immediate consultation with both the treating physician and neurologic surgery is recommended.

2. The differential diagnosis for vertebra plana is very broad. The radiologist must communicate directly with the treating physician to elicit any pertinent clinical history such as known malignancy, prior trauma to that region, and signs of infection.

Answers

1. Biopsy is warranted when the aforementioned classic criteria are not all met, and the diagnosis of EG-induced vertebra plana is uncertain. Such cases include the presence of a soft-tissue mass, neurologic compromise, age over 20 years, extension to posterior elements, and multilevel disease.

2. In EG, disk height is preserved because the disease typically spares cartilage. In osteomyelitis, the disk is often involved either by direct extension or hematogenous spread.

REFERENCES

1. Baghaie M, Gillet P, Dondelinger RF, et al. Vertebra plana: Benign or malignant lesion? *Pediatr Radiol.* 1996;26:431–433.

2. O'Donnell J, Brown L, Herkowitz H. Vertebra plana-like lesions in children: Case report with special emphasis on the differential diagnosis and indications for biopsy. *J Spinal Disord.* 1991;4(4):480–485.

CASE 1.25

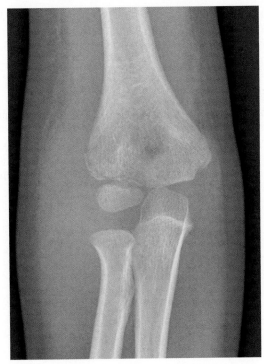

FIGURE **1.25A**

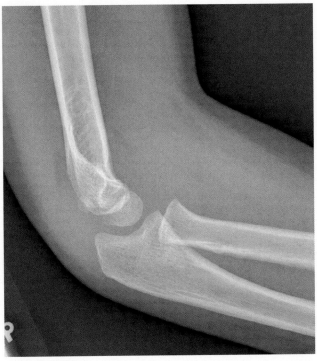

FIGURE **1.25B**

FINDINGS AP radiograph of the elbow demonstrates a fracture line along the lateral condyle (**A**). Lateral radiograph demonstrates an anterior and posterior sail sign indicative of a large joint effusion (**B**).

DIFFERENTIAL DIAGNOSIS Supracondylar fracture, lateral condylar fracture

DIAGNOSIS Lateral condylar fracture

DISCUSSION Lateral condylar fractures are the second most common pediatric elbow fracture. These usually occur after a fall on an outstretched hand with forced varus angulation. Radiographically, lateral condylar fractures may resemble a Salter–Harris type II fracture. However, lateral condylar fractures may often extend to the articular surface and this may only be visible by MRI.[1] Nondisplaced lateral condylar fractures can be treated conservatively with casting. When there is greater than 2 mm displacement, these fractures should be percutaneously pinned to avoid complications such as nonunion, cubitus varus, or cubitus valgus deformity.[2]

Question for Further Thought

1. Name in order the top three pediatric elbow fractures.

Reporting Responsibilities

Differentiating a lateral condylar fracture and supracondylar fracture. Oblique views may be necessary to identify the lateral condylar fracture plane that often is parallel with respect to the medial aspect of the distal humeral physis.

What the Treating Physician Needs to Know

Describe the degree of displacement in millimeters. If there is greater than 2 mm displacement, then surgical reduction and pin fixation is required.

Answer

1. Supracondylar, lateral condylar, and medial epicondylar fractures.

REFERENCES

1. Beltran J, Rosenberg ZS, Kawelblum M, et al. Pediatric elbow fractures: MRI evaluation. *Skeletal Radiol.* 1994;23:277–281.

2. Shrader MW. Pediatric supracondylar fractures and pediatric physeal elbow fractures. *Orthop Clin North Am.* 2008;39: 163–171.

J. Herman Kan

CLINICAL HISTORY *A 14-year-old boy with medial elbow pain*

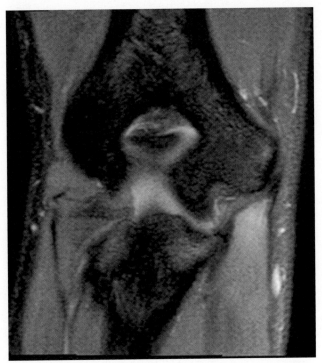

FIGURE **1.26A**

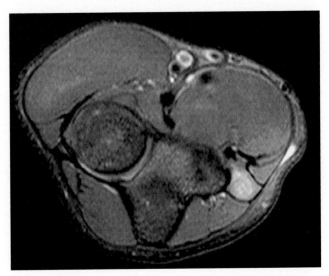

FIGURE **1.26B**

FINDINGS (**A**) PD FS coronal and (**B**) T2 FS axial sequences show myositis of the flexor digitorum superficialis muscle origin. There is also mild osteitis of the sublime tubercle at the insertion of the anterior band of the ulnar collateral ligament.

DIFFERENTIAL DIAGNOSIS Medial epicondylitis, anterior band medial collateral ligament tear

DIAGNOSIS Medial epicondylitis

DISCUSSION Medial epicondylitis represents a chronic overuse injury related to repetitive valgus stress often seen in throwing athletes.[1] It is a misnomer because proximal soft-tissue injuries of the flexor–pronator complex usually are present[2] rather than osteitis of the medial epicondyle. In younger children in whom the medial epicondylar physeal equivalent remains patent, the weakest component of the musculoskeletal unit is the physis. Therefore, in younger children, medial epicondylar avulsion fractures may occur rather than soft-tissue injuries of the flexor–pronator complex origin.

Additional injuries related to repetitive valgus stress include tears of the ulnar collateral ligament and chronic impaction injuries to the lateral compartment of the elbow. The most commonly identified tear of the ulnar collateral ligament by MRI is the anterior band. Chronic impaction injuries of the lateral compartment of the elbow related to repetitive valgus stress may lead to OCD of the capitellum and less commonly the radial head.[3]

Question for Further Thought

1. Which nerve may be inflamed or injured indirectly in the setting of medial epicondylitis?

Reporting Responsibilities

Make sure to evaluate both the medial and lateral compartments of the elbow in children with repetitive valgus injury. Therefore, in addition to evaluating for medial epicondylitis, the lateral compartment should be assessed for changes related to chronic impaction injury, including OCD of the capitellum and radial head.

What the Treating Physician Needs to Know

Must differentiate medial epicondylitis from alternative causes for medial elbow pain, including tears of the anterior band of the ulnar collateral ligament and medial epicondylar avulsion fractures.

Answer

1. Ulnar nerve.

REFERENCES

1. Walz DM, Newman JS, Konin GP, et al. Epicondylitis: Pathogenesis, imaging, and treatment. *Radiographics.* 2010;30:167–184.
2. Martin CE, Schweitzer ME. MR imaging of epicondylitis. *Skeletal Radiol.* 1998;27:133–138.
3. Klingele KE, Kocher MS. Little league elbow: Valgus overload injury in the pediatric athlete. *Sports Med.* 2002;32:1005–1015.

CASE 1.27

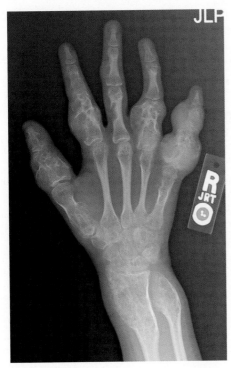

FIGURE **1.27A**

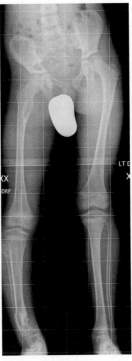

FIGURE **1.27B**

FINDINGS Frontal radiograph of the hand (**A**) shows multiple lobulated lytic lesions with endosteal scalloping involving all five digits as well as the distal radius and ulna. A calcific matrix is noted in the distal radius and ulna. A leg length survey (**B**) shows a foreshortened right lower extremity with multiple lobulated lytic lesions with chondroid matrix in the tibia and fibula as well as the proximal femur. Longitudinal lucent channels are also noted in the distal femur and proximal tibia metadiaphysis.

DIFFERENTIAL DIAGNOSIS Enchondromatosis (Ollier disease), polyostotic FD

DIAGNOSIS Enchondromatosis (Ollier disease)

DISCUSSION Enchondromatosis (Ollier disease) is a nonhereditary condition characterized by multiple enchondromas usually asymmetrically distributed about the skeleton. These children may present with leg length discrepancy (**B**), pathologic fractures, or palpable masses. The most common location for enchondromas is the hand (**A**), particularly the proximal phalanges.[1] These children are at increased risk for chondrosarcomatous transformation of enchondromas (5% to 30%) as well as solid organ neoplasms but usually occur later in life, usually the third or fourth decade. Maffucci syndrome is a related condition in which multiple enchondromas are associated with multiple vascular anomalies. Longitudinal lucent channels within the appendicular bones may be seen in the setting of enchondromas (**B**) and is felt to represent longitudinally oriented enchondromas.

Questions for Further Thought

1. What calcific matrix pattern description is seen with chondroid lesions?
2. What is the name of the syndrome when there are multiple enchondromas and osteochondromas present?

Reporting Responsibilities

- Describe full extent and involvement of affected extremity.
- Recommend MRI if a pathologic fracture is not identified, and the child presents with persistent pain.

What the Treating Physician Needs to Know

1. Identify any pathologic fractures when present.

2. Comment on presence or absence of appendicular length discrepancies and angular deformities when present.

Answers

1. Ring and arc calcifications
2. Metachondromatosis

REFERENCE

1. Flemming DJ, Murphey MD. Enchondroma and chondrosarcoma. *Semin Musculoskelet Radiol.* 2000;4(1):59–71.

CLINICAL HISTORY *A 4-year-old girl with knee bowing*

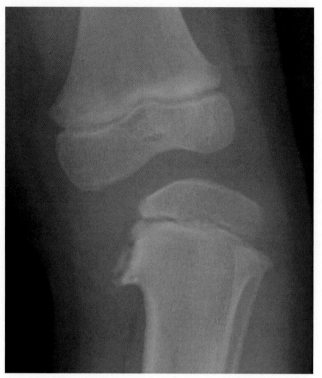

FIGURE 1.28

FINDINGS AP radiograph of the left knee demonstrates proximal tibia medial metaphyseal beaking, fragmentation, and diminished medial epiphyseal height. In addition, there is tibia vara.

DIFFERENTIAL DIAGNOSIS Blount disease, rickets, metaphyseal fracture, physiologic genu varus.

DIAGNOSIS Blount disease

DISCUSSION Blount disease is an idiopathic condition resulting in growth disturbance and angular deformity of the proximal tibia medial metaphysis, physis, and epiphysis resulting in tibia vara. Bilaterality is seen in up to 60% of patients. The radiographic hallmarks include sharp angular metaphyseal beaking, diminished medial epiphyseal height, and fragmentary appearance of the medial tibial epiphysis and metaphysis. The angular deformity related to Blount disease is at the level of the proximal tibia. This should be distinguished from physiologic genu varus where the epicenter of bowing is at the level of the joint line and is not associated with proximal tibial deformity. There are two subtypes of Blount disease: infantile and adolescent Blount. Adolescent Blount disease is a milder form of the disease and presents usually in the second decade of life and is associated with less angular deformity compared with infantile Blount disease.[1] Imaging hallmarks of adolescent Blount disease include diminished medial epiphyseal height of the tibia and medial tibial physeal widening. Unlike infantile Blount disease, medial metaphyseal beaking and epiphyseal fragmentation are usually absent in adolescent Blount disease.

Question for Further Thought

1. At approximately what age does physiologic genu varus resolve?

Reporting Responsibilities

Rule out alternative causes for tibia vara such as rickets or fracture.

What the Treating Physician Needs to Know

The degree of tibia vara is more severe with weight-bearing views. Therefore, quantifying the degree of tibia vara should also account for whether the radiographs were taken with or without weight bearing.

Answer

1. Approximately 2 years of age. Eventually, genu valgus develops and peaks at approximately 4 years.

REFERENCE

1. Do TT. Clinical and radiographic evaluation of bowlegs. *Curr Opin Pediatr.* 2001;13:42–46.

CASE 1.29

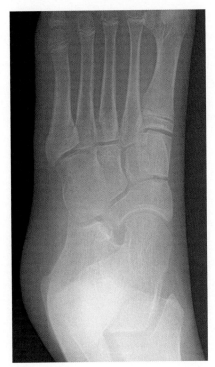

FIGURE **1.29A**

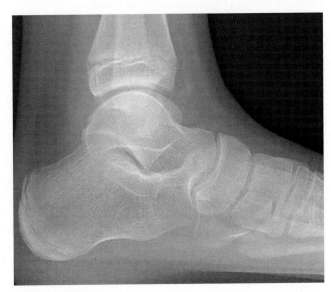

FIGURE **1.29B**

FINDINGS Oblique (**A**) and lateral (**B**) radiographs of the foot show irregularity and narrowing of the talonavicular joint. An "anteater" sign is evident of the lateral radiograph. The longitudinal arch is maintained on the standing lateral view (**B**).

DIFFERENTIAL DIAGNOSIS Calcaneonavicular coalition, anterior process calcaneal fracture

DIAGNOSIS Calcaneonavicular coalition

DISCUSSION The most frequent coalitions found in the foot are at the talonavicular and calcaneonavicular joints.[1] The most common presentation of coalitions is foot pain which usually occurs when coalitions begin to ossify. Talonavicular coalitions tend to ossify at 3 to 5 years, calcaneonavicular coalitions ossify at 8 to 12 years, and talocalcaneal coalitions ossify at 12 to 16 years.[1] Approximately 50% of coalitions will present with a pes planus deformity.[2]

Radiographic features of calcaneonavicular coalitions include pes planus, anteater sign (**B**), and a reverse anteater sign. A reverse anteater sign is seen on the AP view of the foot and is defined as diminished AP height of the lateral portion of the navicular (compared with the medial navicular) and the navicular bone extends far lateral with respect to the talar head.[2]

Radiographic features of talocalcaneal coalitions include C sign (seen on the lateral view), talar beak, dysmorphic sustentaculum tali, blunted lateral process of the talus, and absent middle facet sign.[2] Talar beak associated with talocalcaneal coalitions is a dorsal lip and is an extension of the talar head. Talar beaks should not be confused with the talar ridge that lies along the dorsal aspect of the distal talar neck and represents bony proliferation related to the insertion of the anterior tibiotalar capsule.[2]

CT and MRI may be helpful for identifying coalitions before they are radiographically apparent, particularly in very young children when coalitions are still fibrocartilaginous. CT evaluation of coalitions is superior with respect to MRI in regard to speed of the study and diagnostic ease of identifying coalitions. MRI is also useful for diagnosing coalitions but is diagnostically more challenging and longer to perform compared with CT, but offer superior soft-tissue resolution. MRI may identify alternative etiologies for foot or ankle pain when coalitions are not present.

Question for Further Thought

1. Approximately what percent of patients have coalitions in both feet?

Reporting Responsibilities

- Determine if the coalition is fibrocartilaginous or bony.
- Identify additional coalitions when present in the same foot.

What the Treating Physician Needs to Know

Determine if there are secondary degenerative changes related to altered biomechanics of the foot related to the coalition.

Answer

1. Coalitions occur bilaterally in approximately 50% of patients.

REFERENCES

1. Zaw H, Calder JD. Tarsal coalitions. *Foot Ankle Clin.* 2010; 15:349–364.
2. Crim J. Imaging of tarsal coalition. *Radiol Clin North Am.* 2008; 46:1017–1026, vi.

CLINICAL HISTORY *A 3-year-old girl with chronic forearm swelling*

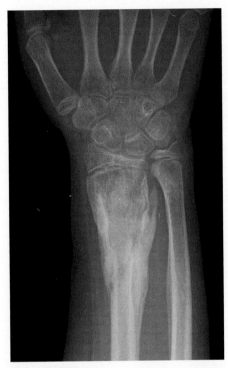

FIGURE **1.30A**

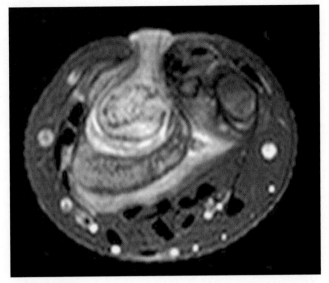

FIGURE **1.30B**

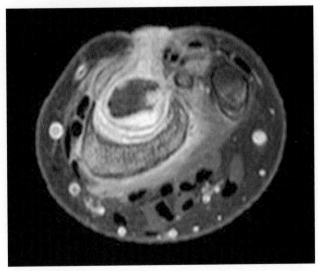

FIGURE **1.30C**

FINDINGS Extensive involucrum surrounds distal radial metadiaphyseal osteolysis with a nondisplaced pathologic fracture present (**A**). Axial T2 FS (**B**) demonstrates a target sign and dorsal sinus tract. Post-Gd T1 FS axial (**C**) demonstrates central nonenhancement and surrounding granulation tissue, consistent with a Brodie abscess.

DIFFERENTIAL DIAGNOSIS Chronic osteomyelitis, Ewing sarcoma

DIAGNOSIS Chronic osteomyelitis

DISCUSSION The most common etiologies for hematogenous osteomyelitis are *Streptococcus pneumoniae* and *Staphylococcus aureus*.[1] In children approximately 18 months and older, hematogenous osteomyelitis usually occurs in the metaphysis where blood flow tends to be sluggish related to terminal sinusoids which loop at the level of the juxtaphyseal metaphysis. In children with open physis, the physis acts as a relative but not absolute barrier for epiphyseal extension of infection. In children younger than 18 months, or in children whose physis have fused, transphyseal extension of infection into the epiphysis is more likely to occur.

Imaging features related to chronic osteomyelitis include sequestrum (necrotic bone centrally located), involucrum (reactive bone formation around a sequestrum), cloaca (fistulous tract between intramedullary abscess and outer cortex), sinus tract (fistulous tract between intramedullary abscess and skin), and Brodie abscess. A Brodie abscess by MRI will have a target appearance.[1] The center of a Brodie abscess contains pus (hyperintense on T2 FS, nonenhancing on T1 post-Gd), surrounding granulation tissue (intermediate on T2 FS, enhancing on T1 post-Gd), and outer sclerotic layer (hypointense on both T2 FS and T1 post-Gd).

Question for Further Thought

1. In the setting of osteomyelitis, approximately when will radiographs become abnormal from the time of onset of infection?

Reporting Responsibilities

- Describe all intra-osseous and soft-tissue abscesses when present.
- Determine if the physis is affected, and if there is transphyseal extension of infection.

What the Treating Physician Needs to Know

If there is coexisting septic arthritis in the setting of osteomyelitis.

Answer

1. Approximately 10 days.

REFERENCE

1. Saigal G, Azouz EM, Abdenour G. Imaging of osteomyelitis with special reference to children. *Semin Musculoskelet Radiol.* 2004;8:255–265.

CLINICAL HISTORY *A 12-year-old boy with chronic shin pain*

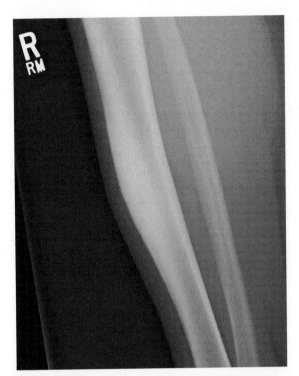

FIGURE **1.31A**

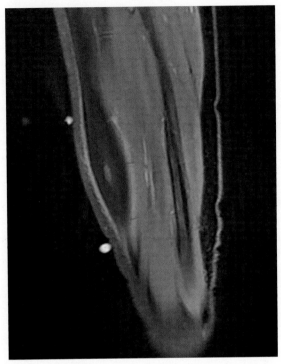

FIGURE **1.31B**

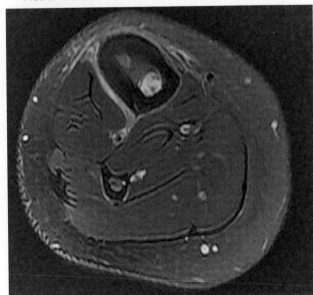

FIGURE **1.31C**

FINDINGS There is diffuse anterior cortical thickening of the mid-tibial shaft (**A**). Fluid-sensitive sequences demonstrate a small hyperintense nidus which is surrounded by mature periosteal and cortical thickening (**B** and **C**). There is diffuse marrow edema and periosteal edema noted (**C**).

DIFFERENTIAL DIAGNOSIS Osteoid osteoma, stress fracture, osteomyelitis

DIAGNOSIS Osteoid osteoma

DISCUSSION Osteoid osteoma is a benign lesion that usually occurs in the second and third decade of life.[1] It usually presents with nocturnal pain that is relieved with nonsteroidal anti-inflammatory medications. On radiography, it presents with diffuse mature periosteal thickening. A nidus may be seen and better delineated by CT or MRI. On MRI, these lesions tend to cause significant juxtalesional soft-tissue and marrow edema (**C**). A nidus may sometimes be identified and will demonstrate increased signal on fluid-sensitive sequences and demonstrate enhancement on post-contrast sequences. On CT, the nidus is radiolucent and surrounded by thick mature periosteal reaction. Osteoid osteomas may be intra- or extra-articular. Intra-articular osteoid osteomas may present as an inflammatory arthritis with a reactive synovitis and effusion present. When osteoid osteomas occur in the spine, they usually present with a painful scoliosis.

The natural history of osteoid osteomas is that they will spontaneously regress. Nonsteroidal anti-inflammatory medications are the first-line agent to treat symptoms. If nonsteroidal medications do not work and the family wishes for a definitive procedure, surgical en bloc resection of the nidus may be performed. Alternatively, thermal or radiofrequency ablation may also be used to destroy the nidus.

Question for Further Thought

1. What is the postulated hormone produced by the nidus of osteoid osteomas that causes regional pain?

Reporting Responsibilities

Identify the nidus when present. Introduce alternative differential considerations including healing stress fracture if a nidus cannot be identified.

What the Treating Physician Needs to Know

Location and size of the nidus, and whether the nidus is intra- or extra-articular.

Answer

1. Prostaglandin E2.

REFERENCE

1. Lee EH, Shafi M, Hui JH. Osteoid osteoma: A current review. *J Pediatr Orthop.* 2006;26:695–700.

CASE 1.32

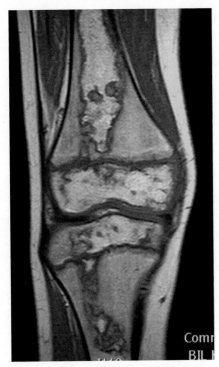

Figure **1.32A**

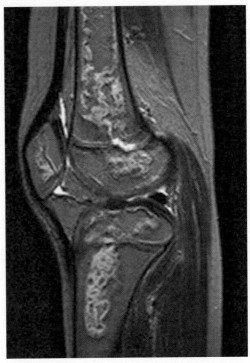

Figure **1.32B**

FINDINGS There are geographic serpiginous lesions affecting the visualized diametaphysis and epiphysis of the distal femur, proximal tibia, and patella (**A** and **B**). Centrally, there is fat signal intensity present, with hyperintensity seen on T1W sequences (**A**) and corresponding decreased signal on FS sequences (**B**).

DIFFERENTIAL DIAGNOSIS Osteonecrosis

DIAGNOSIS Osteonecrosis

DISCUSSION Osteonecrosis results from ischemic injury to bone. This can be due to multiple etiologies, including but not limited to trauma, storage disorders such as Gaucher disease, medications including steroid use, vasculitis, sickle cell disease, and marrow packing disorders such as leukemia.[1] Oftentimes, osteonecrosis is a reversible process. When reversible, MRI will demonstrate central fatty marrow replacement. The area of affected bone will often have reactive changes manifested as the "double-line sign" that will surround the fatty marrow centrally. The double-line sign represents a sclerotic serpiginous outer margin which is dark on all imaging sequences, and an inner lining composed of granulation tissue which will demonstrate increased signal on fluid-sensitive sequences and enhancement on contrasted sequences. When osteonecrosis is irreversible, the center of affected bone will usually be hypointense on all MRI sequences and will demonstrate sclerosis on radiography.

When osteonecrosis involves epiphysis, the term AVN may be applied or alternatively epiphyseal osteonecrosis. Complications related to epiphyseal osteonecrosis include subchondral fracturing, subchondral collapse, and premature degenerative changes.

When an area of osteonecrosis is identified, it is important to determine whether the area is acutely involved, old, or whether there are acute on chronic changes. When osteonecrosis is acute, it may be difficult to discern these changes from early osteomyelitis.[2] An old area of osteonecrosis will show aforementioned MRI changes without associated juxtacortical and juxtalesional edema. An acute on chronic area of osteonecrosis may show juxtacortical and juxtalesional edema around the osteonecrotic elements. However, it may be difficult to distinguish acute on chronic changes of osteonecrosis from superimposed stress reaction and early infection.

Question for Further Thought

1. What is considered the most common etiology of osteonecrosis?

Reporting Responsibilities

- Describe whether the osteonecrotic area is epiphyseal, metaphyseal, or diaphyseal in location.
- For epiphyseal osteonecrosis, describe if there are secondary degenerative changes present, or evidence of subchondral fracturing and/or collapse.

What the Treating Physician Needs to Know

Is the area of osteonecrosis acute on chronic, and is there an etiology for the patient's symptoms unrelated to the identified areas of osteonecrosis.

Answer

1. Traumatic.

REFERENCES

1. Jaramillo D. What is the optimal imaging of osteonecrosis, Perthes, and bone infarcts? *Pediatr Radiol.* 2009;39(suppl 2): S216–S219.
2. Frush DP, Heyneman LE, Ware RE, et al. MR features of soft-tissue abnormalities due to acute marrow infarction in five children with sickle cell disease. *AJR Am J Roentgenol.* 1999; 173:989–993.

J. Herman Kan

CLINICAL HISTORY *A 13-month-old boy with foot deformity*

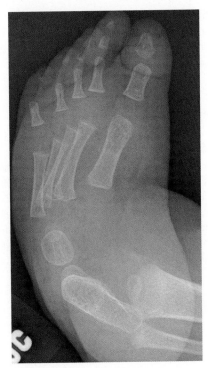

FIGURE **1.33A**

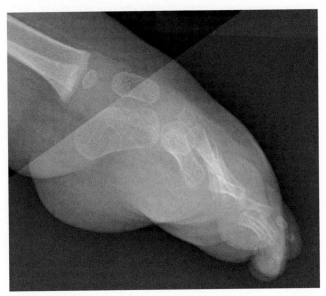

FIGURE **1.33B**

FINDINGS There is severe hindfoot varus, metatarsus adductus, cavus, and equinus deformity of the foot (**A** and **B**).

DIFFERENTIAL DIAGNOSIS Clubfoot deformity, congenital vertical talus, skew foot deformity

DIAGNOSIS Clubfoot deformity

DISCUSSION Clubfoot deformity is one of the most common congenital deformities of the foot. This may occur idiopathically, or may be associated with neurologic sequelae such as cerebral palsy, myelomeningoceles, or may be chromosomal. When left uncorrected, these children will develop premature degenerative changes related to walking on the side of their foot, or even along the dorsum of their foot depending on the severity of the equinus and cavus deformity.

There are four components for a clubfoot deformity: hindfoot varus, metatarsus adductus, cavus, and equinus deformity.[1] Hindfoot varus is when the talocalcaneal angle is narrowed and this can be seen on both the AP and lateral views. With hindfoot varus deformity, the talus and calcaneus assume a more parallel orientation on both the AP and lateral views. Metatarsus adductus is when the meta-

tarsal bones are deviated medially. Invariably, a forefoot varus deformity will coexist. Forefoot varus is when the first metatarsal bone lies medial with respect to the talus. A cavus deformity is when on lateral view a line drawn along the longitudinal length of the talus and the line drawn along the longitudinal length of the first metatarsal form a concavity with the plantar surface. An equinus deformity implies abnormal plantarflexion at the level of the ankle, and this is best seen on the lateral view.

To optimally determine alignment, imaging of the foot should ideally be performed with weight bearing, and this is important particularly when there are subtle features of clubfoot deformity present.

Question for Further Thought

1. True/False: Cavus deformity and equinus deformity refer to the same imaging features of clubfoot seen on lateral radiography.

Reporting Responsibilities

Describe severity of clubfoot deformity, degenerative changes when present, and stress injuries related to abnormal weight bearing.

What the Treating Physician Needs to Know

Describe whether the clubfoot deformity is flexible or not. In the lateral projection, compare neutral non-weight-bearing views with lateral with forced dorsiflexion maneuvers. Make sure to describe flexibility when present both at the level of the ankle and the plantar arch.

Answer

1. False. Cavus deformity describes the exaggerated plantar arch. Equinus deformity describes the fixed plantarflex-ion at the level of the tibiotalar joint, usually related to a tight Achilles tendon.

REFERENCE

1. Dobbs MB, Gurnett CA. Update on clubfoot: Etiology and treatment. *Clin Orthop Relat Res.* 2009;467:1146–1153.

J. Herman Kan

CASE 1.34

CLINICAL HISTORY *A 16-month-old boy with a history of caudal regression syndrome and imperforate anus, with deformity of only his left foot*

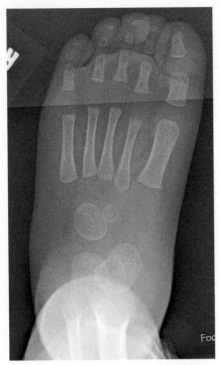

FIGURE **1.34A**

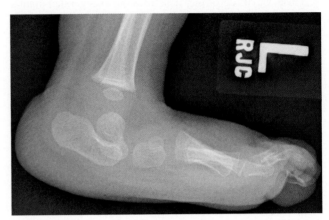

FIGURE **1.34B**

FINDINGS Non-weight-bearing views of the left foot show hindfoot valgus with dorsiflexion deformity of the midfoot resulting in pes planus, and vertically oriented talus (**A** and **B**).

DIFFERENTIAL DIAGNOSIS Vertical talus, pes planovalgus

DIAGNOSIS Vertical talus

DISCUSSION Vertical talus clinically manifests with a rigid flatfoot with a rocker-bottom configuration.[1] The navicular is dorsally dislocated with respect to the talar head. The navicular bone may articulate with the dorsum of the talar head or talar neck. The talar head is downward sloping and may be palpable along the plantar aspect of the foot. The talar head, rather than the calcaneus, becomes the major weight-bearing surface of the foot.

Vertical talus may occur as an isolated deformity. The remainder may occur related to neuromuscular disorders or may be syndromic including entities such as trisomy 13, trisomy 18, nail–patella syndrome, and MPS.[1]

Radiographically, the hindfoot and forefoot are in relative valgus and this is best appreciated on the AP view. Care should be taken to obtain a true AP view because slight obliquity of the AP view may falsely normalize the talocalcaneal angle, or the relationship of the talus and first metatarsal. On the lateral view, the talus is vertically oriented with the navicular dorsally located. In the infant, the navicular is cartilaginous and radiographically difficult to discern, and a dorsal dislocation must be inferred based on the appearance and vertical orientation of the talus.

Question for Further Thought

1. What is the incidence of vertical talus occurring as an isolated entity without coexisting neurologic disease or associated with a syndrome?

Reporting Responsibilities

Distinguish between vertical talus from pes planovalgus. Describe any secondary degenerative changes and remodeling deformities if present.

What the Treating Physician Needs to Know

Is the vertical talus rigid or flexible? Sometimes, forced plantar and dorsiflexion maneuvers in the lateral projection may be helpful.

Answer

1. Approximately 50%.

REFERENCE

1. McKie J, Radomisli T. Congenital vertical talus: A review. *Clin Podiatr Med Surg.* 2010;27:145–156.

J. Herman Kan

CLINICAL HISTORY *A 5-year-old girl with leg weakness*

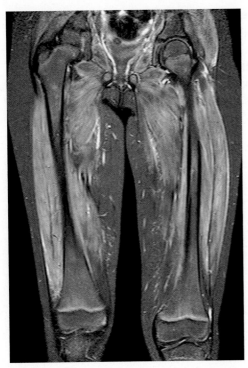

FIGURE **1.35A**

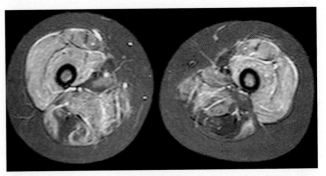

FIGURE **1.35B**

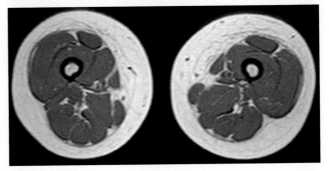

FIGURE **1.35C**

FINDINGS There is diffuse multicompartmental myositis involving the anterior and posterior compartment of the thighs bilaterally (**A** and **B**). T1W sequences (**C**) show symmetric muscle volume of both thighs without evidence of muscular fatty atrophy.

DIFFERENTIAL DIAGNOSIS Dermatomyositis, exercise-induced myositis, viral myositis (e.g., Lyme disease), overlap myositis (myositis associated with any autoimmune disease)

DIAGNOSIS Juvenile dermatomyositis

DISCUSSION Juvenile dermatomyositis is an autoimmune vasculitis which most frequently presents with proximal muscle weakness, elevated serum muscle enzymes, and skin rashes.[1] MRI is helpful for establishing the diagnosis and providing a road map for muscle biopsy if necessary.[2] The characteristic imaging features of dermatomyositis include myositis in a symmetric distribution. Often, there

is also superficial fascial and deep interfascial edema. Both the anterior and posterior compartments of the thigh as well as the pelvic girdle may be affected. Although skin lesions are often present at the time of presentation, subcutaneous edema of the overlying fat is rarely appreciated by MRI.

The thighs and pelvic girdle are an ideal area to image for establishing and following dermatomyositis because this region has the largest muscle volume to sample. In addition, to increase the yield of finding muscle pathology, imaging the proximal extremities is preferred because dermatomyositis usually presents with a proximal myopathy.

Because these children often will undergo serial imaging to follow disease progress, homogeneous fat saturation is helpful. Therefore, STIR imaging is preferred over chemical fat saturation techniques for fluid-sensitive sequences. It may be difficult to compare the relative degree of myositis when chemical fat saturation is used for fluid-sensitive sequences because the areas of inhomogeneous fat saturation may be different on each serial exam. In addition, children with any form of chronic myositis may undergo secondary muscle atrophy and fat infiltration. Therefore, T1W imaging without fat saturation is often helpful to assess muscle volume and presence or absence of intramuscular fatty infiltration.

Question for Further Thought

1. What is the eponym for skin findings on extensor surfaces in patients with dermatomyositis?

Reporting Responsibilities

Report the degree and distribution of myositis, presence or absence of muscle atrophy, and presence or absence of asymmetric muscle volume.

What the Treating Physician Needs to Know

If muscle biopsy is being considered to establish the diagnosis, identify the muscle compartment that is most severely affected to improve biopsy yield.

Answer

1. Gottron papules.

REFERENCES

1. Feldman BM, Rider LG, Reed AM, et al. Juvenile dermatomyositis and other idiopathic inflammatory myopathies of childhood. *Lancet.* 2008;371:2201–2212.
2. Tomasova Studynkova J, Charvat F, Jarosova K, et al. The role of MRI in the assessment of polymyositis and dermatomyositis. *Rheumatology (Oxford).* 2007;46:1174–1179.

CASE 1.36

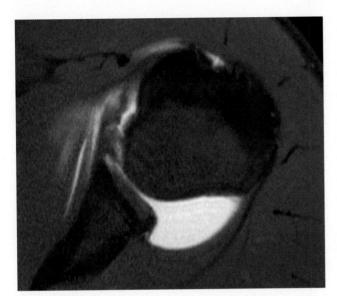

FIGURE **1.36A**

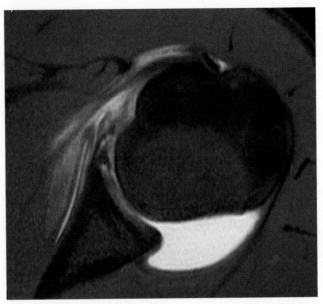

FIGURE **1.36B**

FINDINGS There is contrast insinuation along the anteroinferior glenoid articular cartilage and the anteroinferior labrum is minimally displaced (**A** and **B**). The anterior periosteum of the scapula remains intact.

DIFFERENTIAL DIAGNOSIS Bankart injury, isolated glenoid articular cartilage injury

DIAGNOSIS Bankart injury (Perthes)

DISCUSSION Bankart injuries encompass a spectrum of lesions affecting the anteroinferior glenoid and anteroinferior labrum. This results from a humeral head impaction injury to the anteroinferior glenoid related to anterior shoulder dislocation. The basic subtypes of Bankart injuries include Bankart lesion (displaced anteroinferior labrum from the glenoid rim), anterior labroligamentous periosteal sleeve avulsion (ALPSA; displaced anteroinferior labral tear with intact overlying anterior scapular periosteum), Perthes (ALPSA, but the labrum is nondisplaced), and glenolabral articular disruption (GLAD; anteroinferior labral tear associated with a glenoid articular cartilage injury).[1] Bankart lesions are often associated with a Hill-Sachs fracture, which represents a subchondral depressed

fracture of the posterolateral humeral head related to impaction injury during anterior shoulder dislocation.

When the injury is acute and there is a large glenohumeral joint effusion present, these lesions are best evaluated by MRI without the need for intra-articular contrast. The effusion will have an arthrographic effect.

The earlier in age the first shoulder dislocation occurs, the higher likelihood that there will be future recurrent shoulder dislocations. Dislocations of the shoulder are invariably anterior in direction. Rarely, posterior shoulder dislocations may occur and a reverse Bankart lesion may be seen (glenolabral injury to the posteroinferior quadrant). Traumatic posterior shoulder dislocations are usually related to seizures. Nontraumatic posterior shoulder dislocations may be chronic in nature, and often related to glenohumeral dysplasia related to brachial plexopathy from birth trauma. In this setting, there are often additional telltale signs of glenohumeral dysplasia, including ipsilateral muscle atrophy and a steep, retroverted glenoid.

Question for Further Thought

1. What is an HAGL injury?

Reporting Responsibilities

There is no need to memorize the various subtypes of Bankart injuries. For any Bankart injury, a checklist should be followed to comment on the status of the anteroinferior glenoid articular cartilage, the location of the anteroinferior labrum, status of the anterior scapular periosteum, and if there is extension of injury affecting the anteroinferior glenoid bone.

What the Treating Physician Needs to Know

If there is an associated Hill-Sachs injury.

Answer

1. Humeral avulsion of the glenohumeral ligament. This is an avulsion injury usually by the anterior inferior glenohumeral ligament that may also occur as a result of anterior shoulder dislocation.

REFERENCE

1. Steinbach LS. Magnetic resonance imaging of glenohumeral joint instability. *Semin Musculoskelet Radiol.* 2005;9(1):44–55.

CLINICAL HISTORY *An 11-year-old girl with chronic knee pain*

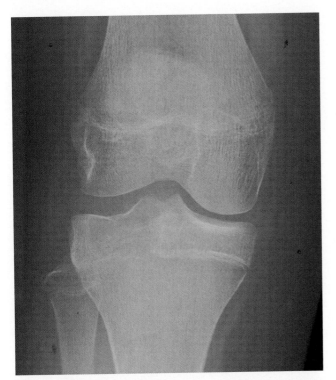

FIGURE **1.37A**

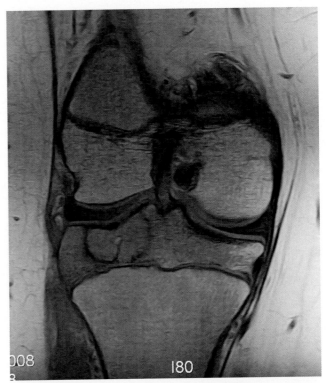

FIGURE **1.37B**

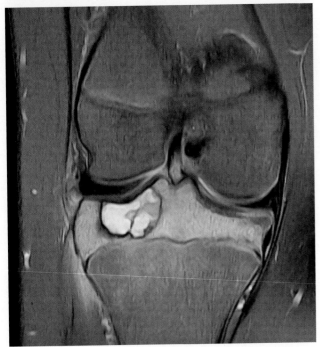

FIGURE **1.37C**

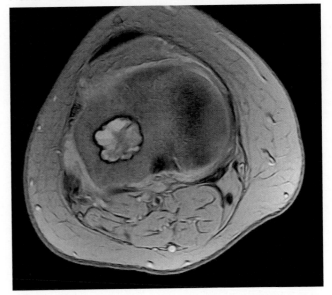

FIGURE **1.37D**

FINDINGS There is an ill-defined lytic lesion located in the lateral tibial epiphysis with relatively well-defined margins (**A**). T1 (**B**) and T2 fat saturated (T2FS) (**C**) sequences show that the lesion is confined to the epiphyseal bone without physeal extension. There is exuberant edema seen throughout the tibial epiphysis. Fluid–fluid levels are also present, best seen on axial sequences (**D**) related to secondary ABC formation.

DIFFERENTIAL DIAGNOSIS Chondroblastoma, epiphyseal Brodie abscess, primary epiphyseal ABC, large subchondral geode

DIAGNOSIS Chondroblastoma

DISCUSSION Chondroblastomas most commonly occur within the epiphysis but will often transgress the physis with metaphyseal extension which is best delineated by MRI.[1] These lesions will often demonstrate characteristic exuberate juxtalesional marrow edema. Secondary ABC development may occur (**D**) manifested with fluid–fluid levels best seen on fluid-sensitive sequences. These lesions have internal chondroid matrix and will often show low signal intensity on all imaging sequences as a result.

Clinically, these lesions may mimic an inflammatory arthritis. A reactive synovitis and effusion may be present because these epiphyseal lesions cause regional inflammation and are intra-articular. Care should be taken to distinguish an epiphyseal Brodie abscess related to osteomyelitis from chondroblastoma, particularly when there is internal cystic change related to secondary ABC formation. The cystic components related to secondary ABC formation should not be confused with abscess related to epiphyseal osteomyelitis.

When the physis are still patent, chondroblastoma should be the top consideration for an epiphyseal lesion with low signal intensity internal matrix. When the physis has fused, GCT should be considered. Both chondroblastoma and GCTs have a propensity to develop secondary ABC formation and may have low signal intensity centrally on all imaging sequences.

Question for Further Thought

1. What percentage of chondroblastomas will extend into the metaphysis?

Reporting Responsibilities

Determine extent of physeal involvement when present and overall size of the lesion.

What the Treating Physician Needs to Know

Distinguish chondroblastoma from an epiphyseal Brodie abscess related to infection.

Answer

1. Approximately 50%.

REFERENCE

1. Wootton-Gorges SL. MR imaging of primary bone tumors and tumor-like conditions in children. *Magn Reson Imaging Clin N Am.* 2009;17:469–487.

CLINICAL HISTORY *A 15-year-old patient with right knee pain after trauma*

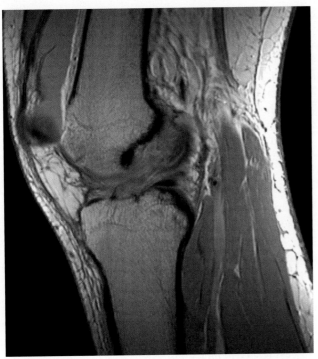

FIGURE 1.38A

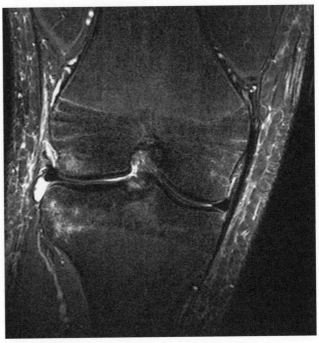

FIGURE 1.38B

FINDINGS (**A**) Sagittal PD sequence through the right knee demonstrates an amorphous anterior cruciate ligament (ACL) with increased signal along the fibers consistent with ACL tear.

(**B**) Coronal STIR image through the right knee shows patchy areas of bright STIR signal in the inferior aspect of the lateral femoral condyle and in the lateral tibial plateau, consistent with "kissing" bone contusions.

DIFFERENTIAL DIAGNOSIS ACL tear, ACL cyst

DIAGNOSIS ACL tear

DISCUSSION ACL tear is rare in children but often seen in adolescents, being the most serious injury in young soccer players.[1] ACL function is primarily limiting tibial anterior translation and to a lesser degree tibial rotation. Mechanism of injury in isolated ACL tear is most often noncontact hyperextension with internal rotation (decelerating during landing or turning), while combined injuries involving other ligamentous and meniscal structures are high-energy impacts on the knee, such as the classic "unhappy triad" of ACL, medial collateral ligament, and medial meniscal tear that occurs with excessive flexion rotation.

Partial ACL tear will show increased intrasubstance signal with intact fibers and unusual undulation in an otherwise intact ACL that is difficult to visualize on T1-weighted images, with fibers visualized on STIR or GRE.[2] Secondary MRI findings suggesting ACL tear are characteristic kissing bony contusions, bony or chondral fractures, and anterior translation of the tibia with respect to the femur. Less than 5 mm anterior subluxation of the tibia can confidently exclude an ACL tear.

Question for Further Thought

1. Which are the clinical and imaging features of an ACL cyst?

Reporting Responsibilities

- Describe the ACL tear (partial or complete).
- Look for associated findings: medial meniscal tear, medial collateral ligament tear, joint effusion, bone bruises on posterolateral tibial plateau, and lateral femoral condyle.

What the Treating Physician Needs to Know

ACL tear is associated with immediate pain and hemarthrosis in 80% to 90% of the cases, usually in associated injuries.

Answer

1. Imaging features of an ACL cyst will show fluid around ACL fibers causing a swollen appearance of the ligament[3] with a drumstick shape; however, patients are usually asymptomatic or may have a minimal knee discomfort while the knee will be stable at clinical examination.

REFERENCES

1. Paterson A. Soccer injuries in children. *Pediatr Radiol.* 2009;39:1286–1298.
2. Vahlensieck M, Genant HK, Reiser M. *MRI of the Musculoskeletal System.* New York, NY: Thieme; 2010:179.
3. Helms CA, Major NM, Anderson MW, et al. *Musculoskeletal MRI.* Philadelphia, PA: Saunders; 2009:367–368.

CLINICAL HISTORY *A 17-year-old patient with left knee pain and effusion*

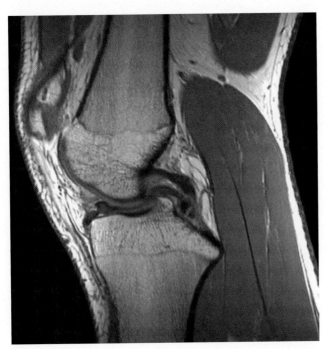

FIGURE **1.39A**

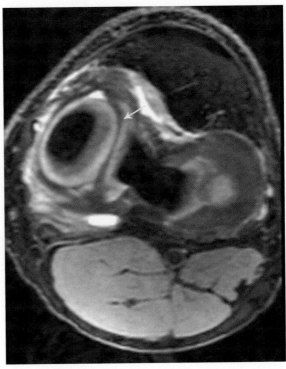

FIGURE **1.39B**

FINDINGS (**A**) Sagittal PD of the left knee shows displaced meniscal fragment anterior and parallel to posterior collateral ligament (PCL), consistent with double PCL sign.

(**B**) Axial dual echo steady state (DESS) image of the left knee demonstrates a flipped meniscal fragment medially (arrow).

DIFFERENTIAL DIAGNOSIS Bucket handle meniscal tear, ring-shaped meniscus

DIAGNOSIS Bucket handle meniscal tear

DISCUSSION Bucket handle tear can be seen in about 10% of meniscal tears and classic appearance is described as a vertical or oblique tear involving the posterior meniscal horn that can extend through the body and anterior horn, with a displaced fragment away from the meniscus. Preferential involvement of the medial meniscus is noted.

Most common and sensitive MR signs in bucket handle tear seen in up to 98% of the cases are the intercondylar notch fragment and absent bow-tie sign, while double PCL sign, flipped meniscus, double anterior horn, and dispro-portional posterior horn sign are less frequently present.[1] Of note, the double PCL sign was found to occur only with medial meniscus tears, likely due to ACL blocking the lateral meniscal fragment access to the intercondylar notch.[2]

A ring-shaped meniscus is a rare entity that can mimic a bucket handle meniscal tear, with fragment present in the intercondylar notch represented by the medial aspect of the ring; however, margins of the free meniscal edge should be smooth.

Questions for Further Thought

1. What is a common associated injury in bucket handle meniscal tear?
2. How can an ACL tear mask a bucket handle meniscal tear?

Reporting Responsibilities

• Describe the findings.
• Evaluate for associated injuries.

What the Treating Physician Needs to Know

1. Is there a free fragment and where has it been displaced.

2. Are there any associated injuries.

Answers

1. There is a frequent association of ACL rupture with bucket handle meniscal tear reported to be up to 48%.[2]

2. The intercondylar fragment can be misinterpreted as ACL tear in cases where the absent bow-tie sign is overlooked.

REFERENCES

1. Aydingoz U, Firat AK, Atay OA, MR imaging of meniscal bucket-handle tears: A review of signs and their relation. *Eur Radiol.* 2003;13:618–625.

2. Wright DH, De Smet AA, Norris M, et al. Bucket handle tears of the medial and lateral menisci of the knee: Value of MR imaging in detecting displaced fragments. *AJR Am J Roentgenol.* 1995;165:621–625.

CLINICAL HISTORY *A 3-year-old child with bone pain*

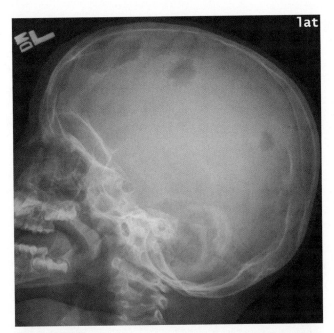

FIGURE **1.40A**

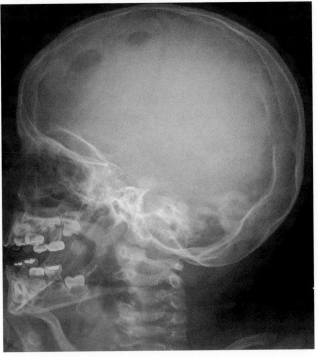

FIGURE **2.40B**

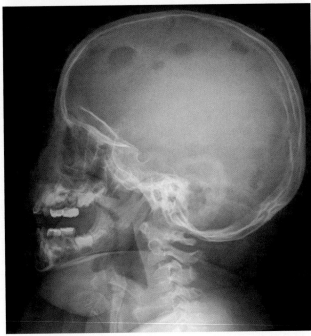

FIGURE **2.40C**

FINDING (**A**) Lateral radiograph of the skull shows multiple well-defined lucent lesions with scalloped borders throughout the bony calvarium, most notably within the frontal and parietal regions.

(**B**) Follow-up radiograph of the skull 8 month later shows significant decrease in size and number of the previously seen lytic lesions throughout the skull that now demonstrate smooth contours, suggesting response to treatment.

(**C**) Follow-up radiograph of the skull 18 month after the first one now shows new ill-defined lytic lesions throughout the calvarium, consistent with disease recurrence.

DIFFERENTIAL DIAGNOSIS For ill-defined lytic lesions: LCH, osteomyelitis, malignancy

DIAGNOSIS LCH

DISCUSSION LCH is defined by monoclonal proliferation of abnormal Langerhans cells, with peak age of manifestation between 1 and 4 years.[1] In pediatric population skeletal lesions are predominant, with most frequent sites being the skull, followed by femur, jaw, pelvis, and spine.[2] Majority of the lesions are typically found in flat bones (up to 70%), most commonly presenting as a pure osteolytic lesion with sharp margins, no reactive sclerosis, and sharp zone of transition.[2] The second most common presentation for bony lesions is represented by ill-defined permeative osteolytic lesions with wide zone of transition. Cortical disruption is often seen, while periosteal reaction is present in only one third of the cases.[2] The wide range of radiologic appearance of LCH lesions is correlated with the stage of disease, with early stage characterized by diffuse bone infiltration and edema with significant periosteal reaction corresponding to the permeative osteolytic pattern, while later in the evolution of the disease decreased bone edema and periosteal reaction will confer a more benign appearance to LCH lesions.[3]

Questions for Further Thought

1. Which is the best initial radiographic modality in a child with suspicion of LCH?
2. What is the most common form of extraskeletal involvement in LCH?

Reporting Responsibilities

- Identify the lesions and describe the radiologic features.
- Evaluate for possible pathologic fractures.

What the Treating Physician Needs to Know

Diagnostic biopsy is needed in LCH suspicious lesions as osteomyelitis and malignant lesions cannot be completely excluded by radiologic features.

Answers

1. Initial assessment in a child with suspicion of LCH should include a radiographic skeletal survey given that skeletal lesions are predominant. Routine chest radiograph and abdominal ultrasound should also be obtained to rule extraskeletal involvement.
2. Most common extraskeletal site of LCH involvement is the pituitary gland, clinically manifested as diabetes insipidus.[1]

REFERENCES

1. Schmidt S, Eich G, Hanquinet S, et al. Extra-osseous involvement of Langerhans' cell histiocytosis in children. *Pediatr Radiol.* 2004;34:313–321.
2. Kilpatrick SE, Wenger DE, Gilchrist GS, et al. Langerhans' cell histiocytosis (histiocytosis X) of bone: A clinicopathologic analysis of 263 pediatric and adult cases. *Cancer.* 1995;76:2471–2484.
3. Diederichs G, Hauptmann K, Schröder RJ, et al. Case 147: Langerhans cell histiocytosis of the femur. *Radiology.* 2009;252:309–313.

CASE 1.41

CLINICAL HISTORY *Status of a 7-year-old child after a fall on outstretched hand*

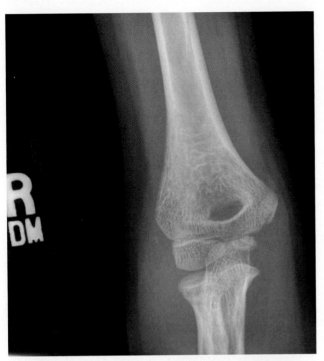

FIGURE **1.41A**

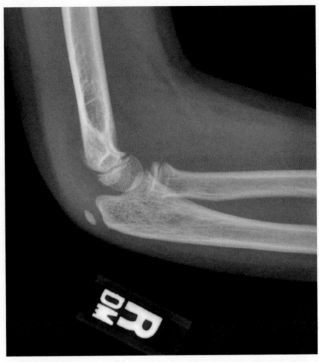

FIGURE **1.41B**

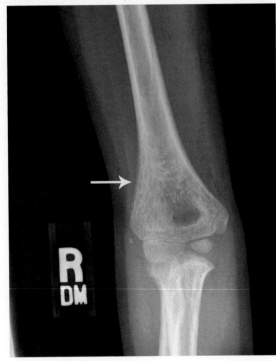

FIGURE **1.41C**

FINDINGS (**A**) AP radiograph of the right elbow shows no evidence for fracture.

(**B**) Lateral radiograph of the elbow shows a large joint effusion with no evidence for fracture. Radiocapitellar alignment and anterior humeral line are maintained.

(**C**) Follow-up radiograph 3 weeks later demonstrates faint periosteal reaction along the distal humerus (arrow) suggestive for healing supracondylar fracture.

DIFFERENTIAL DIAGNOSIS Supracondylar fracture, medial or lateral condyle fracture

DIAGNOSIS Right supracondylar fracture

DISCUSSION Humeral supracondylar fracture is the most common upper extremity fracture in the pediatric population, most often occurring in children 3 to 10 years of age. Mechanism is usually hyperextension of the elbow during fall on an outstretched hand encountered in up to 95% of the cases, and rarely flexion by fall directly on a flexed elbow. Key landmarks in evaluating elbow radiographs for supracondylar fracture are the anterior humeral line and teardrop sign. Anterior humeral line is drawn along the anterior cortex of the distal humeral metaphysis and should intersect the middle third of the capitellum. In children younger than 3, this landmark is not reliable, given that this group of age has usually insufficient or asymmetric calcification of the capitellum.[1] The radiographic teardrop sign is formed by the distal humeral cortices at the olecranon and coronoid process fossae on the lateral view and will be disrupted in a supracondylar fracture.

Questions for Further Thought

1. What is the importance of Baumann angle in evaluating a patient with supracondylar fracture?
2. Which are the neurovascular structures at risk in displaced supracondylar fractures?

Reporting Responsibilities

- If fracture is seen, describe the pattern and the degree of posterior displacement, as well as associated signs (joint effusion, soft-tissue swelling).
- If fracture is not visualized but elbow effusion is present, raise the suspicion of occult fracture (supracondylar or lateral condyle fracture) and recommend follow-up in 10 to 14 days.

What the Treating Physician Needs to Know

Presence of a posttraumatic elbow joint effusion in children is associated in 70% of the cases with an occult fracture, most commonly supracondylar.[1]

Answers

1. Baumann angle is defined as the angle between a line perpendicular to the humeral long axis and a line parallel to the capitellar growth plate measured on the AP view and is useful in the assessment of the carrying angle of the distal fracture fragment.

   More than 10° of varus malalignment as compared to contralateral side is an indication for open reduction and pinning. Angular malunion at the fracture site is a possible complication, with cubitus varus being the most common deformity as a result of malunion and growth arrest of the medial condylar physis.[2]

3. Manipulation at fracture site in displaced fractures increases the risk of median nerve (anterior interosseous nerve) and radial nerve injury, while brachial artery can also be affected with significant posterior displacement of the distal fracture fragment.[2]

REFERENCES

1. Shore RM. Elbow trauma, pediatric. eMedicine. Accessed October 22, 2009.
2. Brubacher JW, Dodds SD. Pediatric supracondylar fractures of the distal humerus. *Curr Rev Musculoskelet Med.* 2008; 1(3–4):190–196.

Luana Stanescu and Mahesh Thapa

CASE 1.42

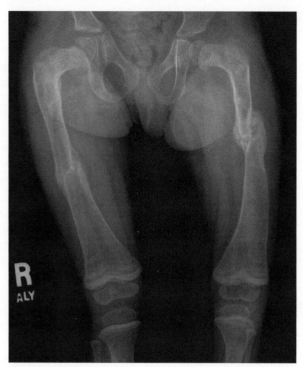

FIGURE **1.42A**

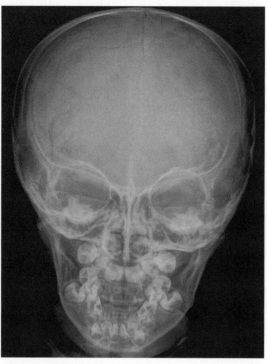

FIGURE **1.42B**

FINDINGS (**A**) AP radiograph of both femurs shows diffuse osteopenia with bilateral coxa vara and bowing consistent with shepherd's crook deformity. Healing bilateral mid shaft fractures with exuberant callus formation also noted. Alternating sclerotic and lucent bands in the distal femur and proximal tibial metaphysis are consistent with bisphosphonate (pamidronate) treatment.

(**B**) Lateral view of the skull demonstrated diffuse osteopenia and innumerable wormian bones.

DIFFERENTIAL DIAGNOSIS Osteogenesis imperfecta (OI), steroid-induced osteoporosis, nonaccidental trauma (NAT)

DIAGNOSIS OI type III

DISCUSSION OI represents a spectrum of inherited disorders characterized by a defective type I collagen synthesis resulting primarily in brittle bones prone to fracture. The most common form and also the mildest is type I characterized by mild osteopenia with minimal bone deformities, blue sclera, brittle teeth, and predisposition for conductive hearing loss, while type III is the most progressive form with multiple fractures causing dwarfism and limb deformities. Type II is the most severe and usually lethal in utero or early infancy.[1]

Typical radiologic features in OI include osteoporosis with gracile, overtubulated bones with relatively few fractures in mild forms and deformed, thickened bones with exuberant callus formation at multiple fracture sites in severe forms. Skull radiographs may demonstrate wormian bones and basilar invagination. Variable degrees of kyphoscoliosis with platyspondyly and typical codfish vertebrae are characteristic findings for OI in spine imaging.[2]

Questions for Further Thought

1. What is "zebra stripe sign" in OI?
2. What is the significance of "popcorn calcifications" in OI?

Reporting Responsibilities

- Identify and describe typical features of OI.
- Multiple fractures in an infant should trigger careful evaluation for typical features of NAT.

What the Treating Physician Needs to Know

Suggest obtaining a skeletal survey as the preferred imaging modality in a neonate with clinical suspicion of OI.

In later presentation of OI, the most common feature is fracture after mild trauma, usually in a patient with increased tendency for bruising.

Answers

1. Cyclic bisphosphonate treatment promotes dense bone formation resulting in dense stripes along the long bones metaphysis in a "zebra stripe" pattern.
2. Scalloped radiolucent areas with sclerotic margins at the metaphyseal–epiphyseal junction are often described as popcorn calcifications and represent a characteristic feature in OI as a result of repeated microfractures at the growth plate.[3]

REFERENCES

1. Kirpalani A, Chew FS. Osteogenesis imperfecta. eMedicine Pediatric Radiology. August 5, 2008. Accessed May 15, 2010.
2. Farooq S. Osteogenesis imperfecta. April 5, 2010. Available at: http://www.Radiopaedia.org. Accessed June 1, 2010.
3. Goldman AB, Davidson D, Pavlov H, et al. "Popcorn" calcifications: A prognostic sign in osteogenesis imperfecta. *Radiology.* 1980;136(2):351–358.

Anisha Desai and J. Herman Kan

CLINICAL HISTORY *A 7-year-old male with a history of intermittent right hip pain and new limp*

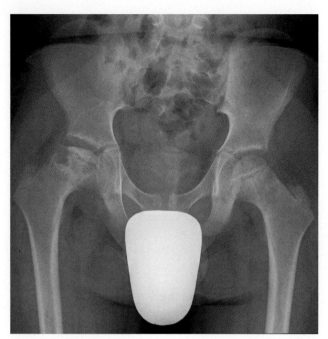

FIGURE 1.43A

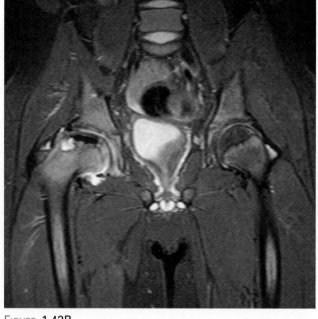

FIGURE 1.43B

FINDINGS AP (**A**) view of the pelvis demonstrates deformity of the right femoral capital epiphysis with subchondral sclerosis, cyst formation, and collapse. The left hip appears normal. A coronal, STIR MRI image (**B**) of the pelvis demonstrates similar finding with a fluid signal subchondral cyst seen in the lateral metaphysis of the right femur. Sclerotic change appears as T2 dark signal in the affected femoral epiphysis.

DIFFERENTIAL DIAGNOSIS Legg-Calve-Perthes disease (LCPD), SCFE with secondary osteonecrosis, septic hip with secondary osteonecrosis, epiphyseal dysplasia

DIAGNOSIS LCPD

DISCUSSION LCPD is classically described as idiopathic AVN of the capital femoral epiphysis. The etiology of LCPD remains unknown but it tends to affect boys between 2 and 14 years old with a peak between 5 and 8 years.[1] The disease may be bilateral in up to 10% to 20% of patients.

Imaging findings of LCPD include delayed appearance or asymmetrically small femoral head, fragmentation and flattening of the femoral head, subchondral fracture and lucency at the epiphysis, and/or metaphyseal irregularity with cystic change. Waldenstrom radiographically staged the findings from an initial stage of increased joint space distance and sclerosis to a final healed stage of collapse with an incongruent hip joint.[2] The radiographic phases of the disease include fragmentation and osteolysis, reparative healing, and healed with remodeling. The lateral pillar and Catterall classification systems can be applied during the fragmentation stage to determine the extent of femoral head involvement.[3] The Herring lateral pillar classification has implications for prognosis in LCPD. The femoral head is divided into three columns on the AP view, with the lateral pillar comprising 15% to 30% of the femoral epiphysis. Herring group A hips have no loss of height at the lateral pillar, group B demonstrates between 50% and 100% normal height, and group C demonstrates less than 50% normal height. The greater the degree of collapse of the lateral pillar (Herring class), the worse the prognosis.[4]

MRI has also become a part of the evaluation of LCPD. Cartilaginous changes at the hip joint and more readily evaluated using MRI. Lateral pillar involvement and transphyseal neovascularity, which may hold prognostic information, is also better seen by MRI.[5] Contrasted MRI in the setting of LCPD may help differentiate it from other entities and show the extent of hypoperfusion or avascularity (subchondral vs central) with nonenhancement.[5,6] Revascularization and reparative phases may demonstrate heterogeneous signal in the epiphysis on fluid-sensitive and contrast-enhanced sequences. Healed LCPD can demonstrate lateral subluxation of coalesced sclerotic fragments with thickening of the cartilage and synovium.[7]

Question for Further Thought

1. How can one differentiate Meyer dysplasia from LCPD?

Reporting Responsibilities

Extent of findings (early vs late stage, involvement of lateral pillar, dislocation/subluxation)

What the Treating Physician Needs to Know

1. Determine the radiographic stage of LCPD, including active fragmentation and osteolysis, reparative healing, and healed with remodeling.
2. When LCPD is healed with remodeling, determine degree of coverage of the femoral head by the acetabulum. Determine if there is secondary DDH because LCPD may heal in relative valgus due to relative growth disturbance of the lateral column of the proximal femoral physis.

Answer

1. Meyer dysplasia tends to occur in younger children compared with LCPD. In addition, Meyer dysplasia usually is an incidental imaging finding in an asymptomatic child (e.g., the hip is imaged incidentally during radiography of the abdomen and pelvis). Radiographically, Meyer dysplasia and an early age presentation of LCPD are difficult to distinguish.

REFERENCES

1. Kim HK. Legg-Calve-Perthes disease. *J Am Acad Orthop Surg.* 2010;18(11):676–686.
2. Waldenström H. The definitive forms of coxa plana. *Acta Radiol.* 1922;1:384.
3. Ritterbusch JF, Shantharam SS, Gelinas C. Comparison of lateral pillar classification and Catterall classification of Legg-Calve-Perthes disease. *J Pediatr Orthop.* 1993;13(2):200–207.
4. Wiig O, Terjesen T, Svenningsen S. Prognostic factors and outcome of treatment in Perthes' disease: a prospective study of 368 patients with five-year follow-up. *J Bone Joint Surg Br.* 2008;90-B(10):1364–1371.
5. Lamer S, Dorgeret S, Khairouni A, et al. Femoral head vascularisation in Legg-Calve-Perthes disease: Comparison of dynamic gadolinium-enhanced subtraction MRI with bone scintigraphy. *Pediatr Radiol.* 2002;32:580–585.
6. Dillman J, Hernandez RJ. MRI of Legg-Calve-Perthes disease. *AJR Am J Roentgenol.* 2009;193:1394–1407.
7. Jaramillo D, Kasser JR, Villegas-Medina OL, et al. Carilaginous abnormalities and growth disturbances in Legg-Calve-Perthes disease: Evaluation with MR imaging. *Radiology.* 1995; 197:767–773.

CLINICAL HISTORY *A 2-month-old female who fell from the changing table*

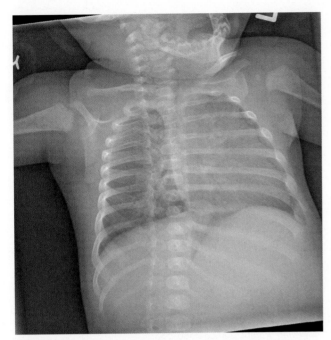

FIGURE **1.44A**

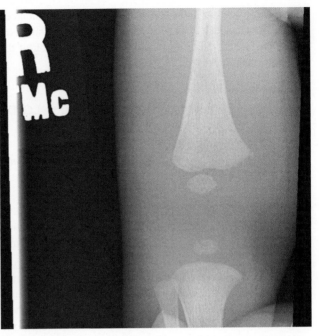

FIGURE **1.44B**

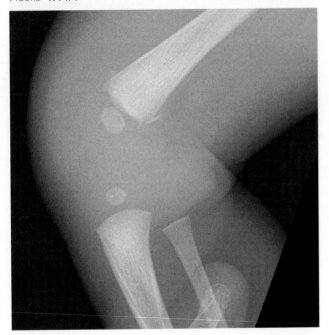

FIGURE **1.44C**

FINDINGS PA view of the chest (**A**) as well as frontal and lateral views of the right femur (**B** and **C**) were obtained as part of a skeletal survey. Multiple healing left rib fractures are seen on the chest film posteromedially (**A**). The postero-medial metaphysis of the right femur demonstrates irregularity (**B**) with a small ossific fragment seen adjacent to the cortex and periosteal reaction (**C**) consistent with metaphyseal corner fractures.

DIFFERENTIAL DIAGNOSIS Child abuse, OI, metaphyseal dysplasia

DIAGNOSIS Child abuse

DISCUSSION The radiologic hallmark of child abuse is multiple fractures in different areas of the body at different stages of healing, more suspicious in a child who is not yet of walking age. Certain radiographic findings, such as classic metaphyseal fracture of child abuse (**B** and **C**) and posteromedial rib fractures (**A**), are considered pathognomonic of child abuse. The classic metaphyseal fracture of child abuse may be subtle. Classic metaphyseal fractures of child abuse appear as small avulsed bone fragments at the distal metaphysis, commonly involving the femora, tibia, and humeri.[1] Classic metaphyseal fractures of child abuse are technically Salter type II injuries associated with shearing force at the growth plate usually from shaking a child.[1] Salter type I injuries may also be present.

Posteromedial rib fractures are caused by AP compression of the chest, as is the case when a child is squeezed while shaken. Rib fractures associated with cardiopulmonary resuscitation (CPR) in children are rare and tend to be anterior.[2] Additional radiologic findings may include subdural hematomas of varying age, skull fractures, and long bone fractures before a child is of walking age, vertebral body compressions, and exuberant callus at an old fracture site (suggesting continued motion at the fracture plane and a lack of medical attention for old injuries).

The diagnosis of NAT is often a team effort between the clinician and radiologist. When possible, it is important to obtain an accurate clinical history and physical exam report. Cutaneous findings or retinal hemorrhages may further support the diagnosis.

Question for Further Thought

1. How do you differentiate child abuse from other entities such as OI?

Reporting Responsibilities

Child abuse falls under the federal required reporting statutes of the Child Abuse Protection and Treatment Act (1996) in all 50 states, and physicians are always mandated to report abuse by law. The reporting responsibilities and techniques vary state by state.

What the Treating Physician Needs to Know

1. Extent and severity of injuries. Possible aging of injuries, but this remains controversial.

2. Additional exams to order for complete evaluation (i.e., complete skeletal survey if diagnosis is suspected on a single extremity film).

Answer

1. The most common way of differentiating child abuse from other entities is osteopenia. Bones are usually normally mineralized in NAT but osteopenic in conditions such as OI and rickets. Clinical scenario, physical exam, and laboratory data may help with distinguishing child abuse from metabolic mimickers.

REFERENCES

1. Kleinman PK, Marks SC, Blackbourne B. The metaphyseal lesion in abused infants: A radiologic-histopathologic study. *AJR Am J Roentgenol.* 1986;146:895–905.

2. Maguire S, Mann M, John N, et al. Does cardiopulmonary resuscitation cause rib fractures in children? A systematic review. *Child Abuse Negl.* 2006;30(7):739–751.

Anisha Desai and J. Herman Kan

CASE 1.45

CLINICAL HISTORY *A 12-year-old male with right ankle pain after twisting ankle while skateboarding*

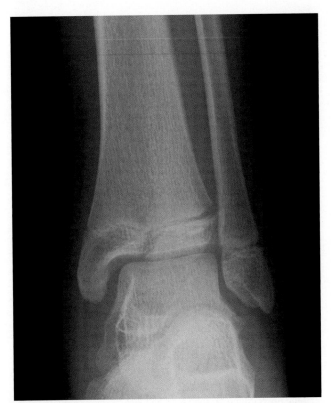

FIGURE **1.45A**

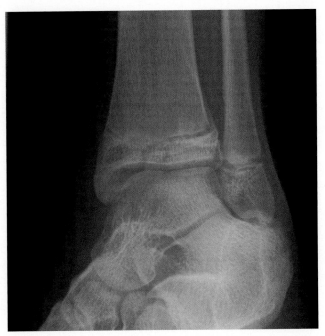

FIGURE **1.45B**

FINDINGS Frontal (**A**) and mortise (**B**) radiographs of the ankle show a vertical fracture plane at the midportion of the tibial epiphysis. The lateral physis is slightly widened compared with the medial physis of the tibia. There is minimal distraction at the epiphyseal fracture plane.

DIFFERENTIAL DIAGNOSIS Salter–Harris type III fracture, Salter–Harris type IV fracture (triplane)

DIAGNOSIS Tillaux fracture

DISCUSSION A Tillaux fracture is a Salter–Harris type III injury of the distal tibia. Distal tibial physeal fusion begins in the midportion. The medial and posterior physis fuse before the anterior and lateral portions. The Tillaux fracture classically occurs at the junction of the fused and unfused physis.[1] By the age of 15, the entire tibial physis is fused, with the process extending over 12 to 18 months. The peak age of incidence of Tillaux fractures is 11 to 14 years.[2] With an open physis, the anterior tibiofibular ligament is relatively more resilient compared with the epiphysis during an external rotation injury of the foot relative to the leg. The additional compressive torque of the talus causes avulsion of the anterolateral tibial epiphysis.

Radiographically, the fracture produces a vertical or oblique line through the midportion of the tibial epiphysis. There may be physeal widening at the lateral growth plate. The findings are best appreciated on the mortise view of the ankle. Multidetector CT is at times advocated in high-impact injuries to rule out additional radiographically occult fractures.[3]

Questions for Further Thought

1. What are the major complications of this fracture being left untreated?
2. When is surgical intervention warranted?

Reporting Responsibilities

Describe location and extent of the fracture with the degree of displacement.

What the Treating Physician Needs to Know

Degree of lateral displacement and physeal widening.

Answers

1. Untreated Tillaux fractures can cause irregular fusion of the lateral physis resulting in pain/stiffness, varus deformity at the tibiotalar joint, early degenerative changes, malunion, and tibiotalar slant.

2. Most common indications for surgical management include incongruity at the ankle mortise and displacement of the lateral epiphyseal fracture fragment by greater than 2 mm.[4]

REFERENCES

1. Felman A. Tillaux fractures of the tibia in (adolescents). *Pediatr Radiol.* 1989;20:87–89.

2. Erlemann R, Wuisman P, Just A, et al. Deformities and trauma sequelae of the ankle joint in children and adolescents. *Radiologe.* 1991;31(12):601–608.

3. Happamaki VV, Kiuru MJ, Koskinen SK. Ankle and foot injuries: analysis of MDCT findings. *AJR Am J Roentgenol.* 2004; 183(3):615–622.

4. Kaya A, Altay T, Ozturk H, et al. Open reduction and internal fixation in displaced juvenile Tillaux fractures. *Injury.* 2007; 38(2):201–205.

CLINICAL HISTORY *A 14-year-old girl on chronic steroids for graft-versus-host disease, currently undergoing bisphosphonate therapy for steroid-induced osteoporosis*

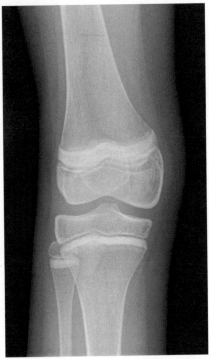

FIGURE **1.46A**

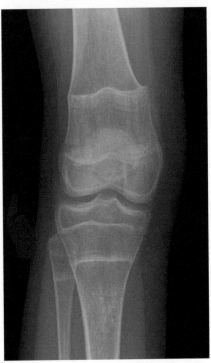

FIGURE **1.46B**

FINDINGS Initial frontal radiograph of the right knee (**A**) demonstrates diffuse sclerosis of the metaphyseal plates. Follow-up radiograph 3 years later (**B**) demonstrates multiple sclerotic metaphyseal bands as well as undertubulation of the distal femoral metaphysis. Incidental note is made of patchy sclerosis in the proximal tibia likely related to medullary infarct.

DIFFERENTIAL DIAGNOSIS Bisphosphonate therapy, heavy metal intoxication, treated leukemia, healing rickets, chronic anemia

DIAGNOSIS Bisphosphonate therapy

DISCUSSION Bisphosphonates are synthetic analogs of inorganic pyrophosphate that are deposited on the surface of bone and ingested by osteoclasts during bone turnover. This results in inhibition of osteoclastic activity and subsequent decreased bone resorption.[1] The use of bisphosphonates in children is currently an off-label use for osteoporotic bone conditions, including OI, juvenile osteoporosis, Gaucher disease, and steroid-induced osteoporosis. Treatment of children with bisphosphonates results in characteristic radiographic findings, which depend on the duration and frequency of medical treatment. Continuous treatment with bisphosphonates results in dense metaphyseal bands, while children undergoing intermittent therapy will develop characteristic thin sclerotic metaphyseal bands with increased bone density. The spacing of these metaphyseal bands will depend on the number of treatments, time period in-between treatments, and the rate of growth of the bone being observed with metaphyseal lines becoming more widely spaced in bones, which demonstrate more rapid growth. Undertubulation of the metaphysis has also been reported as a consequence of bisphosphonate therapy. After discontinuation of therapy, there is a gradual decrease in sclerosis of the metaphysis over time.[2]

Questions for Further Thought

1. Undertubulation of the metaphysis seen in bisphosphonate therapy can be seen in what other disorders?

2. Are there any characteristic fractures that occur in pediatric patients on long-term bisphosphonate therapy?

Reporting Responsibilities

Report the characteristic imaging findings of bisphosphonate therapy in children in order to avoid confusing these findings with pathology.

What the Treating Physician Needs to Know

1. Children undergoing treatment with bisphosphonates can develop characteristic radiologic findings as early as 2 months after initiating therapy.
2. Treatment of children with bisphosphonates has not been shown to inhibit linear growth or result in decreased height potential.[1]

Answers

1. Subtrochanteric diaphyseal fractures are uncommon but have been reported to occur in adult patients undergoing long-term bisphosphonate therapy greater than 5 years. These fractures have not been shown to occur in the pediatric population.[3]

2. Osteoclastic activity is required for the normal development of the metaphysis with inhibition of osteoclastic resorption resulting in undertubulation of the metaphysis. This "Erlenmeyer flask" deformity can also be seen with osteopetrosis, where an osteoclastic deficiency results in a failure of bone resorption. Similar deformities can be seen in disorders with abnormal marrow packing, including Gaucher disease and severe anemia.

REFERENCES

1. Marini JC. Do bisphosphonates make children's bones better or brittle? *N Engl J Med.* 2003;349(5):423–426.
2. van Persijn van Meerten EL, Kroon HM, Papapoulos SE. Epi- and metaphyseal changes in children caused by administration of bisphosphonates. *Radiology.* 1992;184(1):249–254.
3. Park-Wyllie LY, Mamdani MM, Juurlink DN, et al. Bisphosphonate use and the risk of subtrochanteric or femoral shaft fractures in older women. *JAMA.* 2011;305(8):783–789.

CASE 1.47

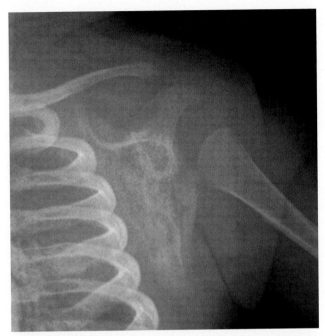

FIGURE **1.47A**

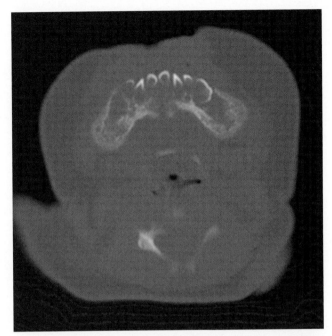

FIGURE **1.47B**

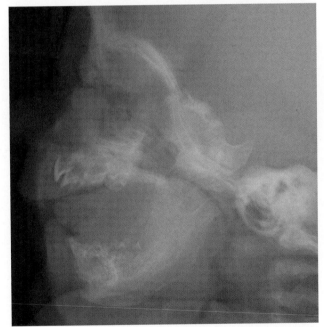

FIGURE **1.47C**

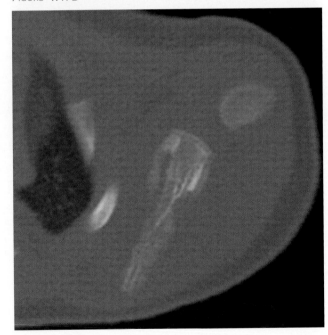

FIGURE **1.47D**

FINDINGS Left shoulder radiograph (**A**) demonstrates diffuse scapular periosteal reaction and permeative appearance, confirmed on CT (**B**). There is additional diffuse periosteal reaction and cortical thickening of the lower mandible seen on plain radiographs and CT (**C** and **D**).

DIFFERENTIAL DIAGNOSIS Osteomyelitis, physiologic periosteal reaction, prostaglandin therapy, infantile cortical hyperostosis, hypervitaminosis A, metastatic neuroblastoma, EG, trauma

DIAGNOSIS Infantile cortical hyperostosis (Caffey disease)

DISCUSSION Infantile cortical hyperostosis (Caffey disease) is a rare, self-limited disorder of early infancy characterized by hyperirritability, soft-tissue swelling, and subperiosteal new bone formation.[1] These findings can often be clinically misdiagnosed as cellulitis, osteomyelitis, or malignancy. The average age of onset is 9 weeks, with no cases reported starting after 5 months of age.[2] Both familial and sporadic forms occur with the familial form inherited in an autosomal dominant manner with variable penetrance.[3] The radiologic hallmark of Caffey disease is periosteal new bone formation and cortical thickening underlying soft-tissue swelling. The distribution of lesions is characteristic, with the mandible most often affected. Mandibular involvement is seen in 75% to 80% of cases with its involvement virtually pathognomonic of Caffey disease.[2] Asymmetric involvement of the diaphysis of long bones, clavicle, ribs, and scapula may also be seen; however, all bones except the phalanges, vertebral bodies, and cuboid bones have been implicated. Treatment is primarily symptomatic with analgesics and prostaglandin inhibitors such as Naproxen or Indomethacin. The disease is ultimately self-limited, usually resolving without treatment within 6 to 9 months.

Questions for Further Thought

1. Caffey disease has been shown to be mediated by a defect in type I collagen. What other disorders are associated with this type of collagen?

2. What role do prostaglandins play in the pathophysiology of periosteal reaction?

Reporting Responsibilities

Describe the location and characteristics of periosteal reaction, including the bones involved and any overlying soft-tissue abnormalities.

What the Treating Physician Needs to Know

1. Consider Caffey disease in the proper clinical setting to facilitate diagnosis and prevent invasive procedures or treatment of suspected osteomyelitis or malignancy.

2. The differential diagnosis of periosteal reaction in infants is broad and varies by age of the patient. Caffey disease and physiologic periosteal reaction occur primarily in newborns and should not be considered in children over 5 to 6 months of age.

Answers

1. Type I collagen is the main collagen of tendon and bone and is a major contributor to the tensile strength of bone. Molecular defects in type I procollagen are seen in OI, Ehlers–Danlos syndrome, and infantile cortical hyperostosis.

2. A potential side effect of prostaglandin therapy is inhibition of osteoclastic bone resorption, which can result in periosteal reaction associated with limb pain and swelling of the extremities.

REFERENCES

1. Parnell SE, Parisi MT. Caffey disease. *Pediatr Radiol.* 2010; 40(suppl 1):S39.

2. Kamoun-Goldrat A, le Merrer M. Infantile cortical hyperostosis (Caffey disease): A review. *J Oral Maxillofac Surg.* 2008; 66(10):2145–2150.

3. Shannon FJ, Murphy M, Atchia I, et al. Caffey's disease: An unusual cause for concern. *Ir J Med Sci.* 2007;176(2):133–136.

CASE 1.48

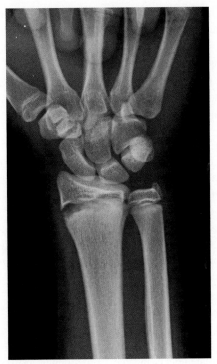

FIGURE **1.48A**

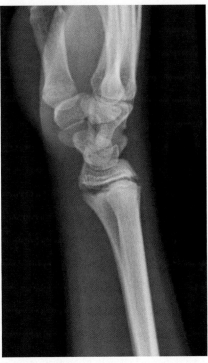

FIGURE **1.48B**

FINDINGS Frontal (**A**) and lateral (**B**) views of the right wrist demonstrate metaphyseal irregularity and widening of the growth plate without evidence of fracture.

DIFFERENTIAL DIAGNOSIS Gymnast wrist, Salter–Harris type I fracture, infection

DIAGNOSIS Gymnast wrist

DISCUSSION Gymnasts are especially prone to overuse injuries of the upper extremities due to the repetitive compressive loading and shearing forces on the growth plate that occur during competition.[1] These forces can lead to chronic stress injuries of the distal radial growth plate, which is often referred to as "gymnast wrist." Radiographic changes of gymnast wrist include asymmetric widening of the growth plate with haziness and irregularity of the physis as well as variable sclerosis and cystic changes within the metaphysis.[1] Additional findings of stress injury may be seen on MRI with high T2 signal intensity associated with widening of the distal radial physis.[2] Long-term sequelae of stress injury to the distal physis may include premature closure of the growth plate with resultant positive ulnar variance.

This positive ulnar variance may then predispose the athlete to ulnar impaction with associated tears of the scapholunate ligaments and triangular fibrocartilage.[2] Treatment of gymnast wrist is largely conservative, requiring a variable amount of inactivity for healing of this stress injury.

Questions for Further Thought

1. Why are the majority of growth plate changes in gymnast wrist seen in the radius?
2. What are the components of the growth plate, and in what portion is it most prone to injury?

Reporting Responsibilities

- Describe the location and extent of growth plate abnormalities, including bilateral findings.
- Report degree of ulnar variance, which may predispose to additional ligamentous injuries.

What the Treating Physician Needs to Know

Gymnasts are prone to overuse injuries of the upper extremities. Wrist pain in this population should prompt evaluation of possible stress injury to the growth plate.

Answers

1. The growth plate of the radius is more commonly involved in gymnast wrist primarily due to differences in weight bearing between the radius and ulna. In neutral position with neutral ulnar variance, 80% of the axial load on the forearm is exerted on the radius. With negative ulnar variance often found in children, this asymmetric loading on the radius increases to 96%.[2]

2. The growth plate is composed of multiple layers of cartilage differentiation. Immediately adjacent to the epiphysis is the resting cell zone which supplies developing cartilage cells. Adjacent to this layer is the zone of proliferating cartilage where bone length is created by active growth of cartilage cells. The hypertrophic cell zone (maturation zone) is next and is the weakest portion of the growth plate where fractures are most likely to occur. The final component of the growth plate is the zone of provisional calcification where the cartilaginous matrix becomes calcified and osteoblastic bone formation occurs.

REFERENCES

1. Davis KW. Imaging pediatric sports injuries: Upper extremity. *Radiol Clin North Am.* 2010;48(6):1199–1211.
2. Dwek JR, Cardoso F, Chung CB. MR imaging of overuse injuries in the skeletally immature gymnast: Spectrum of soft-tissue and osseous lesions in the hand and wrist. *Pediatr Radiol.* 2009;39(12):1310–1316.

CLINICAL HISTORY *A 4-year-old girl with chronic neck pain without history of antecedent trauma*

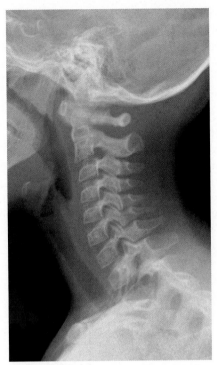

FIGURE **1.49A**

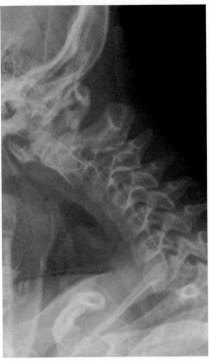

FIGURE **1.49B**

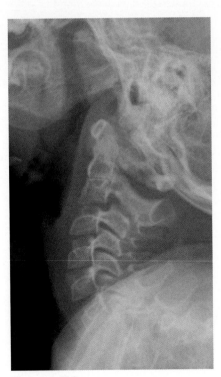

FIGURE **1.49C**

FINDINGS Lateral cervical spine radiograph in neutral position (**A**) demonstrates anterior offset of C2 on C3 with the posterior spinolaminar line maintained. There are no fractures or prevertebral soft-tissue swelling present. Anterior offset of C2 on C3 is reduced with flexion positioning (**B**). There is mild posterior positioning of C2 on C3 on extension lateral view (**C**) likely reflecting ligamentous laxity.

DIFFERENTIAL DIAGNOSIS Pseudosubluxation, true subluxation related to ligamentous injury

DIAGNOSIS Pseudosubluxation

DISCUSSION Pseudosubluxation of the cervical spine is relatively common in the pediatric population, estimated to occur in 19% to 40% of children younger than 8 years.[1] This is seen as an apparent anterior misalignment of C2 relative to C3 on lateral radiographs, which may be accentuated in flexed position. These findings have been attributed to ligamentous laxity as well as a more horizontal orientation of the facet joints in children.[2] Differentiating true subluxation from pseudosubluxation can be difficult, especially if there is a high possibility of true subluxation based on the mechanism of injury. Soft-tissue swelling may suggest true subluxation, although this can be exaggerated depending on phase of swallowing as well as degree of flexion and obliquity.

In order to evaluate cervical spine radiographs for malalignment, three lines should be drawn: the anterior spinal line, the posterior spinal line, and the spinolaminar line. Another spinal line that is less subject to variability in pediatric patients is the Swischuk line. This is a line drawn through the posterior arches of C1 and C3, which should be within 1 to 2 mm of the posterior arch of C2. If there is malalignment of the Swischuk line >2 mm and subluxation persists during extension, or if there are neurologic deficits, a true cervical spine injury should be considered.

Questions for Further Thought

1. Where are cervical spine fractures more likely to occur in children, and what anatomic factors predispose children to injury at these levels?

2. At what age should the pediatric cervical spine assume a more adult appearance?

Reporting Responsibilities

• Report alignment of the cervical spine and recognize pseudosubluxation as a normal developmental variant.

• Report any fractures or secondary findings of cervical spine injury, including prevertebral soft-tissue swelling.

What the Treating Physician Needs to Know

Pseudosubluxation is a relatively common normal variant seen in children under 8 years of age and should not be confused with pathology.

Answers

1. Pediatric cervical spine injuries usually occur in the upper cervical spine between the occiput and C3. A relatively large head and weak neck muscles predispose children to instability of the upper cervical spine with the fulcrum of motion of the pediatric spine occurring at the C2 to C3 level, compared to the C5 to C6 level in adults.[3]

2. By the time a child is 8 to 10 years old, the cervical spine reaches adult proportions. After 10 to 12 years of age, the clinical sequelae of pediatric and adult trauma are similar.[3]

REFERENCES

1. McIntosh A, Pollock AN. Pseudosubluxation. *Pediatr Emerg Care.* 2010;26(9):691–692.

2. Fesmire FM, Luten RC. The pediatric cervical spine: Developmental anatomy and clinical aspects. *J Emerg Med.* 1989; 7(2):133–142.

3. Lustrin ES, Karakas SP, Ortiz AO, et al. Pediatric cervical spine: Normal anatomy, variants, and trauma. *Radiographics.* 2003;23(3):539–560.

CLINICAL HISTORY *A 3-year-old child with arm pain after falling out of an armchair*

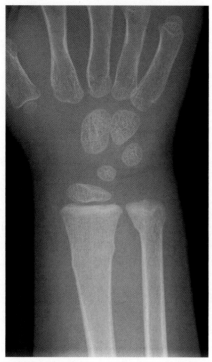

FIGURE **1.50A**

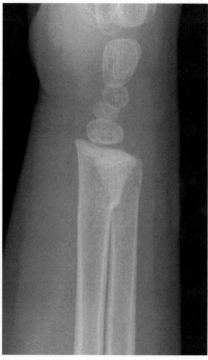

FIGURE **1.50B**

FINDINGS Frontal (**A**) and lateral (**B**) views of the right wrist show cortical buckling of the distal radius and ulna within slight dorsal angulation of the distal radial component.

DIFFERENTIAL DIAGNOSIS Greenstick fracture, buckle (torus) fracture

DIAGNOSIS Buckle (torus) fracture

DISCUSSION Buckle (torus) fractures are common in infants and children, generally occurring in the metaphysis of long bones. They traditionally result from axial loading injuries with resultant buckling of the trabeculae along the fracture line. This leads to bulging of the cortex at either end of the fracture line. Buckle fractures most commonly occur in the wrist, ankle, and elbow but can also occur around the knee and shoulder although less commonly. There are two types of buckle fractures, the classic buckle fracture, in which there is outward buckling of the cortex, and the angled buckle fracture, in which one side of the cortex is mildly angulated.[1] These angled buckle fractures are often subtle; however, in our experience the vast majority of these subtle

buckle fracture occur along the dorsal aspect of the forearm. The management of buckle fractures is usually conservative with a short arm cast or splint used to increase patient comfort during healing and prevent further injury. Buckle fractures are also known as torus fractures, from the Latin (tori) meaning swelling or protuberance.

Questions for Further Thought

1. Why is the metaphysis the most common site for a buckle fracture?
2. Are there any soft-tissue findings that can help in the detection of subtle fractures in the distal forearm and wrist?

Reporting Responsibilities

Describe the anatomic location and configuration of the fracture, including angulation of fracture fragments.

What the Treating Physician Needs to Know

Buckle fractures are best treated with conservative splinting or casting. Follow-up radiographs of simple buckle fractures are controversial but usually not necessary.[2]

Answers

1. The relatively plastic epiphysis serves as a shock absorber transferring the majority of the energy from an axial load to the metaphysis.

2. Elevation of the pronator quadratus fat pad can suggest deep soft-tissue swelling related to subtle fractures of the distal radius and ulna.

REFERENCES

1. Hernandez JA, Swischuk LE, Yngve DA, et al. The angled buckle fracture in pediatrics: A frequently missed fracture. *Emerg Radiol.* 2003;10(2):71–75.

2. Farbman KS, Vinci RJ, Cranley WR, et al. The role of serial radiographs in the management of pediatric torus fractures. *Arch Pediatr Adolesc Med.* 1999;153(9):923–925.

CASE 1.51

CLINICAL HISTORY *A 16-year-old female with 5-year history of joint paint and a positive rheumatoid factor (RF)*

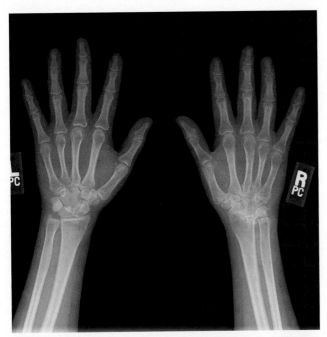

FIGURE **1.51A**

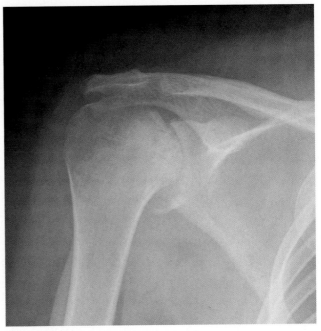

FIGURE **1.51B**

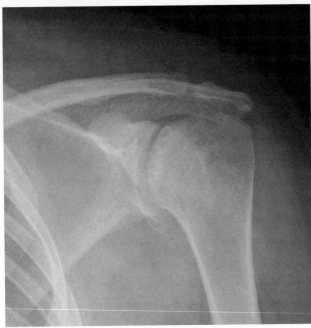

FIGURE **1.51C**

FINDINGS AP radiographs of the bilateral hands (**A**) demonstrate multiple erosions in the right radiocarpal, intercarpal, and carpometacarpal joints with diffuse intercarpal joint space loss and juxtaarticular osteopenia. AP radiographs of the bilateral shoulders (**B** and **C**) demonstrate symmetric joint space narrowing and erosions and of the bilateral glenohumeral joints with remodeling of the glenoid fossae.

DIFFERENTIAL DIAGNOSIS Seropositive polyarticular juvenile idiopathic arthritis (JIA), seronegative polyarticular JIA (PJIA), oligoarticular JIA (OJIA), systemic-onset JIA

DIAGNOSIS Seropositive PJIA

DISCUSSION JIA is a general term encompassing all forms of primary inflammatory arthritis in children. By definition, there must be clinical evidence of joint inflammation lasting greater than 6 weeks, without known cause and with onset at age 16 years or younger. Although there are a number of classification systems for JIA, the most frequently used is that developed by the International League Against Rheumatism (ILAR). In this classification, juvenile arthritis is characterized by number of joints involved within 6 months of presentation, RF status, presence of systemic symptoms, and presence of related clinical findings, including enthesitis or psoriasis. If four or fewer joints are initially involved, the term OJIA is utilized. This form of arthritis has a typical age of onset between 1 and 3 years with a female preponderance.[1] Radiologically, OJIA is characterized by an asymmetric inflammatory arthritis of large joints, most commonly the knee, ankle, elbow, or wrist. The hips are typically spared. Radiographic findings reflect the effect of chronic inflammation on the immature skeleton, and include osteopenia, joint effusion, growth arrest due to premature physeal closure, and epiphyseal overgrowth. Osseous erosions and joint space loss are late and infrequent findings due to the thickness of the epiphyseal and articular cartilage.[2] If five or more joints are involved in the setting of RF positivity, the term seropositive PJIA (RF + PJIA) is employed. This form closely resembles classic rheumatoid arthritis (RA), with a generally symmetric polyarthritis involving both small and large joints. Onset is typically in the early teen years. Distribution and appearance are similar to adult-onset RA, with the exception that distal interphalangeal (DIP) joint involvement is not infrequently seen. Early erosions and joint space narrowing are commoner than in OJIA due to the relatively later age of onset and thinner joint cartilage.[3] In the setting of RF negativity, juvenile polyarthritis is termed seronegative PJIA (RF – PJIA). This form of arthritis has a bimodal age distribution, with an early onset form closely resembling OJIA and later onset form that mimics RF + PJIA.[1] Systemic JIA demonstrates prominent systemic inflammation, including fever, serositis, and rash with relatively minor arthritis. The distribution is variable as is the radiographic appearance, depending largely on the age of onset. Arthritis associated clinically with enthesitis is separately classified as enthesitis-related arthritis (ERA). It typically presents in older children with an asymmetric peripheral arthritis of the hands or feet, often with coexistent dactylitis. Associated involvement of the hips is not uncommon, but unlike in adult spondyloarthropathies, axial involvement is rare. Arthritis associated with psoriasis has a bimodal age distribution, with an early onset form that resembles OJIA and a later onset form similar to ERA.[1]

Questions for Further Thought

1. What is the significance of anti-nuclear antibody (ANA) positivity in JIA?
2. What joint commonly involved in JIA is most difficult to assess clinically, and how is it best evaluated?

Reporting Responsibilities

- Describe the overall pattern of joint involvement.
- Describe the presence or absence of joint space narrowing, osteopenia, erosions, growth disturbance, soft-tissue swelling, and subluxation at each affected joint.

What the Treating Physician Needs to Know

Most forms of JIA are associated with a risk of developing a painless chronic anterior uveitis which can lead to blindness, and ophthalmology referral for periodic screening is required. ANA positivity increases the risk of uveitis substantially.[2]

Answers

1. There is emerging evidence that early onset RF–PJIA, OJIA, and early onset psoriatic arthritis may represent a spectrum of manifestation of the same disease, underscored by similar epidemiology, frequent ANA positivity, and an association with HLA DRw8. All have increased risk of developing chronic anterior uveitis.[1]
2. The temperomandibular joint (TMJ) is difficult to evaluate clinically, and contrast-enhanced MR is the modality of choice if there are suggestive symptoms in a patient with known JIA.

REFERENCES

1. Prakken B, Albani S, Martini A. Juvenile idiopathic arthritis. *Lancet.* 2011;377:2138–2149.
2. Golmuntz EA, White PH. Juvenile idiopathic arthritis: A review for the pediatrician. *Pediatr Rev.* 2006;27(4):e24–e32.
3. Williams RA, Ansell BM. Radiological findings in seropositive juvenile chronic arthritis (juvenile rheumatoid arthritis) with particular reference to progression. *Ann Rheum Dis.* 1985; 44(10):685–693.

CLINICAL HISTORY *A 12-year-old girl with right hip pain*

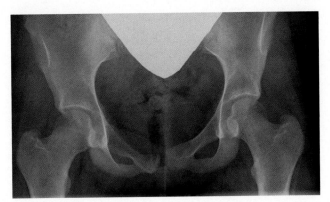

FIGURE **1.52A**

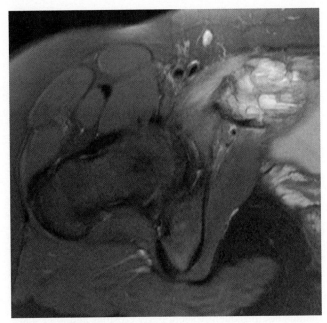

FIGURE **1.52B**

FINDINGS Radiograph (**A**) demonstrates an expanding lucent lesion in the superior ramus of the right obturator ring. The accompanying fat-suppressed, fluid-sensitive axial MRI (**B**) shows a multiseptated lesion with several fluid–fluid levels.

DIFFERENTIAL DIAGNOSIS Telangiectatic osteosarcoma, GCT, osteoblastoma, unicameral bone cyst, ABC

DIAGNOSIS ABC

DISCUSSION ABCs are benign lesions, and as the name implies, they are expansile and cystic. Pathologically, the cysts are filled with blood, and their walls are composed of fibrous tissue. Patients are usually less than 30 years of age at time of presentation, and there is a slight female predominance. ABC may be primary or secondary. Primary lesions arise within normal bone. Secondary lesions develop in bones with preexisting lesions, which may be benign or malignant.[1] Radiographically, ABCs appear as lytic, expansile lesions, often with internal septations. Bony margins, when visible, are often sclerotic. Central calcifications are uncommon. Lesions have a geographic shape with a narrow zone of transition. The hallmark of ABC on MRI is fluid–fluid levels. T1W and T2W images have variable signal intensities depending on the amount and type of fluid, blood products, and proteinaceous material contained within the lesion. ABC may occur in any bone, but favor long tubular bones, pelvis, and the posterior spinal elements. Most occur in the metaphysis (80% to 90%).[2] The lesions typically occupy the intramedullary space, but may be occur within the cortex or in the subperiosteum.

Questions for Further Thought

1. True/False: ABC can affect two contiguous vertebral bodies by crossing the intervertebral disk.
2. What is the hallmark of ABC on MRI?

Reporting Responsibilities

- Describe the location and extent of abnormalities.
- Describe complications such as a pathologic fracture.
- Determine if the lesion is new or a recurrence. If recurrent, careful examination of the prior imaging studies and pathology specimens is recommended to exclude undetected neoplasm.

What the Treating Physician Needs to Know

1. If lesion is in the vertebral elements, the amount of cord compression and nerve root impingement.

2. Associated pathologic fractures.

3. Areas suspicious for malignancy, as ABC may be a secondary lesion.

Answers

1. True

2. Fluid–fluid levels

REFERENCES

1. Kransdorf MJ, Sweet DE. Aneurysmal bone cyst: Concept, controversy, clinical presentation, and imaging. *AJR Am J Roentgenol.* 1995;164(3):573–580.

2. Cory DA, Fritsch SA, Cohen MD, et al. Aneurysmal bone cysts: Imaging findings and embolotherapy. *AJR Am J Roentgenol.* 1989;153(2):369–373.

CASE 1.53

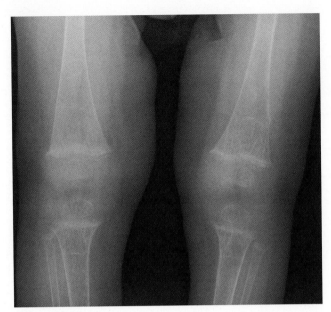

FIGURE 1.53A

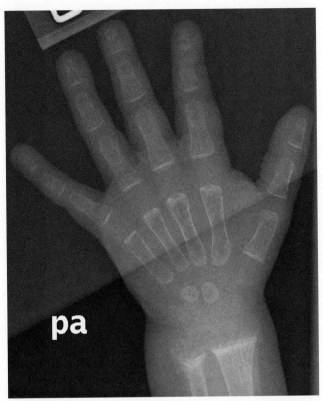

FIGURE 1.53B

FINDINGS Frontal radiographs of the knees (**A**) and left hand (**B**) show widening of the growth plates and metaphyseal irregularity with cupping and fraying. The bones are diffusely osteopenic. There is also a subtle insufficiency fracture at the lateral cortex of the distal left femoral metadiaphysis.

DIFFERENTIAL DIAGNOSIS Rickets, metaphyseal chondrodysplasia

DIAGNOSIS Rickets

DISCUSSION Deficiency in vitamin D, calcium, or phosphorus causes rickets. In the growing skeleton, this results in failure of osteoid mineralization. Radiographically, the changes are most evident in rapidly growing bones, such as the knees and wrists. Frequently, there is widening, cupping, and fraying at the metaphysis. Along the diaphysis, the peri-osteum may appear to be separated from the underlying bone because of the uncalcified osteoid. The bones will appear osteopenic, and the child is prone to insufficiency fractures. Laboratory findings can include hypophosphatemia, hypocalcemia, elevated alkaline phosphatase, and increased parathyroid hormone (PTH) levels. Low levels of 25-hydroxyvitamin D (25(OH)D) establish the diagnosis but may not be needed when other clinical, radiologic, and laboratory findings are highly suggestive.[1] Although MRI is unnecessary for the diagnosis of rickets, typical findings include a widened physis that is most apparent on the T2-weighted images and an absent zone of provisional calcification.[2]

Questions for Further Thought

1. For a child younger than 3 years old, what is the single best radiographic view to obtain if there is a suspicion of rickets?
2. What are Looser zones?

Reporting Responsibilities

• Describe the locations and extent of abnormalities.
• Identify and describe any associated fractures.

What the Treating Physician Needs to Know

1. Offer the most likely alternative diagnosis if not rickets (e.g., metaphyseal chondrodysplasia).
2. If the patient is very young (under 3 years of age) and rickets is suspected by the clinicians, suggest obtaining bilateral frontal radiographs of the knees.

Answers

1. Frontal view of bilateral knees is the single best radiograph to obtain, because the distal femurs and proximal tibias are the sites of most rapid skeletal growth. Ricketic changes will be most pronounced at these locations.
2. Frequently seen in osteomalacia, Looser zones are transverse lucencies within bone, perpendicular to the cortical surface. They represent incomplete fractures that contain unmineralized osteoid.

REFERENCES

1. Misra M, Pacaud D, Petryk A, et al. Vitamin D deficiency in children and its management: Review of current knowledge and recommendations. *Pediatrics*. 2008;122:398–417.
2. Ecklund K, Doria A, Jaramillo D. Rickets on MR images. *Pediatr Radiol*. 1999;29:673–675.

CASE 1.54

CLINICAL HISTORY *Knee pain*

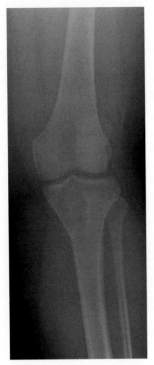

FIGURE **1.54A**

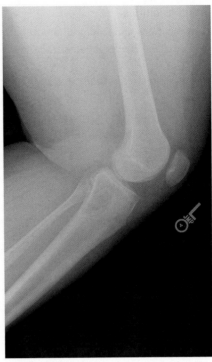

FIGURE **1.54B**

FINDINGS A lucent lesion (**A** and **B**) with well-defined borders within the metaphysis and epiphysis of the posterior tibia is visualized.

DIFFERENTIAL DIAGNOSIS ABC, chondroblastoma, infection, GCT, brown tumor

DIAGNOSIS GCT

DISCUSSION GCT is a lytic lesion that usually affects the epiphyses of bones. Most of these tumors involve the metaphysis as well. Metaphyseal involvement without epiphyseal involvement is rare (about 1%). Patients are skeletally mature, and most patients (80%) are usually between the age of 20 and 50, with a majority in their 20s, and GCTs are slightly more common in females than in males.[1]

GCTs are solitary and involve the long bones. Most common locations for GCTs are knee (distal femur and proximal tibia, at least half all GCTs occur in this location), distal radius, sacrum, proximal humerus, and distal tibia. Multiple lesions are rare, more aggressive, and are seen in smaller bones in younger patients.[2]

The most common clinical presentation of GCTs is pain, while approximately 30% GCTs present with fracture of the bone. While GCTs usually are benign, they can cause bone destruction, recur locally, and metastasize to other areas. The common location for metastases is the lung, while occasionally

GCTs can spread to other locations, such as lymph nodes, bone, skin, and breast.[3] Malignant transformation is rare.

On plain films and CT, GCTs present as a well-defined expansile lucent lesion with an eccentric location, intraarticular extension, narrow zone of transition, and soft-tissue expansion. While GCTs usually do not demonstrate a rim of sclerosis, calcifications, or adjacent periosteal reaction, peripheral calcifications are common in lesions that involve the soft tissue. Lesions of the soft tissue usually tend to be seen in recurrent or aggressive lesions. The appearance of the cortex varies, from very thin to thick. CT is particularly helpful in demonstrating an absence of bone/mineralization within the lesion.[1]

A grading system exists: grade 1 lesions have well-circumscribed radiopaque margins and intact cortex, grade 2 lesions have well-circumscribed margins that are not radiopaque with thinning/expansion of cortex, and grade 3 lesions have ill-defined borders with cortical destruction. While this grading system has no relevance to whether a GCT recurs or metastasizes, it helps direct treatment options for the patient.[4]

MRI is used to evaluate tumor involvement of adjacent soft tissues, vessels, and nerves. The central portions of the GCTs tend to demonstrate low to intermediate signal on T1 sequences and intermediate to high signal on T2 sequences. The peripheral rim on GCTs is hypointense on both T1- and T2-weighted images. Bone scans demonstrate increased uptake in the peripheral rim with decreased uptake in the center portions, on delayed imaging.[1]

Several treatment options for GCT exist. Grade 1 and 2 tumors in the lower limbs are treated with intralesional curettage, adjunctive therapy with cryosurgery, and either filling the curettage site with bone graft, cement (polymethylmethacrylate), or performing a total knee arthroplasty (in older patients). This treatment is also recommended in grade 3 tumors, but wide resection should also be considered. If the tumor recurs, treatment involves wide resection with placement of bone graft or cement. In the upper limb, curettage and cryosurgery are also performed, but calcium phosphate or bone graft is placed in the surgical site. As in the lower limb, wide resection is performed in recurrent upper limb GCTs, and bone graft is placed. Radiation therapy is usually avoided because of possible malignant degeneration of tumor, although no documented cases in literature have been identified. For pulmonary lesions, surgical resection is considered.[5]

Prognosis with GCT is usually good. Recurrence risk is also low and patients who receive wide resection of the tumor have a lower recurrence risk than those who receive intralesional surgery. Some studies have also shown that cement has lower recurrence risk than bone graft.[6] However, in patients with malignant tumor and pulmonary metastases (which is usually rare), mortality rate can be as high as 25%.[7]

While GCTs and ABCs are radiographically similar and can coexist, most ABCs occur in patients younger than 20 years of age,[8] while most patients with GCT are older. Chondroblastomas usually occur in patients who are skeletally immature, unlike GCTs, and are epiphyseal in location. Infection usually presents with soft-tissue abnormality with irregular bone destruction, unlike the expansile well-circumscribed lesion seen in GCT, and WBC usually is abnormal in infection. Brown tumors can also present as expansile well-circumscribed tumors, but patients with brown tumors have hyperparathyroidism secondary to renal failure, while patients with GCT do not have either condition.

Questions for Further Thought

1. At what location is GCT more aggressive?
2. Do you continue with the above treatment options if a fracture is present?

Reporting Responsibilities

- If there is any break through the cortex, because that could alter treatment options.
- If the tumor demonstrates invasion of the local soft tissues.

Answers

1. Distal radius.
2. No, you treat the fracture first and once healed, the above treatment options can be pursued.

REFERENCES

1. Lewis V, Peabody T, Raymond AK, et al. Giant cell tumor. Diseases & Conditions—Medscape Reference. Adler J, et al. February 6, 2012.
2. Hoch B, Inwards C, Sundaram M, et al. Multicentric giant cell tumor of bone. Clinicopathologic analysis of thirty cases. *J Bone Joint Surg Am.* 2006;88(9):1998–2008.
3. Viswanathan S, Jambhekar NA. Metastatic giant cell tumor of bone: Are there associated factors and best treatment modalities? *Clin Orthop Relat Res.* 2010;468(3):827–833.
4. Campanacci M, Baldini N, Boriani S, et al. Giant-cell tumor of bone. *J Bone Joint Surg Am.* 1987;69(1):106–114.
5. Muramatsu K, Ihara K, Taguchi T. Treatment of giant cell tumor of long bones: Clinical outcome and reconstructive strategy for lower and upper limbs. *Orthopedics.* 2009;32(7):491.
6. Klenke FM, Wenger DE, Inwards CY, et al. Giant cell tumor of bone: Risk factors for recurrence. *Clin Orthop Relat Res.* 2011;469(2):591–599.
7. Gong L, Liu W, Sun X, et al. Histological and clinical characteristics of malignant giant cell tumor of bone. *Virchows Arch.* 2012;460(3):327–334.
8. Eastwood B. Aneurysmal bone cyst. Diseases & Conditions—Medscape Reference. Adler J, et al. November 15, 2011.

Kalyan Tatineny and Mahesh Thapa

CLINICAL HISTORY *Back pain*

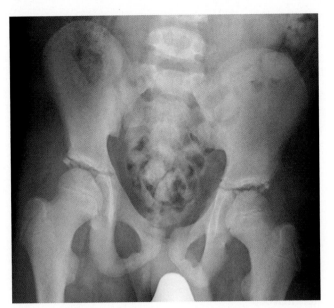

FIGURE **1.55A**

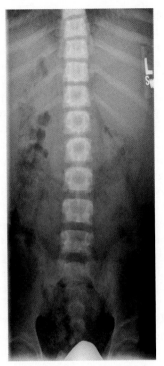

FIGURE **1.55B**

FINDINGS There is diffusely increased density of bone on frontal radiograph (**A**). AP radiograph of the thoracolumbar spine (**B**) demonstrates increased density of the thoracic and lumbar vertebral bodies as well as increased density of the ribs bilaterally.

DIFFERENTIAL DIAGNOSIS Renal osteodystrophy, osteopetrosis, mastocytosis, lymphoma, Paget disease

DIAGNOSIS Renal osteodystrophy

DISCUSSION Renal osteodystrophy is the phrase used to describe any musculoskeletal manifestations of chronic renal failure. In this case, we will talk about the imaging characteristics of renal osteodystrophy in the pediatric population, which includes rickets and osteomalacia. Patients tend to present with a variety of symptoms, including pain, mobility problems, or multiple fractures.

To understand the radiologic effects of renal osteodystrophy, we need to go over a basic overview of the pathophysiology of renal failure. Renal failure induces retention of phosphate within the kidneys, which causes a decrease in blood levels of calcium. This decrease in calcium causes the parathyroid glands to respond, which in turn leads to hyperparathyroidism. The hyperparathyroidism then causes a release of calcium store from the bones.[2]

This leads us into our discussion of the plain film findings seen in renal osteodystrophy. Plain films are the best test to evaluate for renal osteodystrophy. The most common areas of calcium stores within the body are distal clavicles, distal tufts and subperiosteal phalanges, and proximal aspects of the humerus, femur, and tibia. The release of calcium from these stores is what causes the sharpened pencil appearance to the distal clavicles and resorption of the distal tufts and subperiosteum of the phalanges on radiographs. The release of calcium can also be seen in adjacent soft tissues, this is the reason for the soft-tissue calcifications seen around the femur, hip, and phalanges as well as calcifications of ligaments, tendons, and cartilage on radiographs.[1,2]

High phosphate levels also decrease absorption of calcium from the bowel, this type of calcium is called 1α,25-dihydroxycholecalciferol. Intestinal calcium is important in differentiating between osteoblast and osteoclast production in bone remodeling. This imbalance of osteoblasts and osteoclasts with increased bone turnover is thought to cause a coarsened trabecular pattern to the bone, osteopenia, and osteosclerosis (the latter seen in our patient above). This is what explains some of the other plain film findings seen in renal osteodystrophy. Lucent lines can be seen in areas of sclerosis within the bone, called pseudofractures. Within the joints such as the wrist and knee, there is cupping and fraying of the metaphysis with irregularity of the epiphyseal margins, terms used to describe rickets. Anterior bowing of the long bones can also be visualized. AVN within the epiphyses of long bones is sometimes seen.[1,2]

In addition to distal clavicle resorption, in the chest widening of the anterior ribs at the costochondral junction can be seen, called a rachitic rosary. The imbalance of cells can also lead to development of well-circumscribed lytic lesions within bone called brown tumors. Within the spine, irregular end-plate sclerosis, or a "rugger jersey" spine, is visualized. Within the skull, the imbalance can cause a punctuate pattern to the bone, called a "salt-and-pepper" appearance to the skull. Plain films of the abdomen demonstrate areas of calcification in the region of the kidneys, compatible with nephrocalcinosis.[1,3]

Ultrasound evaluation for renal osteodystrophy is very limited. Sonographic imaging of the joints may detect periarticular echogenic foci, suggesting the periarticular calcifications seen on plain films. Within the neck, ultrasound may detect well-circumscribed homogeneously hypoechoic lesions located outside the thyroid adjacent to vessels, compatible with adenomas. Within the kidney, echogenic renal pyramids can be seen, compatible with medullary nephrocalcinosis.

CT is very similar to plain films in detecting changes seen in renal osteodystrophy. It can help further delineate changes to bone described above. It is not as helpful in detecting parathyroid adenomas as ultrasound. Calcifications within the kidney can also be visualized on CT.

MRI can detect changes to bones not easily seen on plain films or CT. Areas of osteosclerosis, including the end plates of the vertebral bodies on the spine, present as decreased T1 signal surrounding normal hyperintense marrow. Abnormal signal within bone marrow, compatible with coarsened trabecula or osteopenia, can sometimes be more easily appreciated on MRI than on plain film. Sometimes plain films can miss fractures given the extensive amount of osteopenia, and these can be better evaluated on MRI, as demonstrated by hypointense lines on PD sequences with increased T2 edema. Soft-tissue calcifications present as areas of low signal on MR sequences.[4]

On bone scan, there is diffusely increased uptake of radiotracer within the extremities without uptake within the kidneys, compatible with a "superscan" appearance. Pseudofractures can present as focal areas of increased uptake within the extremities. Soft-tissue calcifications can present as increased radiotracer uptake surrounding the joint spaces. For evaluation of the parathyroid glands, Tc-99m sestamibi SPECT is useful to looking for adenomas, which present as punctuate areas of increased radiotracer uptake in the thyroid gland region, when no radiotracer should persist on delayed imaging. Sestamibi is not as useful for detecting parathyroid hyperplasia.[1,5]

With regard to therapy, the main goal is to maintain blood levels of calcium and phosphate. Treatment options include dietary restriction of phosphate, phosphate binders such as aluminum hydroxide, and calcium supplementation. Treating the underlying renal disease may also work, but skeletal abnormalities from renal failure can still persist even after renal transplant. Parathyroidectomy is also another treatment option. In the case of brown tumors, if medical treatment of hypercalcemia and hyperparathyroidism does not help, then curettage of the lesion may be performed.[2,6,7]

The best way to differentiate renal osteodystrophy from the other entities is best made by looking at serum calcium, phosphate, creatinine, and PTH levels; abnormal levels not seen in the other differentials. One can also look at the spine films: in renal osteodystrophy the end plates demonstrate irregular sclerosis. The end-plate sclerosis is smooth in patients with osteopetrosis. Thin sclerosis is seen surrounding the vertebral body, in a "picture frame" distribution, in Paget disease.

Question for Further Thought

1. Beside renal osteodystrophy, and what other pathologic processes are included in the differential of a superscan?

Reporting Responsibilities

The most important responsibility for the radiologist is to look for fractures or pseudofractures, including vertebral body height in patients with back pain, because these are the most common complications of osteodystrophy. Even if plain films and CT do not detect fracture, MRI must be performed to evaluate for subtle fractures. This also includes looking for fractures in brown tumors.

What Treating Physician Needs to Know

1. If there is a fracture or pseudofracture.
2. Serum creatinine, PTH, calcium, and phosphorus levels

Answer

1. Metastatic prostate and breast cancer, lymphoma, multiple myeloma, osteomalacia, mastocytosis.

REFERENCES

1. Kline MJ. Imaging in osteomalacia and renal osteodystrophy. Available at: Diseases & Conditions – Medscape Reference. Adler J, et al. May 18, 2011.
2. Hruska KA, Teitelbaum SL. Renal osteodystrophy. *N Engl J Med.* 1995;333:166–175.
3. Wittenberg A. The rugger jersey spine sign. *Radiology.* 2004; 230:491–492.
4. Olmastroni M, Seracini D, Lavoratti G, et al. Magnetic resonance imaging of renal osteodystrophy in children. *Pediatr Radiol.* 1997;27:865–868.
5. Nguyen BD. Parathyroid imaging with Tc-99m sestamibi planar and SPECT scintigraphy. *Radiographics.* 1999;19:601–614.
6. Wesseling-Perry K, Bacchetta J. CKD-MBD after kidney transplantation. *Pediatr Nephrol.* 2011;26(11):2143–2151.
7. Khalil PN, Heining SM, Huss R, et al. Natural history and surgical treatment of brown tumor lesions at various sites in refractory primary hyperparathyroidism. *Eur J Med Res.* 2007;12(5):222–230.

Kalyan Tatineny and Mahesh Thapa

CLINICAL HISTORY *Left-sided neck pain*

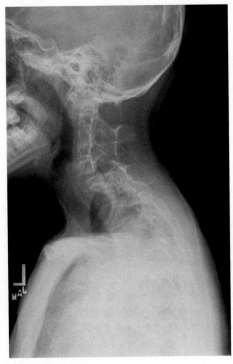

FIGURE **1.56A**

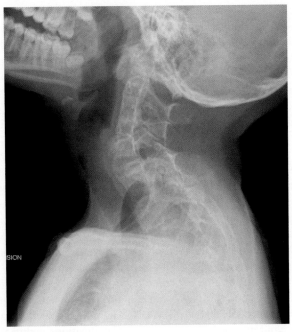

FIGURE **1.56B**

FINDINGS Lateral neutral (**A**) and lateral extension (**B**) radiographs of the cervical spine demonstrate anterior fusion of the C1 to C3 vertebrae.

DIFFERENTIAL DIAGNOSIS Klippel–Feil syndrome, juvenile rheumatoid arthritis (JRA)

DIAGNOSIS Klippel–Feil syndrome

DISCUSSION Klippel–Feil syndrome is used to describe a disorder that involves fusion of at least two spine segments.[1] The exact etiology is unknown, but many theories have been proposed as to possible causes, including subclavian artery disruption.[2]

Klippel–Feil syndrome may occur at any pediatric age, but upper cervical spine involvement tends to occur more commonly in younger patients and lower cervical spine involvement is seen in older patients. The most common clinical symptom is decreased range of motion, with rotational loss more common than flexion or extension. Other less common symptoms and signs include short neck, low hairline, torticollis, or facial asymmetry. Neurologic involvement can also be seen and can include a range of symptoms from sensory problems to hemiplegia, depending on spinal cord involvement.[1] The two most sensitive regions for neurologic injury are the craniocervical junction and the cervical spinal cord.[3] The biggest risk factors for neurologic symptoms are

degenerative changes in the unfused portions and a narrow bony canal.[4]

Klippel–Feil syndrome is categorized into three types based on fusion and location: type 1 involves a single fused segment within the cervical spine, type 2 involves multiple separate fused segments within the cervical spine, and type 3 is a combination of type 1 or 2 with thoracolumbar spine anomalies. This classification system was particularly helpful in correlating the type of symptoms with type of Klippel–Feil syndrome: patients with type 1 tended to have axial neck symptoms, while those with type 2 and type 3 tended to have radicular and myelopathic symptoms.[5]

Initial imaging screening includes AP and lateral radiographs of the cervical spine. Once fusion of two or more vertebrae is visualized, then flexion/extension radiographs are recommended to determine if there is craniocervical instability or if an open segment separates the fused segments. In addition to fusion anomalies, basilar invagination through the skull can also be visualized. Radiographs of the chest and thoracolumbar spine should also be obtained to evaluate for anomalies in these regions, such as rib fusion. CT is used for delineating the vertebral anatomy before surgery, as well as determining if there is spinal stenosis. If neurologic problems are seen clinically, MRI is warranted to determine if there is spinal cord involvement or to look for a syrinx.[5]

Klippel–Feil syndrome is associated with a broad variety of different anomalies within the body, including scoliosis (most common), upward displacement of the scapula (Sprengel deformity), hearing loss, cardiovascular anomalies such as septal defects, renal anomalies such as horseshoe kidney and renal agenesis, craniosynostosis, and limb problems.[6] Problems with intubation can also occur, given the limited mobility of the cervical spine secondary to fusion.[7]

Treatment of Klippel–Feil syndrome depends on symptomatology and associated anomalies. Obviously, if renal and cardiovascular anomalies exist, referrals to the respective subspecialists must be made to treat those conditions. If patients are asymptomatic, no treatment is needed. Mild pain can be medically treated with pain management. However, for asymptomatic and mildly symptomatic patients, periodic flexion/extension films should be obtained to assess for craniocervical instability. Also, patients must avoid contact sports and occupations that have a high risk of head injury given their increased risk of neurologic injury, secondary to craniocervical instability, with minor trauma. If there is persistent pain and neurologic problems, a compensatory scoliosis curve is visualized, then surgical treatment is indicated.[1]

JRA may also present with fusion anomalies and basilar invagination. However, soft-tissue erosions (pannus formation) are seen in patients with JRA but not in those with Klippel–Feil syndrome. Another way to differentiate the two entities is by laboratory testing with lab tests such as erythrocyte sedimentation rate (ESR) and RF.

Question for Further Thought

1. What clinical tests must be performed on all patients with Klippel–Feil syndrome?

Reporting Responsibilities

- On radiograph, it is important to describe the levels and segments of vertebral fusions. In addition, flexion/extension radiographs are needed to determine change in position.
- On CT, anatomy and specific locations of the fusions should be described. The spinal canal diameter should also be determined.
- On MRI, spinal cord diameter and signal should be evaluated. Nerve root impingement should also be assessed.

What the Treating Physician Needs to Know

1. On flexion/extension views, if there is change in position of an upper cervical vertebra, there is increased risk of neurologic abnormalities. If positional changes are present in the lower cervical vertebra, there is increased risk of degenerative changes.[1]
2. If there is cord compression.

Answer

1. Otosopy, audiologic testing, and if these are positive, CT of the temporal bones, because patients with Klippel–Feil syndrome can also have external, middle, and inner ear anomalies, reason unknown.[8]

REFERENCES

1. Sullivan JA, Lewis TR. Klippel-Feil syndrome. Diseases & Conditions – Medscape Reference. Adler, J et al. February 7, 2012. Available at: <http://emedicine.medscape.com/article/1264848-overview>. Accessed February 18, 2012.
2. Bavinck JN, Weaver DD. Subclavian artery supply disruption sequence: Hypothesis of a vascular etiology for Poland, Klippel-Feil, and Mobius anomalies. *Am J Med Genet.* 1986;23(4): 903–918.
3. Nagib MG, Maxwell RE, Chou SN. Identification and management of high-risk patients with Klippel-Feil syndrome. *J Neurosurg.* 1984;61(3):523–530.
4. Baba H, Maezawa Y, Furusawa N, et al. The cervical spine in the Klippel-Feil syndrome. A report of 57 cases. *Int Orthop.* 1995;19(4):204–208.
5. Samartzis DD, Herman J, Lubicky JP, et al. Classification of congenitally fused cervical patterns in Klippel-Feil patients: Epidemiology and role in the development of cervical spine-related symptoms. *Spine (Phila Pa 1976).* 2006;31(21): E798–E804.
6. Hensinger RN, Lang JE, MacEwen GD. Klippel-Feil syndrome; a constellation of associated anomalies. *J Bone Joint Surg Am.* 1974;56(6):1246–1253.
7. Khawaja OM, Reed JT, Shaefi S, et al. Crisis resource management of the airway in a patient with Klippel-Feil syndrome, congenital deafness, and aortic dissection. *Anesth Analg.* 2009; 108(4):1220–1225.
8. Yildirim N, Arslanoğlu A, Mahiroğullari M, et al. Klippel-Feil syndrome and associated ear anomalies. *Am J Otolaryngol.* 2008;29(5):319–325.

CASE 1.57

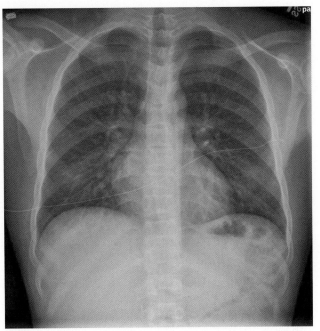

FIGURE **1.57A**

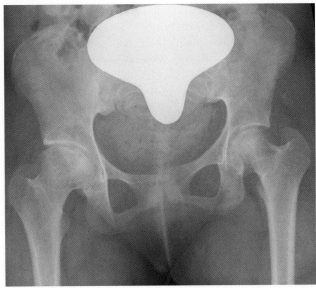

FIGURE **1.57B**

FINDINGS AP radiograph of the chest (**A**) demonstrates loss of height of the vertebral bodies in their superior and inferior end plates, demonstrating an "H-shaped" configuration to the vertebral bodies. AP radiograph of the pelvis (**B**) demonstrates flattening, irregularity, and sclerosis of the right femoral head. The left femoral head is normal.

DIFFERENTIAL DIAGNOSIS

- "H-shaped vertebra" differential: sickle cell disease, Gaucher disease
- Femoral head abnormality (AVN) differential (ASEPTIC GF):
  - Alcoholism, atherosclerosis
  - Sickle cell disease, steroids
  - Environmental (frostbite, thermal injury)
  - Pancreatitis, pregnancy
  - Trauma
  - Idiopathic (LCPD), irradiation
  - Collagen vascular disease, Caisson disease
  - Gaucher disease
  - Fat embolism

DIAGNOSIS Sickle cell disease.

DISCUSSION Sickle cell disease results from an abnormal mutation in hemoglobin. About 10% of African Americans have the gene for sickle cell, and less than 1% of African American have sickle cell anemia. Sickle cell anemia causes an abnormal shape to red blood cells (RBCs), which causes occlusion of small blood vessels, leading to infection, infarction, and necrosis.[1] In this case, we will address the musculoskeletal manifestations of sickle cell anemia.

To understand the radiologic manifestations of sickle cell disease, one needs to understand the basic formation of bone marrow. In the prenatal period, the skeleton is composed of red marrow. At birth, red marrow converts to yellow marrow, starting peripherally in the distal extremities and moving proximally to the central part of the skeleton. In adults without sickle cell disease, conversion to yellow marrow has taken place within the extremities, with normal red marrow seen in axial skeleton, such as the spine, sternum, ribs, and pelvis. However, in patients with sickle cell disease, the conversion to yellow marrow is decreased with the demand of increased RBC production. This causes the increased presence of red marrow in the extremities, affecting all bones in younger patients. As the patient ages, yellow marrow conversion is seen in areas such as the hands and feet, but areas such as the ankles, wrists, and long bone shafts still contain red marrow.[1]

The above abnormal presence of red marrow in the extremities causes the findings of intramedullary expansion of bone with coarsened trabecular pattern and thinning of the cortex, best seen on plain film radiographs. In addition, the increased red marrow causes osteopenia. These findings are seen on all bones, including long bones and ribs. Another pathophysiologic process in sickle cell disease involves the abnormal sickled cells causing occlusion of blood vessels, leading to infarction/necrosis of bone tissue. This leads to areas of bone destruction and sclerosis within long bones. The sclerosis usually occurs after multiple episodes of infarction to bone, and on radiographs presents as diffuse or patchy areas of sclerosis. The bone destruction and sclerosis are also most notable within the epiphyses of long bones such as the femoral and humeral. Patients can present asymptomatically or with hip/shoulder pain. A staging system exists to describe AVN, and this will be discussed later.[1,2]

In the calvarium, red marrow hyperplasia presents as intramedullary expansion with "hair-on-end" appearance of the skull and thinning of the inner and outer table. Within the spine, the thinning and coarsened trabecular pattern causes the "H-shaped" appearance to the vertebral bodies, as seen in our patient, which can lead to vertebral body collapse. Thickening of the paravertebral stripe can also be visualized on radiograph, secondary to the development of a paraspinal mass. Although the exact mechanism of this finding is unknown, a possible explanation is that the red marrow breaks through the cortex and causes a soft-tissue expansion along the spine.[1,3]

CT findings of sickle cell disease are very similar to radiographic findings, but can be more useful in detecting the degree of medullary expansion or bone destruction. CT can also detect areas of sclerosis not well visualized on plain film imaging. Although the "hair-on-end" appearance is not seen on CT of the calvarium, other findings of intramedullary expansion and thinning of the inner and outer tables is visualized. Like plain films, extramedullary

hematopoiesis can present as soft-tissue densities along the spine. Not well visualized on plain films, extramedullary hematopoiesis can also present as soft-tissue masses along multiple ribs.[1,3]

MRI is the best modality for imaging of patients with sickle cell disease, with a very high sensitivity and specificity. Slightly increased T1 and T2 signals are visualized in early bone marrow hyperplasia, secondary to red marrow replacement. Acute changes of sickle cell disease present with diffuse areas of T1 hypointensity and T2 hyperintensity, the hyperintensity secondary to bone marrow edema. The diffuse process becomes more focal as healing takes place. Chronic bone infarcts present as diffuse or patchy areas of serpentine T1 and T2 hypointensity within the bone, corresponding with areas of sclerosis seen on plain films and CT. Paraspinal masses demonstrate intermediate signal intensity on T1 and T2 images. Increased T2 signal can also be seen in adjacent muscles and soft tissues, secondary to occlusion of vessels from the sickled cells leading to decreased perfusion.[1,2]

On bone scan, acute changes of sickle cell disease present as areas of increased uptake. Once the process is chronic and infarcts develop, decreased methylene diphosphonate (MDP) uptake is seen in infarcted areas. Increased MDP activity in a small spleen is also seen in sickle cell, secondary to autosplenectomy from the sickled RBCs. Red marrow hyperplasia can be best visualized as increased uptake on indium-111 imaging.[1,2]

In patients between 6 months and 2 years of age, the infarction combined with abnormally increased red marrow production causes medullary expansion with areas of bone destruction and new bone formation ("mothy appearance" to the bones), called sickle cell dactylitis. While it can occur in any portion of the bone, the most common locations are the diaphysis of metacarpals, metatarsals, and phalanges. This is seen on both plain films and CT, and can eventually lead to deformity of the affected bones. Dactylitis is exacerbated by cold weather leading to vasoconstriction. Clinically, patients present with fever as well as swelling and decreased range of motion in the hands and feet. Given its early presentation, dactylitis can lead to premature closure of growth plates and shortening of bone.[2,4]

Other than AVN, another major complication of sickle cell disease is osteomyelitis. Other less common complications include hyperuricemia, cartilage destruction likely secondary to infection or infarct, and acetabular protrusio, possibly secondary to infarction of the triradiate cartilage.[1]

Treatment of the musculoskeletal manifestations of sickle cell disease involves treating the underlying sickle cell as well as any complications. Such treatment can include pain management with oxygen therapy, hydroxyurea (increases production of normal RBCs), transfusion, or BMT.[5] Osteomyelitis is treated with antibiotics. For complete destruction of femoral or humeral heads (stage 5 as discussed below), total hip or shoulder replacement can be performed.

Questions for Further Thought

1. What are the stages of AVN?
2. What is the most common organism found in sickle cell patients with osteomyelitis?

Reporting Responsibilities

- Appearance to the vertebral bodies.
- Appearance of the humeral and femoral heads.
- Presence of bone infarcts.

What Treating Physician Needs to Know

1. Degree of involvement of the vertebral bodies and femoral/humeral heads (using classification system), the latter to determine if hip or shoulder arthroplasty is needed.

Answers

1. Two commonly used classification systems for AVN are the following[6]:
   a. Steinberg classification system, based on plain film radiographs:
      i. Stage 0: Patients are asymptomatic, the head is normal but contralateral head is abnormal;
      ii. Stage 1: Patient is mildly symptomatic, the radiographs are normal but abnormal signal is visualized on MRI;
      iii. Stage 2: Areas of sclerosis and lucency are visualized in the femoral head, in the superolateral aspect;
      iv. Stage 3: A crescent-shaped density is visualized within the superolateral humeral head, compatible with early collapse, with increased sclerosis and lucency, but the femoral head is still preserved;
      v. Stage 4: While the joint space and acetabulum are still normal, the femoral head has collapsed and patient experiences pain with attempted movement of the femoral head;
      vi. Stage 5: Patient experiences rest pain, the acetabulum is affected, and joint space narrowing is visualized.
   b. MRI classification system:
      i. Class A: In the superolateral femoral head, central necrotic focus that demonstrates fat characteristics with increased T1 signal and intermediate to increased T2 signal. Can use fat suppression to differentiate between class A and class B;
      ii. Class B: Same location, central necrotic focus which demonstrates blood characteristics, increased T1 and T2 signal;
      iii. Class C: Same location, central necrotic focus which demonstrates fluid characteristics, with decreased T1 and increased T2 signal;
      iv. Class D: Same location, central necrotic focus with fibrous tissue characteristics, with decreased T1 and T2 signal.
2. *Salmonella* species is the most common organism detected in osteomyelitis, with *Staphylococcus aureus* the second most common.[1]

REFERENCES

1. Ejindu VC, Hine AL, Mashayekhi M, et al. Musculoskeletal manifestations of sickle cell disease. *Radiographics.* 2007;27:1005–1021.

2. Ramirez I. Sickle cell anemia skeletal imaging. Diseases & Conditions – Medscape Reference. Adler J, et al. July 15, 2011.

3. Gumbs RV, Higginbotham-Ford EA, Teal JS, et al. Thoracic extramedullary hematopoiesis in sickle cell disease. *AJR Am J Roentgenol.* 1987;149(5):889–893.

4. Babhulkar SS, Pande K, Babhulkar S, et al. The hand-foot syndrome in sickle-cell haemoglobinopathy. *J Bone Joint Surg Br.* 1995;77B(2):310–312.

5. Maakaron JE. Sickle cell anemia treatment & management. Diseases & Conditions – Medscape Reference. Adler J, et al. January 3, 2012.

6. Aiello MR. Imaging in avascular necrosis of the femoral head. Diseases & Conditions – Medscape Reference. Adler J, et al. May 25, 2011.

Stephen Darling and Mahesh Thapa

CASE 1.58

CLINICAL HISTORY *A 15-month-old child evaluated for painful soft-tissue swelling of the chest and neck with a history of abnormal orientation of the first toe bilaterally.*

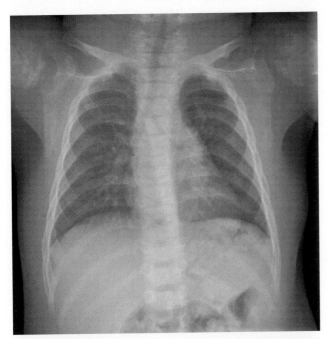

FIGURE 1.58A

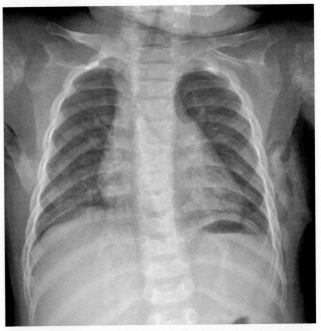

FIGURE 1.58B

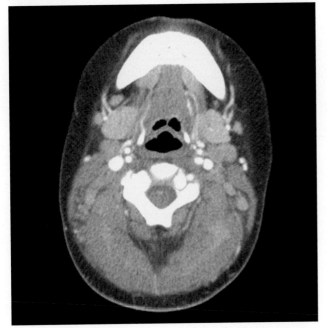

FIGURE 1.58C

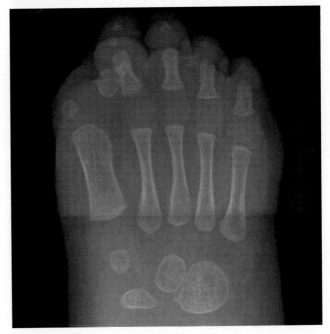

FIGURE 1.58D

FINDINGS Initial frontal chest radiograph (**A**) shows soft-tissue swelling over the lateral thoracic cage. Follow up chest radiograph 4 months later (**B**) demonstrates new soft-tissue ossification within the right axilla, left lateral chest, and posterior to the spine. Bilateral humeral heads demonstrate metaphyseal irregularity with sclerosis and stippled calcifications. CT of the neck with contrast (**C**) demonstrates soft-tissue swelling and abnormal enhancement within the fascia of the posterior paraspinal musculature. Frontal radiograph of the right foot (**D**) demonstrates valgus deformity of the first metatarsophalangeal joint with shortening of the first metatarsal as well as a hypoplastic proximal phalanx and dysplastic distal phalanx.

DIFFERENTIAL DIAGNOSIS Acquired heterotopic ossification (HO), extraskeletal osteosarcoma, fibrodysplasia ossificans progressiva (FOP), dermatomyositis, multiple exostosis (Ollier disease).

DIAGNOSIS FOP

DISCUSSION FOP is a rare hereditary disorder characterized by ossification of striated muscle and connective tissue as well as congenital osseous deformities. Onset is typically in childhood with 50% of patients with FOP presenting during the first 2 years of life and most patients developing soft-tissue calcifications by age 10.[1]

Congenital anomalies of the feet are an early sign of the disorder. Skeletal abnormalities typically occur bilaterally with 75% to 90% of patients demonstrating microdactyly of the toes or fingers, especially the first toe.[1] Painful inflammatory soft-tissue masses are common presenting clinical features of FOP. Trauma to a region of the body may precede the development of these masses; however, there is often no preceding event. Spinal and paraspinal soft-tissue involvement is also common in FOP, often leading to complete fusion mimicking ankylosing spondylitis.

Early radiographs at the site of inflammatory masses may be normal or show only soft-tissue swelling. Ectopic calcification of these masses may progress over weeks with calcification typically developing along tissue planes in muscle.[1] Calcification may also bridge joint spaces resulting in ankylosis. CT is useful in the early diagnosis of FOP given the increased sensitivity of subtle calcification with this modality. Radionuclide imaging also has a role in the imaging of FOP and is helpful in detecting new bone formation and determining extent of disease.[2]

MRI is not particularly useful in diagnosis of FOP. Early in disease, soft-tissue masses will appear hyperintense on T2, giving a similar appearance to other soft-tissue neoplasms. In the later phases of disease, MRI will show low T1 and T2 signal associated with fibrosis or calcification of soft-tissue masses. Angiography of early soft-tissue lesions may show hypervascularity similar to malignant soft-tissue masses; however, the morphology of vessels in FOP is uniform compared to the disordered vasculature and arteriovenous shunting seen in malignant lesions.[1] Well-developed lesions are relatively avascular on angiography.

There is no known effective therapy for FOP. Manipulation of calcium homeostasis has not been shown be effective in long-term treatment.[1] Surgical treatment is hazardous because excision of ectopic bone is often followed by accelerated ossification at the operative site. Prognosis is poor with the most common cause of death due to cardiorespiratory failure secondary to calcification of costochondral joints resulting in restrictive lung disease.[1]

Questions for Further Thought

1. What is the genetic mode of inheritance of FOP?
2. What are other forms of non-inherited HO?

Reporting Responsibilities

Describe the location and characteristics of soft-tissue lesions including associated calcifications. Be familiar with and report skeletal deformities that may be associated with FOP.

What the Treating Physician Needs to Know

Early diagnosis of FOP is important to avoid unnecessary and harmful diagnostic procedures. Clinical suspicion of FOP can be raised in early life on the basis of the preence of malformed great toes and tumorous soft-tissue swelling.

Answers

1. The acquired forms of HO are much more common than the rare hereditary form.[2] In the acquired form, HO is often preceded by trauma such as fracture, total hip arthroplasty, or direct muscular trauma. Neurogenic causes such as spinal cord or central nervous system injury are also known to cause HO.
2. Most cases of FOP are the result of a spontaneous new mutation. However, it is inherited as an autosomal dominant trait with complete penetrance and variable expressivity. Genetic testing is available related to a recurrent single nucleotide substitution of the *ACVR1* gene.[3]

REFERENCES

1. Bridges AJ, Hsu K-C, Singh A, et al. Fibrodysplasia (myositis) ossificans progressiva. *Semin Arthritis Rheum.* 1994;24(3): 155–164.
2. Shehab D, Elgazzar AH, Collier BD. Heterotopic ossification. *J Nucl Med.* 2002;43(3):346–353.
3. Kaplan FS, Xu M, Glaser DL, et al. Early diagnosis of fibrodysplasia ossificans progressiva. *Pediatrics.* 2008;121(5): e1295–e1300.

CLINICAL HISTORY *A 16-year-old female with fever, chills, and back pain*

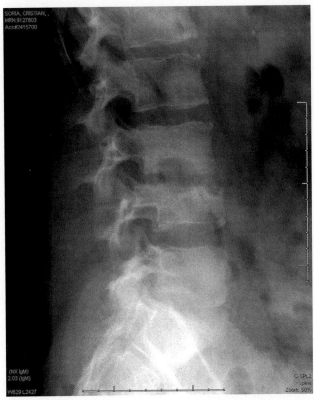

FIGURE **1.59A**

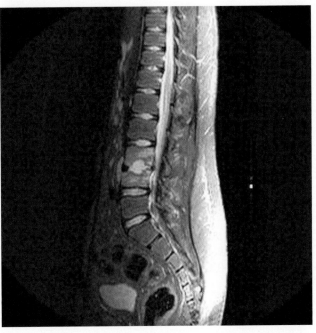

FIGURE **1.59B**

FINDINGS Lateral spine radiograph shows reduced intervertebral disk height at L3-L4 level with irregularity of the end plates (Fig. 1.59A). MRI shows T2 hyperintense signal in the adjacent vertebral bodies, suggesting edema with abnormal signal within the intervertebral disk representing discitis (Fig. 1.59B).

DIFFERENTIAL DIAGNOSIS Pyogenic versus tuberculous etiology

DIAGNOSIS Discitis at L3 to L4 level

DISCUSSION This is typically caused by hematogenous spread of infection. Immunodeficient children are at greater risk. Discitis can be seen in neonates, toddlers, and adolescents; however, the mean age is around 7 to 8 years in the pediatric population. The commonest organism isolated is *Staphylococcus aureus*. A sudden onset of back pain, refusal to walk, and irritability are the most common symptoms with fever accompanied by local tenderness and limited back motion. Plain films of the lumbar spine are obtained initially and they may show changes of reduced disc height, irregularity of the end plates, and displaced paraspinal stripe in case of paraspinal abscess. MRI is sensitive in making the diagnosis, with T2-weighted images demonstrating abnormal T2 hyperintense signal within the involved disc with edema in the surrounding vertebral bodies. T1-weighted images also show the marrow abnormality and after the administration of IV gadolinium the abnormal disc shows enhancement. The presence of phlegmonous soft tissue versus abscess is important. In addition, epidural extension and impingement on the cord should be ruled out. Subsequent radiographs will show end-plate sclerosis and reduced disc height.

Question for Further Thought

1. What is the role of nuclear bone scan?

Reporting Responsibilities

Abscess formation, cord compression from epidural spread

What the Treating Physician Needs to Know

1. Level and extent of involvement
2. Local complications such as paravertebral abscess
3. Epidural extension

Answers

1. It is helpful when multifocal infection is being considered.

REFERENCES

1. Numaguchi Y, Rigamonti D, Rothman MI, et al. Spinal epidural abscess: evaluation with gadolinium-enhanced MR imaging. *Radiographics.* 1993;13(3):545–559; discussion 559–560.
2. Brown R, Hussain M, McHugh K, et al. Discitis in young children. *J Bone Joint Surg Br.* 2001;83(1):106–111.

Prakash Masand

CLINICAL HISTORY *A 15-year-old male with history of trauma while playing soccer*

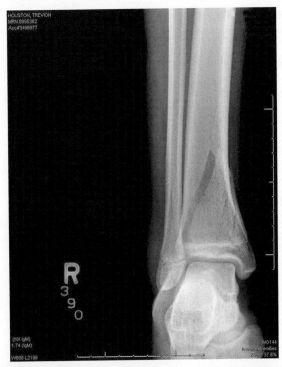

FIGURE **1.60A**

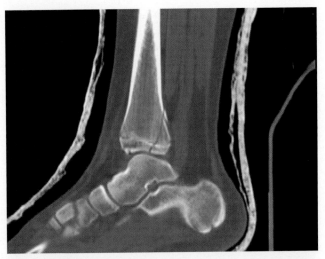

FIGURE **1.60B**

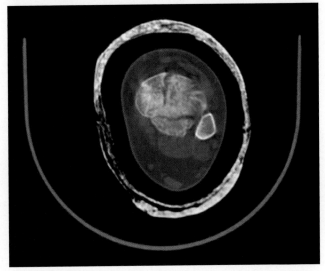

FIGURE **1.60D**

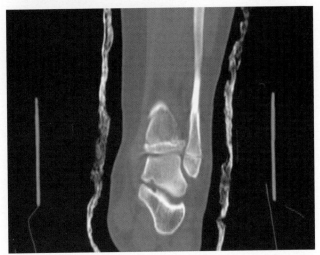

FIGURE **1.60C**

FINDINGS Frontal radiograph of ankle shows distal tibial fracture (Fig. 1.60A). CT images show distal tibial fracture with extension through growth plate, epiphysis, and distal tibial metaphysis, and intra-articular extension (Salter–Harris type IV fracture) (Fig. 1.60B–D).

DIFFERENTIAL DIAGNOSIS Tillaux fracture, triplane fracture

DIAGNOSIS Triplane fracture

DISCUSSION This fracture is classically seen before complete closure of the distal tibial physis, in adolescents. The three types include a 2-part, 3-part, and 4-part depending upon the number of fracture fragments. The 2-part involves a fracture line in the horizontal plane through the physis, leaving the anteromedial portion of the physis attached to the distal tibia. The second fracture line is in the sagittal plane through the epiphysis, lateral to the original formation of the epiphyseal fusion hump. The third fracture line is in the coronal plane, coursing superiorly through the posterior metaphysis. The resulting two fragments are[1] the posteromedial and lateral portions of the epiphysis attached to a posterior metaphyseal spike and[2] the distal tibia, with the anteromedial epiphysis attached. In a 3-part fracture, the fracture line in the coronal plane is complete in its course through the epiphysis, and the posterior metaphysis. The 4-part triplane fracture includes an additional fracture of the medial malleolus. If fracture fragments are displaced by <2 mm, immobilization in a cast is sufficient; however, if displacement is >2 mm, open reduction and internal fixation are preferred.

Question for Further Thought

1. Can there be an associated fibular fracture?

Reporting Responsibilities

Adequately define the fracture.

What the Treating Physician Needs to Know

1. All three components of the triplane fracture
2. Type of triplane fracture
3. Degree of displacement of the fracture fragments

Answer

1. Each type may have a coexisting fibular fracture as well, but is not counted as a component of the triplane.

REFERENCES

1. Schnetzler KA, Hoernschemeyer D. The pediatric triplane ankle fracture. *J Am Acad Orthop Surg.* 2007;15(12):738–747.
2. Patel S, Haddad F. Triplane fractures of the ankle. *Br J Hosp Med (Lond).* 2009;70(1):34–40.

CLINICAL HISTORY *A 10-year-old male with incidental finding on radiograph of hand*

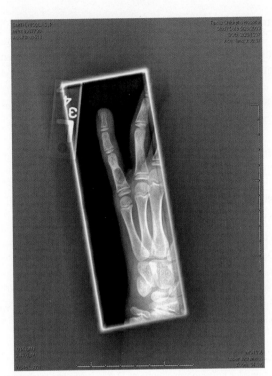

FIGURE **1.61A**

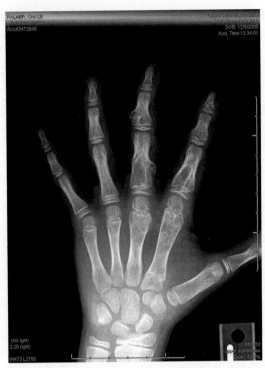

FIGURE **1.61B**

FINDINGS Radiographs of the hand show an intramedullary lytic lesion in the phalanges, suggesting enchondromas. Multiple enchondromas are seen in Ollier disease (Fig. 1.61A and B).

DIFFERENTIAL DIAGNOSIS Osteomyelitis, EG, metastasis, tuberous sclerosis

DIAGNOSIS Enchondroma (Ollier disease when multiple and Maffucci syndrome when associated with soft-tissue hemangiomas)

DISCUSSION Enchondroma is a benign chondroid tumor, which is usually seen incidentally on imaging. About a third of these occur in tubular bones of the hands and feet, with rare occurrence in the pelvis and other areas in the axial skeleton. These benign lesions are oval shaped, well defined with narrow zone of transition, intramedullary, and cause mild endosteal scalloping. They can demonstrate cartilaginous matrix, with popcorn-like appearance however cortical

disruption, and soft-tissue extension is strongly suggestive of chondrosarcomatous change. Multiple enchondromas are seen in a host of syndromes, with the two common ones being Ollier disease and Maffucci syndrome. Patients with Ollier disease tend to present in childhood, and malignant transformation is estimated to occur in 5% to 50% of patients. Also, there is a higher incidence of extraskeletal malignancies, especially glial neoplasms. Maffucci syndrome has multiple soft-tissue hemangiomas (venous malformation) and also carries a higher risk of malignant transformation of enchondromas as well as neoplasms in other locations such as the brain.

Question for Further Thought

1. Is there a higher chance of malignancy in multiple enchondromatosis syndromes?

Reporting Responsibilities

Well-defined intramedullary lesion with chondroid matrix suggests enchondroma.

What the Treating Physician Needs to Know

1. Solitary or multiple enchondromas
2. Presence of cortical break, and associated soft-tissue mass on advanced imaging to suggest chondrosarcoma
3. Associated venous or lymphatic malformation in the soft tissues

Answer

1. Yes.

REFERENCES

1. Murphey MD, Flemming DJ, Boyea SR, et al. Enchondroma versus chondrosarcoma in the appendicular skeleton: Differentiating features. *Radiographics*. 1998;18(5):1213–1237.

CLINICAL HISTORY *Adolescent male with low back pain*

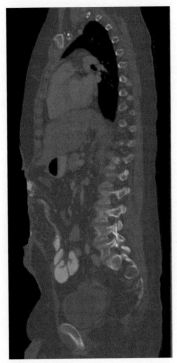

FIGURE **1.62A**

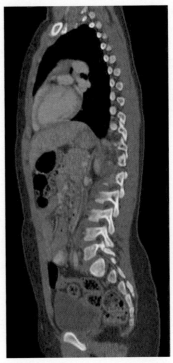

FIGURE **1.62B**

FINDINGS Lateral lumbar spine CT reconstructions showing radiolucent defects involving the left-sided L5 pars interarticularis in two different patients with back pain (**A** and **B**).

DIFFERENTIAL DIAGNOSIS None

DIAGNOSIS Pars interarticularis fracture (aka spondylolysis)

DISCUSSION One of the commonest reasons for low back pain in the adolescent population, especially those involved in athletic activities, is unilateral or bilateral pars interarticularis fracture. This anatomic region is where the lamina, pedicle, and articular facet of the vertebral body join. The fracture occurs almost exclusively in the lumbar spine, and the L5 vertebra is involved in greater than 90% of cases. This tends to occur in younger patients (<16 years) because the weakest portion is in-between the vertebral bodies, when the skeleton is not entirely mature. The etiologic factors proposed include acute or chronic repetitive trauma, congenitally weak pars, spini bifida occulta, and a strong family history of pars fractures. Spondylolysis can lead to slippage of the vertebral bodies causing spondylolisthesis. Plain radiographs demonstrate the break through the pars with associated listhesis. Multiplanar CT reformats are superior in resolution and MRI can show marrow edema in the affected region on the fluid-sensitive sequences from stress reaction, before the break is actually seen. The presence of a sclerotic margin indicates a chronic fracture and smooth, non-sclerotic margins indicate an acute fracture which would benefit from immediate immobilization. The treatment is generally conservative.

Question for Further Thought
1. What is postulated as being an important risk factor in the occurrence of pars fracture?

Reporting Responsibilities
Level of involvement and unilateral/bilateral.

What the Treating Physician Needs to Know
1. Presence of pars fracture with or without spondylolisthesis

2. Presence of sclerotic margins around the defect, suggesting chronicity
3. Associated spina bifida occulta

Answer

1. Hereditary predisposition.

REFERENCES

1. Leone A, Cianfoni A, Cerase A, et al. Lumbar spondylolysis: A review. *Skeletal Radiol.* 2011;40(6):683–700.
2. Harvey CJ, Richenberg JL, Saifuddin A, et al. The radiological investigation of lumbar spndylolysis. *Clin Radiol.* 1998; 53(10):723–728.

CLINICAL HISTORY *A 12-year-old male with fracture of the right femoral shaft*

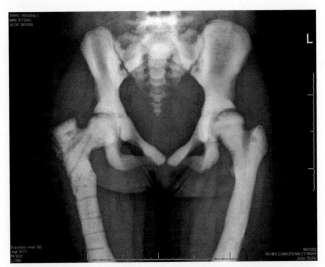

FIGURE **1.63A**

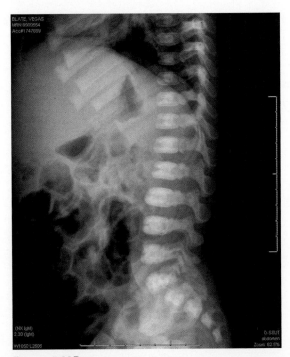

FIGURE **1.63B**

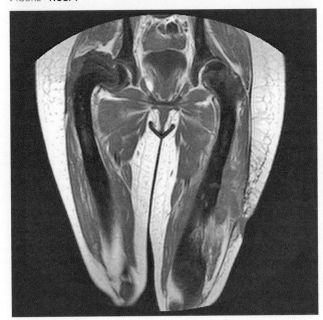

FIGURE **1.63C**

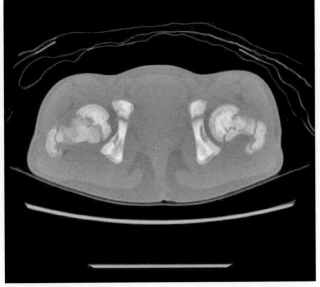

FIGURE **1.63D**

Figure 1.63 (**A** and **B**) Diffuse osteosclerosis on plain films with typical sandwich vertebrae on lateral spine film. (**C**) Coronal MRI image shows low T1 signal intensity involving all the bones, representing osteosclerosis. (**D**) Axial CT image demonstrates lucent and sclerotic bands in femoral head with generalized increase in bone density.

FINDINGS Diffusely increased bone density, vertebral end-plate sclerosis resulting in so-called "sandwich vertebrae" (**A and B**). CT scan shows characteristic bone within bone appearance (Fig. 1.63D), and T1-weighted MRI demonstrates sclerosis (Fig. 1.63C).

DIFFERENTIAL DIAGNOSIS Pycnodysostosis, fluoride poisoning, sickle cell disease, myeloproliferative disease, osteoblastic metastases

DIAGNOSIS Osteopetrosis (aka Albers–Schönberg or marble bone disease)

DISCUSSION The term osteopetrosis is derived from the Greek words "osteo" meaning bone and "petros" meaning stone. Osteopetrosis is variably referred to as "marble bone disease" and "Albers–Schönberg disease." Osteopetrosis comprises a clinically and genetically heterogeneous group of conditions that share the hallmark of increased bone density. The autosomal recessive type presents earlier in life (osteopetrosis congenita), often in infancy and 75% die before 6 years of age, due to complications of infection. There is increased propensity for fractures, osteomyelitis, and even short stature. The autosomal dominant type presents in adults (osteopetrosis tarda). The other clinical associations include cranial neuropathies, dental abscess, spontaneous fractures, scoliosis, hip osteoarthritis, and osteomyelitis. The radiographs show increased sclerosis of the skull base, vertebral end-plate sclerosis leading to a sandwich vertebra, or rugger jersey appearance, in addition to diffusely increased bone density.

Question for Further Thought

1. What is the cause for increase in bone density?

Reporting Responsibilities
Associated complications

What the Treating Physician Needs to Know

1. Diagnosis.
2. Complications arising from the same, such as fractures, osteomyelitis, dental abscesses, as well as cranial nerve compression.

Answer

1. The increase in bone density results from abnormalities in osteoclast function or differentiation.

REFERENCES

1. Stark Z, Savarirayan R. Osteopetrosis. *Orphanet J Rare Dis.* 2009;4:5.
2. Rajathi M, Austin RD, Mathew P, et al. Autosomal-dominant osteopetrosis: an incidental finding. *Indian J Dent Res.* 2010;21:611–614.(**A** and **B**)

CHAPTER 2

Neuroimaging

Gisele E. Ishak

CASE 2.1

CLINICAL HISTORY *A 17-month-old girl with myelomeningocele treated surgically at birth*

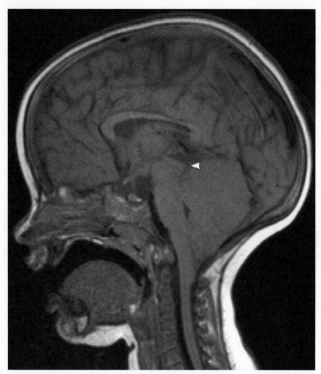

FIGURE **2.1A**

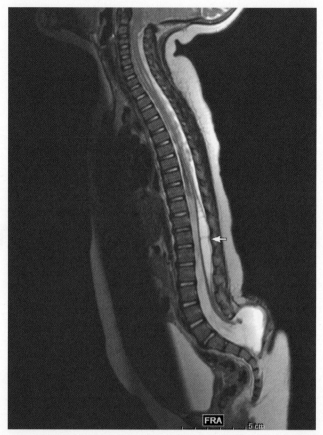

FIGURE **2.1B**

FINDINGS Midline sagittal T1-weighted image of the brain (**A**) shows small posterior fossa with inferior cerebellar ectopia and slight superior towering of cerebellum, beaking of the tectum (*arrowhead*), and a stretched appearance of the pons, medulla, and fourth ventricle with scalloping of the clivus. There is thinning of posterior aspect of the corpus callosum. Sagittal T2-weighted image of the spine (**B**) obtained when the patient was 1 year of age shows lumbosacral spinal dysraphism with low-lying cord and neural placode seen within an enlarged subarachnoid cerebrospinal fluid (CSF) cystic space which extends to near the skin surface (myelomeningocele repair had been performed at birth). There is also syringohydromyelia (*arrow*) extending from T9 to L3, a finding which was new at the time of imaging, and believed to be related to dysfunction of a ventriculoperitoneal (VP) shunt.

DIFFERENTIAL DIAGNOSIS Chiari II malformation with lumbosacral myelomeningocele

DIAGNOSIS Chiari II malformation with lumbosacral myelomeningocele

DISCUSSION Chiari II malformation is a complex malformation of the hindbrain virtually always with myelomeningocele. Typically, the posterior fossa is very small; hence, the cerebellum, which is of normal size, tends to wrap around the brainstem anteriorly, herniates inferiorly below the foramen magnum and superiorly through a widened tentorial incisura, referred to as "superior towering," which causes beaking of the tectum. The fourth ventricle, pons, and medulla are stretched craniocaudally and are narrowed in anteroposterior (AP) dimension. The clivus may be scalloped. Corpus callosal dysgenesis is seen in 70% to 90% of cases with associated colpocephaly. Fenestration of the falx cerebri is seen with interdigitation of the cerebral gyri. Lateral ventricles are usually dilated, often from a combination of colpocephaly, as well as isolated fourth ventricle due to aqueductal narrowing and obstruction of the fourth ventricular outflow.[1]

The myelomeningocele is often discovered in utero or at birth. This is defined as an open neural tube defect where the neural placode herniates with the meninges through the bony defect in the midline of the back.[2] Alteration of CSF flow dynamics, such as with an isolated fourth ventricle or a nonfunctioning VP shunt, can result in syringohydromyelia.

Questions for Further Thought

1. Is myelomeningocele an open or closed neural tube defect?
2. Why is the untreated myelomeningocele rarely imaged?

Reporting Responsibilities

- Report intracranial and spinal abnormalities.
- Report presence of hydrocephalus and identify any signs of VP shunt dysfunction.

What the Treating Physician Needs to Know

Signs of VP shunt failure, such as hydrocephalus or syringohydromyelia. Signs of overshunting, such as presence of subdural hematoma.

Answers

1. Myelomeningocele is an open neural tube defect as it is exposed to the environment and is not skin covered.
2. Shortly after birth, a child with myelomeningocele must have a repair of the open neural tube as ulceration of the exposed placode and infection are leading causes of mortality in the untreated newborn.

REFERENCES

1. Barkovich AJ, Raybaud CA. Congenital malformations of the brain and skull. In: Barkovich AJ, Raybaud C, eds. *Pediatric Neuroimaging.* 5th ed. Philadelphia, PA: Lippincott Williams & Wilkins; 2012:367–568.
2. Tortori-Donati P, Rossi A, Biancheri R, et al. Magnetic resonance imaging of spinal dysraphism. *Top Magn Reson Imaging.* 2001;12(6):375–409.

CASE 2.2

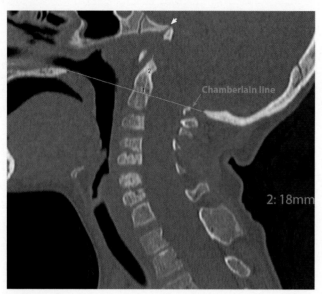

FIGURE **2.2A**

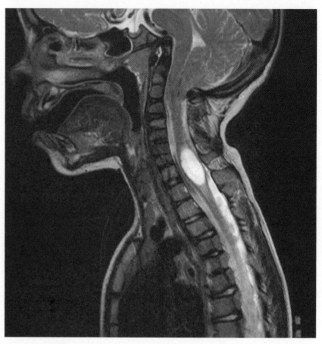

FIGURE **2.2B**

FINDINGS Midline sagittal computed tomography (CT) bone window image (**A**) shows basilar invagination (tip of the odontoid process extends 18 mm above Chamberlain's line) with platybasia and segmentation anomalies of the clivus (*arrow*). In addition, there are multiple segmentation anomalies of the cervical and upper thoracic spine. Midline sagittal T2-weighted magnetic resonance imaging (MRI) image (**B**) shows same findings as on CT as well as focal syringohydromyelia from C6/7 to T2 and kinking of the pontomedullary junction anteriorly with inferior cerebellar ectopia.

DIFFERENTIAL DIAGNOSIS Basilar invagination associated with Klippel–Feil syndrome, platybasia, syringohydromyelia, and Chiari I malformation

DIAGNOSIS Basilar invagination associated with Klippel–Feil syndrome, platybasia, syringohydromyelia, and Chiari I malformation

DISCUSSION Basilar invagination is a primary developmental anomaly in which the vertebral column is abnormally high and prolapsed into the skull base.[1] This is due to failure of segmentation of the occipital sclerotomes and is seen with basiocciput hypoplasia, occipital condyle hypoplasia, and various atlanto-occipital assimilations. Basilar impression is

an acquired or secondary form of this abnormality, resulting from softening of the skull base, and may be seen in association with osteogenesis imperfecta, Hurler syndrome, rickets, Paget disease, osteomalacia, hyperparathyroidism, and skull base infection.[2,3] Chamberlain's line is used to diagnose basilar invagination or basilar impression. This line extends from the posterior margin of the hard palate to the opisthion (posterior margin of the foramen magnum), and is considered abnormal if the tip of the odontoid process projects more than 5 mm above Chamberlain's line.[2,3]

Basilar invagination may be associated with platybasia, which is defined as flattening of the skull base, or with dorsal displacement of the odontoid process, which typically results in a decreased AP dimension of the foramen magnum and severe compression of the underlying cervicomedullary junction.

Questions for Further Thought

1. What is the line used to diagnose basilar invagination and when is it considered abnormal?

2. What is the difference between basilar invagination and basilar impression?

Reporting Responsibilities

Basilar invagination is a radiographic finding and not a diagnosis in and of itself. Report associated anomalies including other bony segmentation anomalies such as Klippel–Feil syndrome, and signs of neural dysgenesis such as Chiari I malformation and syringohydromyelia (reported to occur in 25% to 35% of these patients).

What the Treating Physician Needs to Know

- Whether one is dealing with a primary or secondary form of basilar invagination.
- Associated anomalies such as Chiari I malformation, syringohydromyelia, or platybasia.
- Presence of kinking and compression of the cervicomedullary junction which places the patient at high risk for development of progressive neurologic deficits and may result in sudden death.

Answers

1. Chamberlain's line, which extends from the posterior margin of the hard palate to the opisthion (posterior margin of the foramen magnum), and is considered abnormal if the tip of the odontoid process projects more than 5 mm above this line.

2. Basilar invagination is a primary disorder. Basilar impression is a secondary form, due to softening of the base of the skull.

REFERENCES

1. Smith JS, Shaffrey CI, Abel MF, et al. Basilar invagination. *Neurosurgery.* 2010;66(3 suppl):39–47.

2. Smoker WR, Khanna G. Imaging the craniocervical junction. *Childs Nerv Syst.* 2008;24(10):1123–1145.

3. Smoker WR. MR imaging of the craniovertebral junction. *Magn Reson Imaging Clin N Am.* 2000;8(3):635–650.

Gisele E. Ishak

CLINICAL HISTORY *A 16-year-old child with atonic epilepsy, developmental delay, and diabetes insipidus*

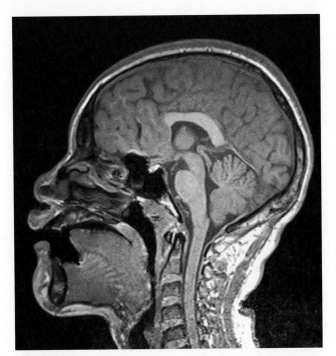

FIGURE **2.3A**

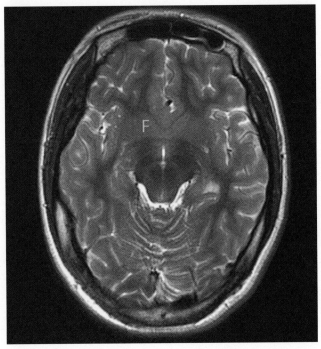

FIGURE **2.3B**

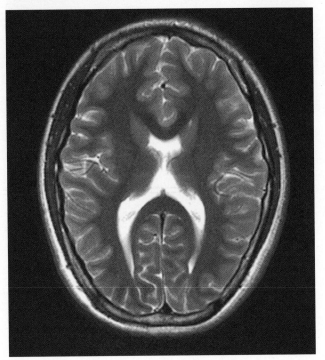

FIGURE **2.3C**

FINDINGS Sagittal T1-weighted midline MRI image (**A**) shows dysgenesis of the genu of the corpus callosum in a region of anterior cerebral fusion. The cerebral fusion involves the hypothalamus with deformity of the pituitary stalk. Axial T2-weighted image at the level of anterior commissure of the brain (**B**) demonstrates a focal area of interhemispheric cerebral fusion along the inferior frontal lobes (where F is the right side of region of fusion), anterior to the anterior commissure. Note the azygous anterior cerebral artery (ACA). Axial T2-weighted image at the level of lateral ventricles (**C**) demonstrates that frontal horns are deficient and septum pellucidum is absent.

DIFFERENTIAL DIAGNOSIS Holoprosencephaly (HPE; lobar)

DIAGNOSIS HPE (lobar)

DISCUSSION HPE is a spectrum of congenital structural forebrain anomalies, defined by lack of formation of midline structures and variable degree of interhemispheric cerebral fusion. It is divided into three major types from most to least severe: alobar, semilobar, and lobar. Absence of the septum pellucidum is seen in all types with variation in the absence of the falx cerebri.[1,2] For example, in lobar HPE, the falx is absent only anteriorly just anterior to the anterior commissure with focal fusion of the frontal lobes and hypoplasia of the genu of the corpus callosum at this level. On the other hand, in alobar HPE, the falx cerebri is completely absent with pancake-like configuration of anterior cerebral tissue and monoventricle. It may be challenging to distinguish lobar from semilobar HPE. However, if the posterior half of the body of the corpus callosum is formed, fusion is classified as lobar HPE. In patients with HPE, the basal ganglia, thalami, and hypothalami may also have variable extent of fusion.[2] Olfactory nerves may be absent and myelination may be delayed, predominantly in more severe cases of fusion. Absent or azygous ACA may also occur. The findings of septo-optic dysplasia (SOD) may overlap with lobar HPE and it has been considered as a forme fruste of HPE.

Questions for Further Thought

1. Where is the level of cerebral fusion in the mildest form of HPE?
2. What is the middle interhemispheric variant of HPE?

Reporting Responsibilities

- Identify severity of midline defects, including absence of the septum pellucidum, falx cerebri, olfactory bulbs, basal ganglia and hemispheric fusion, and dysgenesis of corpus callosum.

- Identify and describe any associated craniofacial malformations which correlate with severity of disease and include metopic suture synostosis, cyclopia, and midline facial clefting.

What the Treating Physician Needs to Know

- Assess degree of hemispheric and deep gray nuclei fusion, which relates to clinical severity of disease.
- Assess for hypothalamic fusion, which may correlate with pituitary/hypothalamic dysfunction and necessitates hormone replacement therapy.

Answers

1. In lobar-type HPE, fusion is most pronounced anteriorly, just anterior to the level of the anterior commissure, respecting a gradient of development in which the normal separation of the cerebral hemispheres progresses from posterior to anterior.
2. The middle interhemispheric variant of HPE is characterized by middle interhemispheric fusion of the posterior frontal and parietal lobes associated with callosal dysgenesis at the level of the fusion.

REFERENCES

1. Barkovich AJ, Raybaud CA. Congenital malformations of the brain and skull. In: Barkovich AJ, Raybaud C, eds. *Pediatric Neuroimaging*. 5th ed. Philadelphia, PA: Lippincott Williams & Wilkins; 2012:367–568.
2. Hahn JS, Barnes PD. Neuroimaging advances in holoprosencephaly: Refining the spectrum of the midline malformation. *Am J Med Genet C Semin Med Genet*. 2010;154C(1):120–132.

CASE 2.4

CLINICAL HISTORY *A 10-year-old child with trauma*

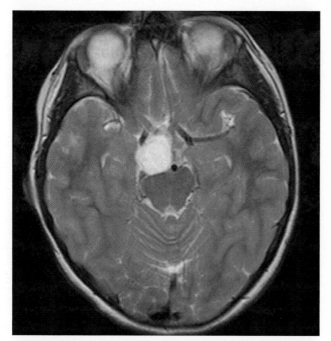

FIGURE 2.4A

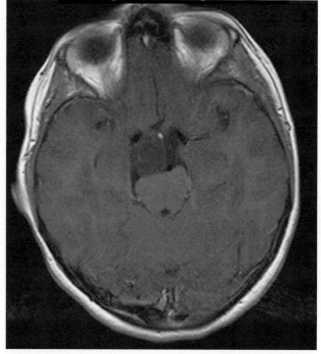

FIGURE 2.4B

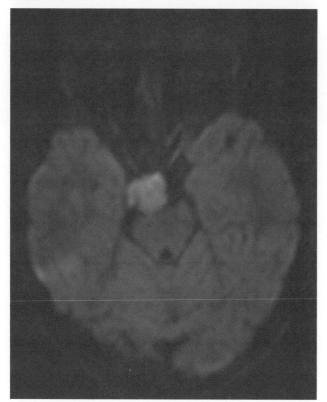

FIGURE 2.4C

FINDINGS Axial T2-weighted (**A**), T1-postcontrast (**B**), and diffusion-weighted imaging (DWI) (**C**) from an MRI demonstrate a right-sided nonenhancing suprasellar mass showing low T1 and high T2 signal with restricted diffusion (bright on the DWI image). There is effacement of brain stem.

DIFFERENTIAL DIAGNOSIS Epidermoid cyst, dermoid cyst, arachnoid cyst, neurenteric cyst, craniopharyngioma

DIAGNOSIS Epidermoid cyst

DISCUSSION Epidermoid and dermoid cysts develop from congenital rests as a result of incomplete separation from the cutaneous ectoderm at the time of closure of the neural tube.[1] Most are intracranial, but extracranial location, such as skull and spine, can occur. Epidermoids consist of squamous epithelium while the rarer demoid also contains associated dermal appendages.[1,2] Intracranially, both epidermoid and dermoid are extra-axial in location. Epidermoid has a greater tendency to deviate from the midline. The most frequent location for epidermoid is the cerebellopontine angle, followed by pineal region, suprasellar region, and middle cranial fossa.[1,3]

Epidermoids usually appear as a fluid density mass on CT and are similar to CSF on T1- and T2-weighted MRI. However, epidermoids are generally brighter than CSF on fluid-attenuated inversion recovery (FLAIR) imaging and show diffusion restriction, thus having signal similar or higher than brain parenchyma on DWI. Dermoids are usually well-circumscribed and contain some tissue of fat signal. After contrast administration, epidermoids and dermoids do not enhance or show just minimal marginal enhancement. Craniopharyngiomas usually show at least some enhancement. In contradistinction to an epidermoid cyst, arachnoid and neurenteric cysts have fluid signal (dark) on DWI.[3]

Questions for Further Thought

1. What is the key sequence for the diagnosis of epidermoid cyst?
2. How does an epidermoid cyst appear on postcontrast T1-weighted images?

Reporting Responsibilities

Describe the location and check for any complication.

What the Treating Physician Needs to Know

Epidermoid in the occipital and nasofrontal regions may be associated with a dermal sinus tract which should be completely resected. Epidermoid in the suprasellar or pineal region may cause hydrocephalus. Patients with epidermoid in the cerebellopontine angle may present with cranial neuropathy, and with epidermoid in the middle cranial fossa may present with chemical meningitis.

Answers

1. DWI, which will show diffusion restriction (signal higher than CSF). FLAIR imaging will generally also show signal higher than CSF, but some FLAIR sequences can be difficult to interpret as normal CSF can appear to have signal higher than CSF, especially in areas of pulsatility.
2. Epidermoid cyst should appear as a nonenhancing mass or possibly show just minimal marginal enhancement unless there is superimposed infection. Enhancing components may also indicate presence of a teratoma.

REFERENCES

1. Raybaud C, Barkovich AJ. Intracranial, orbital, and neck masses of childhood. In: Barkovich AJ, Raybaud C, eds. *Pediatric Neuroimaging*. 5th ed. Philadelphia, PA: Lippincott Williams & Wilkins; 2012:637–807.

2. Jones BV. Dermoid and epidermoid cysts. In: Donnelly LF, ed. *Diagnostic Imaging: Pediatrics*. 2nd ed. Salt Lake City, UT: Amirsys; 2012;7:36–37.

3. Osborn AG, Preece MT. Intracranial cysts: Radiologic-pathologic correlation and imaging approach. *Radiology*. 2006; 239(3):650–664.

CLINICAL HISTORY *A 5-year-old male with history of severe developmental delay*

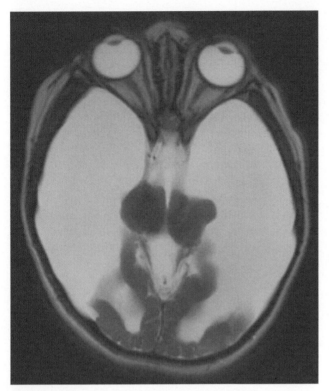

FIGURE 2.5A

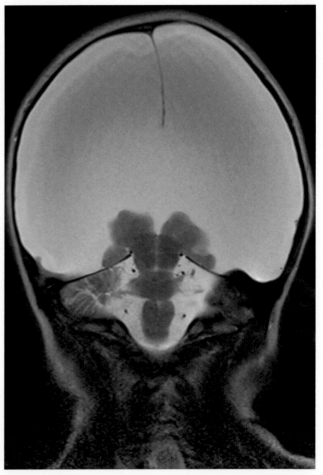

FIGURE 2.5B

FINDINGS Axial (**A**) and coronal (**B**) T2-weighted sequences through the brain demonstrate a largely CSF-filled supratentorial compartment with absent cortical mantle of the bilateral frontal, temporal and parietal lobes. The falx cerebri is present. There is relative sparing of bilateral occipital lobes, brain stem, and posterior fossa structures. The thalami are unfused.

DIFFERENTIAL DIAGNOSIS Hydranencephaly, severe hydrocephalus, HPE, bilateral, large open-lipped schizencephaly

DIAGNOSIS Hydranencephaly

DISCUSSION Hydranencephaly is thought to occur at about 25 weeks of gestation, from intrauterine compromise of the supraclinoid internal carotid arteries bilaterally with an intact posterior circulation, resulting in liquefactive necrosis and destruction of bilateral cerebral hemispheres with relative sparing of the structures supplied by the posterior circulation (occipital lobes, thalami, brain stem, and posterior fossa structures). Patients are generally born with macrocephaly and demonstrate severe failure to thrive, hyperreflexia, and seizures. MRI demonstrates a largely CSF-filled supratentorial compartment with relative sparing of structures supplied by posterior

circulation. The falx cerebri is at least partially present. In the neonatal period, ultrasound can be effectively used to make this diagnosis. Oftentimes, diagnosis has already been made using prenatal ultrasound.[1] Hydranencephaly is usually sporadic in occurrence but rarely can be autosomal recessive. Patients generally do not survive infancy. Rarely, a unilateral form, hemihydranencephaly, can be seen.

DIFFERENTIAL DIAGNOSTIC CONSIDERATIONS

Severe hydrocephalus: Cerebral mantle is present, although thinned.

HPE: Absent or deficient falx cerebri, with fused thalami in the alobar form.

Bilateral, large open-lipped schizencephaly: Portions of cerebral hemisphere are seen and the large CSF clefts are usually lined by dysplastic gray matter.

Questions for Further Thought

1. In hydranencephaly, do the occipital lobes show changes of ischemic insult?
2. What features of hydranencephaly besides the presence of a falx differentiate hydranencephaly from alobar HPE?

Reporting Responsibilities

- Describe features which may suggest other differential diagnoses.
- An MR angiogram may be performed to look for the anterior circulation vessels.

What the Treating Physician Needs to Know

The correct diagnosis. Hydrocephalus is usually treatable with early shunting.[2]

Answers

1. The occipital lobes may show atrophy. Gliotic changes are not seen as a gliotic response is not expected if the ischemic insult occurs before about 32 weeks of gestation.
2. Patients with hydranencephaly typically have unfused thalami and relatively spared occipital lobes.

REFERENCES

1. Byers BD, Barth WH, Stewart TL, et al. Ultrasound and MRI appearance and evolution of hydranencephaly in utero: A case report. *J Reprod Med.* 2005;50(1):53–56.
2. Sutton LN, Bruce DA, Schut L. Hydranencephaly versus maximal hydrocephalus: An important clinical distinction. *Neurosurgery.* 1980;6(1):34–38.

CLINICAL HISTORY *A 16-year-old male with history of hearing loss*

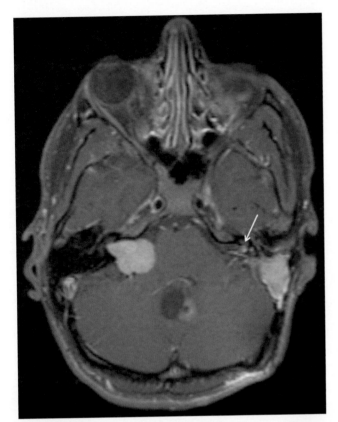

FIGURE 2.6A

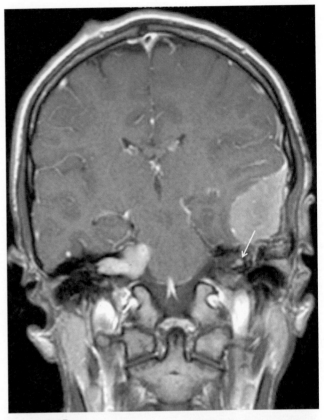

FIGURE 2.6B

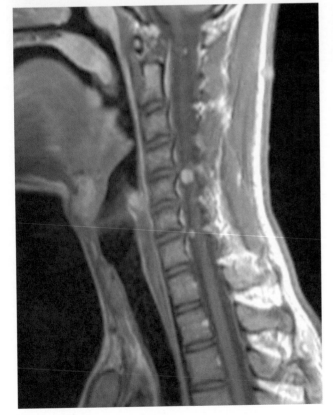

FIGURE 2.6C

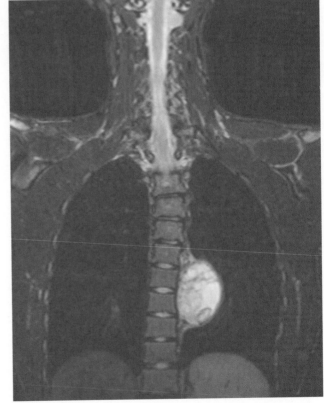

FIGURE 2.6D

FINDINGS Axial (**A**) and coronal (**B**) T1-weighted fat-suppressed postcontrast MR images of the brain demonstrate an enhancing mass in the right cerebellopontine angle that extends into the internal auditory canal, as well as a small enhancing focus in the left internal auditory canal (*arrow*). There is also a dural-based enhancing mass in the left middle cranial fossa as well as an ill-defined mass in the vermis, posterior to the partially effaced fourth ventricle, that has both cystic and enhancing solid components. Sagittal T1-weighted postcontrast image of the cervical spine (**C**) demonstrates extramedullary enhancing lesions within the cervical spinal canal. Coronal short-tau inversion recovery (STIR) image (**D**) demonstrates a heterogeneous left paraspinal mass in the thoracic region.

DIFFERENTIAL DIAGNOSIS Neurofibromatosis type 2 (NF2), multiple metastases, multiple meningiomas, multiple schwannomas, inflammatory disease such as sarcoidosis

DIAGNOSIS NF2

DISCUSSION The patient presented in this case had bilateral vestibular schwannomas, a left middle cranial fossa meningioma, a posterior fossa ependymoma, multiple intraspinal schwannomas as well as a large left paraspinal schwannoma. Also known as MISME syndrome (multiple inherited schwannomas, meningiomas, and ependymomas), NF2 is associated with an abnormality of the long arm of chromosome 22. Patients typically become symptomatic in the late second to third decades of life. Younger age at presentation frequently implies a poorer prognosis. Patients characteristically have bilateral vestibular schwannomas. They may also have other craniospinal schwannomas, meningiomas, and posterior fossa and cord ependymomas. Other infrequent central nervous system (CNS) abnormalities include cerebral calcifications and meningioangiomatosis. CT may demonstrate a widened porus acusticus and internal auditory canal in a patient who has vestibular schwannomas. Overall, however, MRI is better for evaluation of the brain parenchyma, extra-axial lesions, and spinal cord. Acoustic or vestibular schwannomas typically enhance homogeneously and may rarely be necrotic. Meningiomas typically have intense enhancement, may be en plaque in configuration, and, especially if large, can cause vasogenic edema in subjacent brain due to capillary obstruction. Contrast MRI is the best tool for baseline and follow-up imaging.[1]

Questions for Further Thought

1. What are some of the clinical presentations of patients with NF2?
2. Are neurofibromas a frequent occurrence in NF2?

Reporting Responsibilities

Extent of disease, cord compression. Stability or change in size of intracranial and intraspinal lesions over serial exams.

What the Treating Physician Needs to Know

Change in size of intracranial and intraspinal lesions over serial exams. Presence of new lesions.

Answers

1. About one-third of patients present with hearing loss.[2] Other presentations include cranial neuropathies, cataracts, scoliosis, and cord compressive symptoms from intraspinal lesions.
2. No, neurofibromas are rarely seen with NF2.

REFERENCES

1. Baser ME, R Evans DG, Gutmann DH. Neurofibromatosis 2. *Curr Opin Neurol.* 2003;16(1):27–33.
2. Bance M, Ramsden RT. Management of neurofibromatosis type 2. *Ear Nose Throat J.* 1999;78(2):91–92, 94, 96.

CASE 2.7

CLINICAL HISTORY *A 15-year-old male recently involved in a motor vehicle accident*

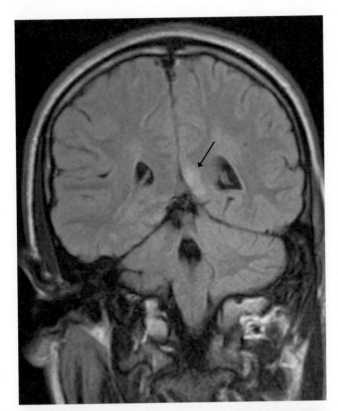

FIGURE **2.7A**

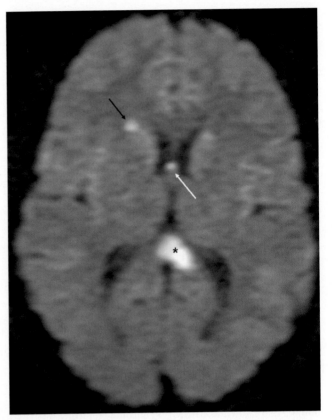

FIGURE **2.7B**

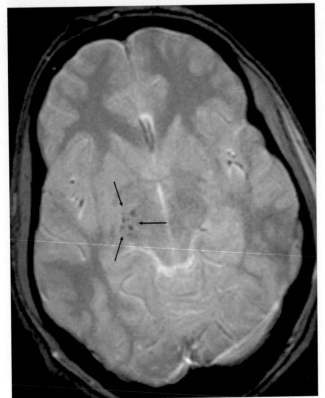

FIGURE **2.7C**

FINDINGS Coronal FLAIR MR image of the brain (**A**) demonstrates signal abnormality along the left aspect of the splenium of the corpus callosum (*arrow*). Axial diffusion image (**B**) demonstrates restricted diffusion in this area (*asterisk*) as well as within the right anterior caudate head (*black arrow*) and fornix (*white arrow*). Axial gradient-recalled echo (GRE) image (**C**) depicts punctate microhemorrhages (low-signal foci) at the margin of right cerebral peduncle (*arrows*).

DIFFERENTIAL DIAGNOSIS Diffuse axonal injury (DAI), vasculitis (infectious, inflammatory, autoimmune)

DIAGNOSIS DAI

DISCUSSION DAI is a type of traumatic axonal stretch/shear injury resulting from forces of deceleration. MRI is considerably better than CT in the detection of DAI and shows findings of DAI in about 40% of children imaged for traumatic brain injury.

T2-weighted and FLAIR sequences may identify small parenchymal abnormalities. Lesions may or may not be hemorrhagic,[1,2] and may demonstrate restricted diffusion. Common sites of imaged DAI include the gray–white interface, corpus callosum, and brainstem.[3] Multifocal punctate hemorrhages are a good clue to the diagnosis. Although not universally available, susceptibility-weighted MRI is a more sensitive technique than GRE technique for the detection of hemorrhagic foci.

The Adams and Gennarelli grading or staging of DAI are as follows:

I. Lesions at frontotemporal gray–white interface.

II. Lesions in lobar white matter and corpus callosum.

III. Lesions in dorsolateral midbrain and upper pons.

The findings in this case represent a grade III DAI.

Questions for Further Thought

1. What are findings at CT in patients with DAI?
2. What is the significance of grading of DAI?

Reporting Responsibilities

• Distribution of signal abnormality and assignment of grade.
• Description of nature of lesions, including whether restricted on diffusion imaging or hemorrhagic.

What the Treating Physician Needs to Know

Presence and grade of DAI and important ancillary findings such as cerebral edema, and impending herniation.

Answers

1. In 50% to 80%, CT scan in a patient with DAI will be normal at time of initial examination. There may be hypodense foci likely representing edema at site of injury or hyperdense petechial foci.[3]

2. Grading is a prognostic indicator. Higher grade signifies deeper brain involvement and usually implies poorer prognosis.

REFERENCES

1. Tong KA, Ashwal S, Holshouser BA, et al. Hemorrhagic shearing lesions in children and adolescents with posttraumatic diffuse axonal injury: Improved detection and initial results. *Radiology.* 2003;227(2):332–339.

2. Hofman PA, Stapert SZ, van Kroonenburgh MJ, et al. MR imaging, single-photon emission CT, and neurocognitive performance after mild traumatic brain injury. *AJNR Am J Neuroradiol.* 2001;22(3):441–449.

3. Katzman GL. Diffuse axonal injury (DAI). In: Osborn AG, Salzman KL, Barkovich AJ, eds. *Diagnostic Imaging: Brain.* 2nd ed. Salt Lake City, UT: Amirsys; 2010;I:2:36–39.

Paritosh C. Khanna

CASE 2.8

CLINICAL HISTORY *A 2-year-old male who presents with masses on the head*

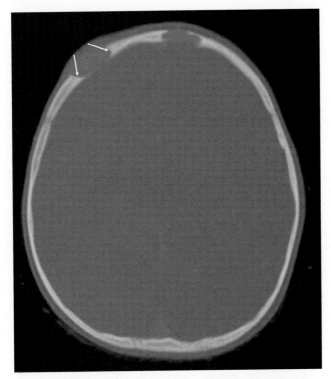

FIGURE **2.8A**

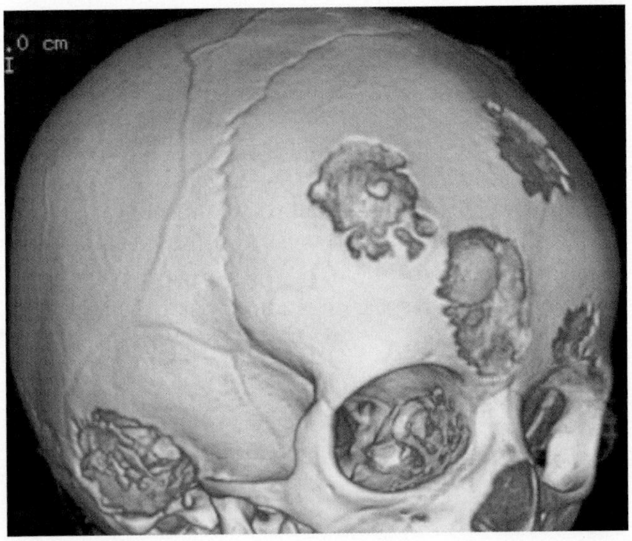

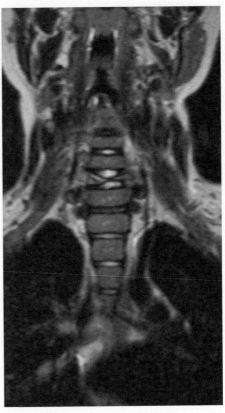

FIGURE **2.8B**

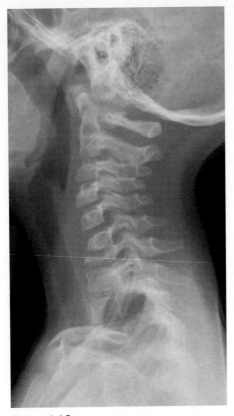

FIGURE **2.8C**

FIGURE **2.8D**

FINDINGS Axial bone-window CT image (**A**) and three-dimensional (3D) surface-shaded reconstruction (**B**) demonstrate lytic frontal bone lesions with beveled edges (*arrows,* **A**). Lateral radiograph (**C**) and coronal T2-weighted MRI (**D**) of the cervical spine demonstrate C7 vertebra plana.

DIFFERENTIAL DIAGNOSIS

Calvarium: Langerhans cell histiocytosis (LCH), osteomyelitis, neuroblastoma metastases, lymphoma, leukemia, iatrogenic (burr-hole), epidermoid and dermoid, leptomeningeal cyst.

Spine: LCH, infection, trauma, metastases, leukemia, lymphoma, radiation therapy.

DIAGNOSIS LCH

DISCUSSION Also known as eosinophilic granuloma and histiocytosis X, the pathologic hallmark of this disease process is focal or multifocal involvement with granuloma formation from abnormal proliferation of Langerhans cell histiocytes. Virtually any organ system can be involved. Patients may present with hepatosplenomegaly. The etiology is unknown with peak incidence within the first decade of life. *Findings in calvarium and brain:* Skull is the most frequently involved osseous structure. Sharply marginated, geographic lytic skull defects with beveled edges are characteristic. Infrequently noted is a central island of dead bone referred to as the "button sequestrum". The bony lesions may be associated with soft-tissue masses. Other findings include inflammatory thickening and enhancement of the pituitary stalk with or without absent posterior pituitary bright spot on MRI. Rarely, LCH may manifest with choroid plexus, basal ganglia, hypothalamic, cerebellar, and leptomeningeal lesions. *Findings in spine:* LCH starts off as a lytic vertebral body lesion which subsequently collapses, sparing adjacent discs and posterior elements. There may be small prevertebral and epidural soft-tissue components. With healing, the vertebra may regain some of its height with residual sclerosis and coarsening of trabeculae and sometimes, scoliosis. Management may involve chemotherapy with surgical intervention in select cases.[1,2]

Questions for Further Thought

1. What is the most common clinical presentation in patients with pituitary involvement?
2. What is the prognosis of this disease?

Reporting Responsibilities

Extent of involvement. Description of changes suggestive of healing on serial follow-up imaging.

What the Treating Physician Needs to Know

LCH is often multifocal. Discovery of an abnormality suggesting this diagnosis usually warrants further imaging to evaluate for other sites of involvement.

Answers

1. The most common clinical presentation is diabetes insipidus, visual disturbances, and hypothalamic dysfunction.
2. Prognosis is worse with younger age at onset and multifocality. Although some lesions may spontaneously regress, others may become aggressive over time with a mortality approaching 20% in severe cases.

REFERENCES

1. Resnick D. Lipidoses, histiocytoses, and hyperlipoproteinemias. In: Resnick D, ed. *Diagnosis of Bone and Joint Disorders.* 4th ed. Philadelphia, PA: Saunders; 2002:2233–2290.
2. Steiner M, Prayer D, Asenbaum S, et al. Modern imaging methods for the assessment of Langerhans' cell histiocytosis-associated neurodegenerative syndrome: Case report. *J Child Neurol.* 2005;20(3):253–257.

Paritosh C. Khanna

CLINICAL HISTORY *A 13-year-old female with Cushing disease and hypertension*

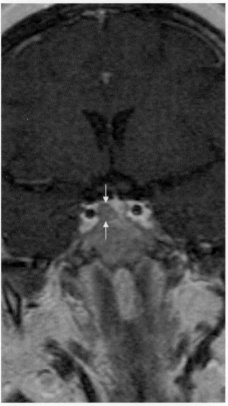

FIGURE **2.9A**

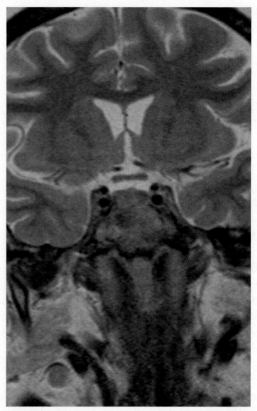

FIGURE **2.9B**

FINDINGS Coronal dynamic contrast-enhanced T1-weighted image (**A**) demonstrates a hypoenhancing, well-circumscribed area within the right aspect of the anterior pituitary (*arrows*). On the coronal T2-weighted image (**B**), this area is slightly brighter than surrounding pituitary but isointense to gray matter. The lesion measured less than 10 mm in maximal dimension. Remainder of the pituitary demonstrated normal enhancement and T2 signal characteristics.

DIFFERENTIAL DIAGNOSIS Pituitary microadenoma, pituitary hyperplasia, Rathke cleft cyst, pars intermedia cyst, intrasellar craniopharyngioma

DIAGNOSIS Pituitary microadenoma

DISCUSSION Pituitary microadenoma is a well-circumscribed pituitary mass less than 10 mm in maximal dimension, as distinct from the macroadenoma that typically is more than 10 mm. Microadenomas, depending on their size, may cause an asymmetric bulge of the superior aspect of the pituitary gland. Gland tissue surrounding this mass is compressed. Microadenomas generally do not enhance as rapidly as

surrounding normal pituitary tissue. This differential enhancement is best appreciated during the dynamic phase of a contrast-enhanced MRI study.[1,2] On standard postcontrast images, the microadenomas may not be appreciated; up to one-third are only seen with dynamic imaging. On coronal T2-weighted imaging, microadenomas are iso- to hyperintense to the surrounding gland. Rarely, this tumor can have an extrasellar location, for example, pituitary infundibulum. Uncommonly, microadenomas may have hemorrhage, necrosis, and calcification, especially seen with prolactinomas in males. The most common microadenoma is a prolactinoma, followed by growth hormone and adrenocorticotrophic hormone (ACTH)-secreting microadenomas. Microadenomas may be considered an "incidentaloma" if nonfunctioning. MRI is the best diagnostic modality; CT and angiography with petrosal sinus sampling are rarely used.

DIFFERENTIAL DIAGNOSTIC CONSIDERATIONS

Pituitary hyperplasia: Entire gland is usually involved.

Rathke cleft cyst: Nonenhancing; may be T1 hyperintense and T2 variable due to proteinaceous content and/or blood product.

Pars intermedia cyst: T1 hypointense, small, located between the anterior and posterior lobes of the pituitary gland. Nonenhancing.

Intrasellar craniopharyngioma: Rare, can be calcified, compresses and displaces pituitary.

Questions for Further Thought

1. How do patients with microadenomas present and how does this differ from macroadenoma presentation?
2. What is the difference in MRI protocol for micro- versus macroadenomas?

Reporting Responsibilities

Describe presence and location of pituitary mass.

What the Treating Physician Needs to Know

Cause of underlying endocrine abnormality.

Answers

1. Prolactinoma: Young female, primary or secondary amenorrhea with galactorrhea and infertility. Growth hormone-secreting tumor: Gigantism. ACTH-oma: Cushing syndrome. Macroadenoma: Typically mass effect resulting in visual field defects and panhypopituitarism.
2. Dynamic contrast-enhanced coronal thin-section T1-weighted imaging for microadenoma whereas standard postcontrast T1-weighted imaging is sufficient for macroadenoma.

REFERENCES

1. Hirsch W, Zumkeller W, Teichler H, et al. Microadenomas of the pituitary gland in children with and without hypophyseal dysfunction in magnetic resonance imaging. *J Pediatr Endocrinol Metab.* 2002;15(2):157–162.
2. Rand T, Lippitz P, Kink E, et al. Evaluation of pituitary microadenomas with dynamic MR imaging. *Eur J Radiol.* 2002; 41(2):131–135.

Paritosh C. Khanna

CASE 2.10

CLINICAL HISTORY *A 17-year-old female with history of posterior fossa ependymoma resection*

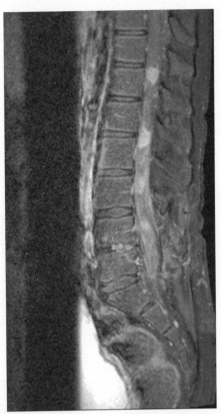

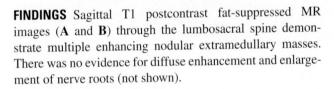

FIGURE 2.10A

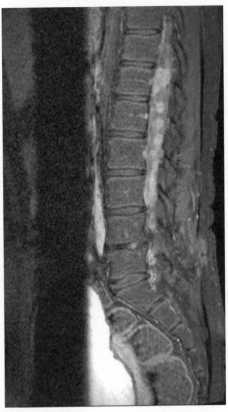

FIGURE 2.10B

FINDINGS Sagittal T1 postcontrast fat-suppressed MR images (**A** and **B**) through the lumbosacral spine demonstrate multiple enhancing nodular extramedullary masses. There was no evidence for diffuse enhancement and enlargement of nerve roots (not shown).

DIFFERENTIAL DIAGNOSIS Drop metastases, multifocal primary tumor, pyogenic meningitis, granulomatous meningitis, chemical meningitis

DIAGNOSIS Drop metastases from posterior fossa ependymoma

DISCUSSION Drop metastases or leptomeningeal carcinomatosis typically results from spread of malignant CNS tumors through the subarachnoid space and is seen in advanced cases of malignancies of the neural axis. In children, this most often occurs from spread of medulloblastoma, ependymoma, and germinoma with choroid plexus carcinoma (CPC) being a less frequent cause. MRI demonstrates a variable pattern with either a single or multiple enhancing nodular masses or with linear enhancement (sugar-coating) of the spinal cord,

conus, and dorsal and ventral nerve roots, including the filum terminale and cauda equina, which may appear thickened, clumped, or peripherally adherent ("empty sac" sign). Rarely, round or ovoid intramedullary masses, often with a ringlike pattern may be noted, presumably resulting from CSF seeding of the central canal of the spinal cord. For this reason, the entire neural axis should be imaged following the administration of contrast. Patients with drop metastases generally have a history of CNS malignancy and may be asymptomatic or present with pain and polyradiculopathy or symptoms of myelopathy.[1] Within the intracranial compartment, patients with drop metastases may show abnormal FLAIR signal and a leptomeningeal pattern of enhancement along the pia-arachnoid membranes, following the sulci.[2]

DIFFERENTIAL DIAGNOSTIC CONSIDERATIONS

Multifocal primary tumor: Rare; multiple nerve sheath tumors may mimic intradural nodular drop metastases.

Pyogenic and chemical meningitis: Generally demonstrate smooth enlargement and enhancement of nerve roots.

Granulomatous meningitis: Smooth or nodular enhancing nerve roots.

Questions for Further Thought

1. What are additional findings on non-contrast T1 and T2 sequences?
2. What are some other entities to consider in the differential for nodular or linear enhancement?

Reporting Responsibilities

- Presence and extent or absence of drop metastases.
- Presence or absence of cord compression from intradural mass.

What the Treating Physician Needs to Know

- Presence or absence of drop metastases.
- Presence or absence of cord compression from a large intradural mass.
- Response to treatment.

Answers

1. Occasionally noted is a subtle T1 hyperintensity of CSF. Nodules tend to be isointense to cord and nerve roots on T2 imaging.
2. Guillain–Barre syndrome, subarachnoid hemorrhage, sarcoidosis (less common in the pediatric age group).

REFERENCES

1. Gomori JM, Heching N, Siegal T. Leptomeningeal metastases: Evaluation by gadolinium enhanced spinal magnetic resonance imaging. *J Neurooncol.* 1998;36(1):55–60.
2. Khanna PC, Shaw DWW. Neuroimaging. In: Fuhrman BP, Zimmerman J, eds. *Pediatric Critical Care.* 4th ed. Philadelphia, PA: Elsevier; 2011:759–782.

CASE 2.11

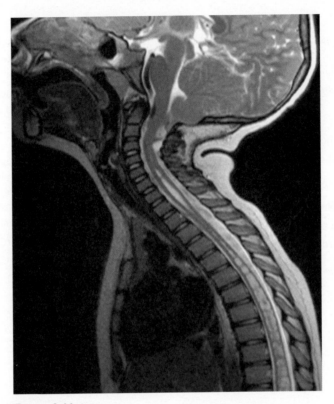

FIGURE 2.11

FINDINGS Sagittal T2-weighted MRI image of the upper spinal cord demonstrates multiseptated CSF intensity area extending from the upper cervical cord caudally through the thoracic cord. Craniocervical junction demonstrates tonsillar ectopia with extension of peg-shaped cerebellar tonsils into the upper cervical spinal canal with effacement of dorsal CSF space at the level of foramen magnum. Posterior fossa is crowded.

DIFFERENTIAL DIAGNOSIS Syringohydromyelia, intramedullary tumor, myelomalacia

DIAGNOSIS Syringohydromyelia

DISCUSSION Syringomyelia is a longitudinally oriented CSF-filled space/cavity within cord parenchyma that is not lined by ependyma and in most cases is difficult to distinguish from hydromyelia, which represents a dilation of the central canal itself and therefore, by definition, is lined by ependyma. Often the term syringohydromyelia or syrinx is used to encompass both these entities. Surrounding cord parenchyma, especially with syringomyelia, may demonstrate T2-hyperintense edema and cord expansion in the acute phase or myelomalacia in the subacute or chronic phase. It may be difficult to differentiate punctate prominence of the central canal from syringohydromyelia. This is especially true at the level of the conus where minimal prominence of the central canal, in the absence of other abnormality, is termed a ventriculus terminalis and considered a normal variant. Both axial and sagittal images are useful to quantify size and extent of a syrinx. Large syringes may often have a septated, lobulated appearance, but are usually a single cavity. Cranial extension into the medulla is referred to as syringobulbia.

The associated causes of syrinx are quite varied, including Chiari I and II malformations, tumor, and idiopathic. Since tumor is one of the underlying causes (and differentials) of a syrinx, first-time evaluation with MRI, in the absence of other obvious causes, should include imaging after administration of contrast to exclude nodular enhancement.[1]

DIFFERENTIAL DIAGNOSTIC CONSIDERATIONS

Intramedullary tumor: May have mixed enhancing solid and variable cystic components.

Myelomalacia: Can be seen in the absence of syrinx as a result of cord infarct, trauma, or hemorrhage. In general, myelomalacia is not as bright on T2-weighted imaging as cord syrinx.

Questions for Further Thought

1. What are some of the underlying processes that result in syringohydromyelia?
2. What is the pathophysiology of a syrinx?

Reporting Responsibilities

Underlying cause, extent of syrinx, changes within cord parenchyma.

What the Treating Physician Needs to Know

- Any changes in syrinx with treatment of underlying cause.
- Any progression of syrinx in the absence of known cause.

Answers

1. Chiari I and II malformations, scoliosis,[2] spinal dysraphism, cord tumor, spontaneous or traumatic hemorrhage, idiopathic.
2. Altered CSF flow dynamics, typically secondary to obstruction at some level within the spinal canal. Cord cavitation is less frequent and is seen in cases of trauma and hematoma.

REFERENCES

1. Piatt JH Jr. Syringomyelia complicating myelomeningocele: Review of the evidence. *J Neurosurg.* 2004;100(2 Suppl Pediatrics):101–109.
2. Ozerdemoglu RA, Denis F, Transfeldt EE. Scoliosis associated with syringomyelia: Clinical and radiologic correlation. *Spine (Phila Pa 1976).* 2003;28(13):1410–1417.

Paritosh C. Khanna

CLINICAL HISTORY *A 14-year-old female who presents with visual field defect (Fig. 2.12A)*

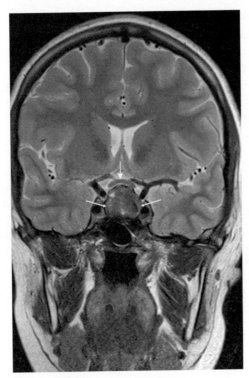

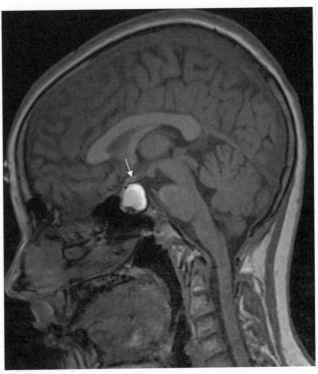

FIGURE **2.12A**

FIGURE **2.12B**

FINDINGS Coronal T2-weighted MRI image (**A**) demonstrates a heterogeneous mass (*oblique white arrows*) replacing the entire pituitary, filling the sella, and extending into the suprasellar cistern. Maximum dimension was 18 mm. Mass enhanced intensely on the postcontrast T1-weighted images (not shown). Sagittal T1-weighted non-contrast MRI image (**B**) in a different 16-year-old female patient with visual field defects demonstrates a predominantly T1-hyperintense mass in expected location of pituitary which showed low-signal blooming on gradient sequence (not shown) suggesting hemorrhage, with lower signal foci along its inferior aspect. Peripheral portions of this mass enhanced on postcontrast T1-weighted imaging (not shown). The masses in both images demonstrate mass effect with superiorly displaced optic chiasm (*vertical white arrows*).

DIFFERENTIAL DIAGNOSIS Pituitary macroadenoma, pituitary hyperplasia, Rathke cleft cyst, craniopharyngioma

DIAGNOSIS Pituitary macroadenoma without (**A**) and with (**B**) hemorrhage (pituitary apoplexy)

DISCUSSION Pituitary macroadenoma by definition is a pituitary mass more than 10 mm in maximal dimension,

derived from anterior pituitary cells called pituicytes. Giant adenomas, rare in children, are more than 40 mm in greatest dimension. The tumor replaces and fills the sella with suprasellar extension often assuming a snowman configuration. This results in mass effect on surrounding structures. Large tumors can expand and erode the sella, and aggressive tumors may invade sphenoid sinus, clivus, and one or both cavernous sinuses. The rare ectopic pituitary macroadenoma may originate in these above-mentioned locations, the infundibulum, or within the third ventricle. The posterior pituitary bright spot may be superiorly displaced or absent.[1] Pituitary macroadenomas usually enhance intensely but heterogeneously and are heterogeneous on T2-weighted imaging. Nearly always benign (WHO grade I), they can have hemorrhage (see **B**) and/or necrosis from infarction, resulting in a clinical syndrome termed "pituitary apoplexy." A small percentage of these tumors calcify. Patients with pituitary macroadenoma may have multiple clinical presentations, including headaches, visual field defects, various endocrinologic abnormalities[2] such as panhypopituitarism, and apoplexy.

DIFFERENTIAL DIAGNOSTIC CONSIDERATIONS

Pituitary hyperplasia: May be difficult to differentiate on basis of imaging alone.

Rathke cleft cyst: Nonenhancing, generally T1 hyperintense and T2 variable due to proteinaceous content and/or blood product.

Craniopharyngioma: Can be calcified, usually suprasellar location, can extend into sella and compress or displace the pituitary. Can rarely be purely intrasellar in location.

Questions for Further Thought

1. What is the most common visual field defect with macroadenomas and why?
2. What is the difference in management for macroadenomas versus microadenomas?

Reporting Responsibilities

Size and extent of mass, invasive features, visualized mass effect (especially on the optic chiasm), hemorrhage if present, and location of the posterior pituitary bright spot.

What the Treating Physician Needs to Know

The likely diagnosis, extent, and mass effect.

Answers

1. Bitemporal hemianopsia due to midline mass effect on the chiasm.
2. Macroadenoma: Surgical resection is the mainstay. Stereotactic radiosurgery and medical therapy may be used. Microadenoma: When functional, medical therapy is the mainstay. Surgery is employed in some cases.

REFERENCES

1. Bonneville F, Narboux Y, Cattin F, et al. Preoperative location of the pituitary bright spot in patients with pituitary macroadenomas. *AJNR Am J Neuroradiol.* 2002;23(4):528–532.
2. Maeder P, Gudinchet F, Rillet B, et al. Cushing's disease due to a giant pituitary adenoma in early infancy: CT and MRI features. *Pediatr Radiol.* 1996;26(1):48–50.

CLINICAL HISTORY *An 8-year-old male with 5-week history of worsening headache*

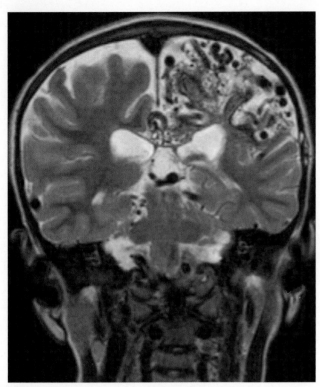

FIGURE 2.13A

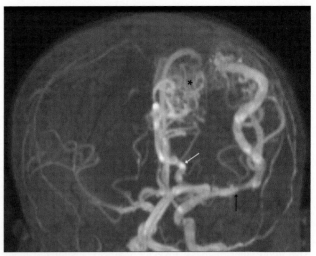

FIGURE 2.13B

FINDINGS Coronal T2-weighted MRI image (**A**) demonstrates multiple flow voids of varying sizes representing a large tangle of vessels which involved much of the left frontal and parietal lobes with some underlying volume loss. 3D time-of-flight (TOF) MR angiogram (**B**) demonstrates that the tangle of vessels (*asterisk*) is supplied by hypertrophic feeders from the anterior (*white arrow*) and middle cerebral (*black arrow*) arteries. No intracranial hemorrhage was identified in this patient.

DIFFERENTIAL DIAGNOSIS Arteriovenous malformation (AVM), dural arteriovenous fistula

DIAGNOSIS Cerebral AVM.

DISCUSSION Cerebral AVMs are vascular malformations with a variably sized tangle of vessels (termed the nidus) without intervening capillary network and direct arteriovenous shunting. Intranidal aneurysms often occur. AVMs are usually sporadic and solitary. Multiple AVMs in children are rare and usually syndromic such as with hereditary hemorrhagic telangiectasia (Osler–Weber–Rendu syndrome). Typical MRI demonstrates a tangle of flow voids on T1 and T2 sequences with flow-related enhancement on 3D TOF MR angiogram. Early draining vein(s) are seen on dynamic, time-resolved contrast-enhanced MR angiogram or conventional cerebral angiography.[1] Hemorrhage from an AVM may occur, generally due to rupture of a thrombosed, kinked, or otherwise obstructed and dilated draining vein. Intranidal aneurysm rupture is rare in children. Gradient-echo sequences are helpful in detecting subacute or old bleeds. In patients with AVM, adjacent parenchymal volume loss is often noted, secondary to arterial steal phenomenon from shunting. Definitive evaluation, particularly for endovascular therapy, is achieved with conventional angiography. Treatment is by surgical resection, endovascular embolization, radiosurgery, or a combination of these options.

DIFFERENTIAL DIAGNOSTIC CONSIDERATION

Dural arteriovenous fistula: These are typically supplied by meningeal arteries (look for an enlarged external carotid artery as a clue) and usually drain into meningeal veins or dural venous sinus(es).

Questions for Further Thought

1. What might be the presentation of patients with AVM?
2. What are the criteria used to determine prognosis and guide management?

Reporting Responsibilities

Size, location, feeding and draining vessels, associated bleed.

What the Treating Physician Needs to Know

Spetzler–Martin grade (see Answer 2).

Answers

1. Congestive cardiac failure in infancy with large volume shunting, headaches, seizures, neurologic deficits, and coma from hemorrhage.

2. The Spetzler–Martin grading system which assigns points to the AVM depending on size (<3 cm, 3 to 6 cm, and >6 cm), whether it involves an eloquent area of brain, and whether it drains into the superficial or deep venous systems.[2]

REFERENCES

1. Khanna PC, Shaw DWW. Neuroimaging. In: Fuhrman BP, Zimmerman J, eds. *Pediatric Critical Care.* 4th ed. Philadelphia, PA: Elsevier; 2011:759–782.
2. Spetzler RF, Martin NA. A proposed grading system for arteriovenous malformations. *J Neurosurg.* 1986;65(4):476–483.

CASE 2.14

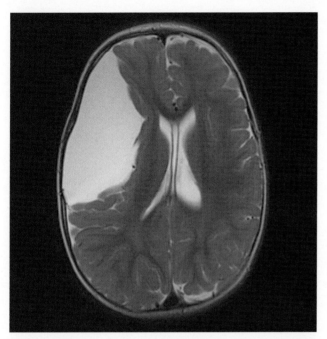

FIGURE 2.14A

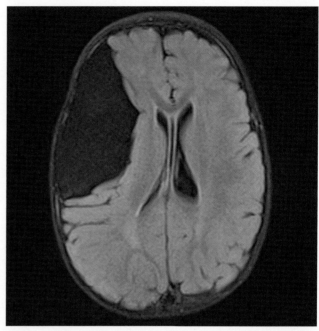

FIGURE 2.14B

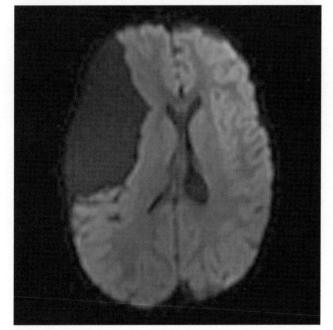

FIGURE 2.14C

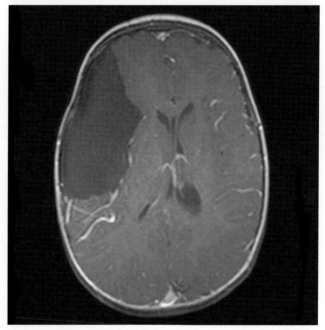

FIGURE 2.14D

FINDINGS Axial T2-weighted (**A**), FLAIR (**B**), diffusion (**C**), and postcontrast T1-weighted (**D**) MRI images demonstrate a large extra-axial cystic lesion arising within the right middle cranial fossa with adjacent mass effect and resultant midline shift. This cystic lesion follows CSF signal on all sequences demonstrating T2 hyperintensity (**A**), FLAIR suppression (**B**), and no diffusion restriction (**C**). The lesion is T1 hypointense with no contrast enhancement demonstrated (**D**).

DIFFERENTIAL DIAGNOSIS Arachnoid cyst, epidermoid cyst, cystic astrocytoma, neuroepithelial cyst, porencephalic cyst

DIAGNOSIS Arachnoid cyst

DISCUSSION Intracranial arachnoid cysts are benign development anomalies that may be clinically asymptomatic. They are often discovered as incidental findings found on imaging, although they may produce symptoms because of expansion or bleeding. If symptoms are present, they are often dependent on size and location of the lesion with common neurologic features in symptomatic patients, including headache, seizure, hydrocephalus, developmental delay, and focal neurologic symptoms related to compression. Arachnoid cysts arise within the supratentorial brain in 90% of cases, most commonly occurring in the middle cranial fossa and sylvian fissure, with other sites including the quadrigeminal plate, sellar region, and supratentorial convexities.[1] On CT, arachnoid cysts typically appear as extra-axial collections with density similar to CSF and no contrast enhancement. Adjacent calvarial remodeling is common. Characteristic MRI findings include an extra-axial cystic lesion that follows CSF signal intensity on all imaging sequences. Arachnoid cysts do not show diffusion restriction on MRI, which helps in the differentiation from epidermoid cysts.[2] Conservative management is recommended for patients who do not demonstrate signs of increased intracranial pressure, progressive hydrocephalus, or focal neurologic signs. When surgery is required, the two most commonly used procedures for treatment include cystoperitoneal shunting and cyst fenestration. Total cyst excision is usually not possible.

Questions for Further Thought

1. What differentiates primary versus secondary arachnoid cysts?

2. Are arachnoid cysts associated with particular syndromes?

Reporting Responsibilities

Report the size, anatomic location, and adjacent mass effect.

What the Treating Physician Needs to Know

- Arachnoid cysts are a relatively common incidental finding, occurring in approximately 3% of the population.[3]
- Arachnoid cysts are more commonly asymptomatic but may demonstrate symptoms related to mass effect and CSF obstruction.

Answers

1. Primary or true arachnoid cysts are congenital, possibly related to splitting and duplication of the arachnoid membrane. Secondary arachnoid cysts result from postinflammatory accumulation of CSF related to scarring after head injury, intracranial hemorrhage, or infection.

2. Arachnoid cysts are seen with higher incidence in polycystic kidney disease, Down syndrome, mucopolysaccharidosis, schizencephaly, and neurofibromatosis.[2]

REFERENCES

1. Wang PJ, Lin HC, Liu HM, et al. Intracranial arachnoid cysts in children: Related signs and associated anomalies. *Pediatr Neurol.* 1998;19(2):100–104.

2. Gosalakkal JA. Intracranial arachnoid cysts in children: A review of pathogenesis, clinical features, and management. *Pediatr Neurol.* 2002;26(2):93–98.

3. Al-Holou WN, Yew AY, Boomsaad ZE, et al. Prevalence and natural history of arachnoid cysts in children. *J Neurosurg Pediatr.* 2010;5(6):578–585.

CLINICAL HISTORY *A 3-year-old male with scoliosis and clubfoot deformity*

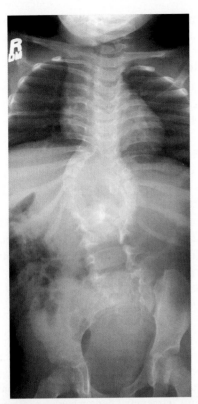

FIGURE **2.15A**

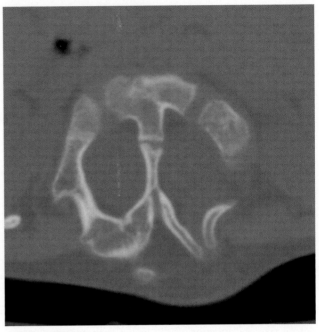

FIGURE **2.15B**

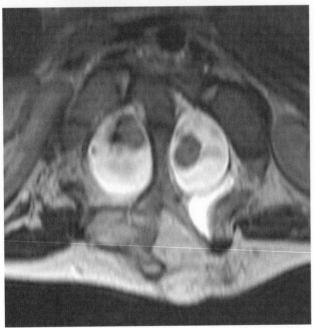

FIGURE **2.15C**

FINDINGS Frontal radiograph of the spine (**A**) demonstrates splaying of thoracolumbar vertebral bodies with posterior dysraphism and evidence of a bony septum. Findings are confirmed on axial CT (**B**), demonstrating a bony septum splitting a widened spinal canal and deficient posterior elements. Axial T2-weighted MRI (**C**) demonstrates similar findings as well as two hemicords separated by a bony septum. There is a small T2-hyperintense extradural fluid collection posterior to the left thecal sac.

DIFFERENTIAL DIAGNOSIS Diastematomyelia, spinal segmental dysgenesis, neurenteric cyst

DIAGNOSIS Diastematomyelia

DISCUSSION Diastematomyelia, or split cord malformation, is a closed spinal dysraphism characterized by two hemicords split by a dividing septum. Each hemicord contains its own central canal as well as its own ventral and dorsal horn. There are two main types of diastematomyelia: Type I is the less common of the two types, accounting for 25% of cases.[1] This occurs when two hemicords are encased in their own dural sacs and separated by a bony septum. Cord separation usually occurs in the thoracolumbar region with 85% occurring below the T8-T9 vertebral body level. Severe vertebral segmentation and fusion anomalies with resultant scoliosis are commonly observed with Type I diastematomyelia. Type II diastematomyelia occurs when two hemicords are encased in a single dural sac separated by a fibrous septum. Cutaneous stigmata of both type I and type II are similar with cutaneous birthmarks, hemangiomas, or hairy tufts often indicating the underlying malformation.[1]

Patients with Type II diastematomyelia are less likely to have symptoms than those with Type I. Symptoms, when present, usually relate to cord tethering and/or hydromyelia. Orthopedic problems of the foot, particularly clubfoot, are not uncommon.[2]

Questions for Further Thought

1. What is considered a normal level of the conus medullaris, and at what age does it reach its mature level?
2. When in embryologic development do spinal dysraphisms occur?

Reporting Responsibilities

- Report the extent of split cord malformation as well as the presence or absence of an osseous or fibrous septum and any other spinal cord abnormalities such as syringohydromyelia.
- Report the presence and extent of vertebral body anomalies and resultant scoliosis.

What the Treating Physician Needs to Know

- Diastematomyelia can be associated with severe segmentation and fusion anomalies of the thoracolumbar spine with resultant scoliosis.
- Cutaneous stigmata in the sacral region including birthmarks, hemangioma, or hairy tufts can indicate underlying malformations and should prompt evaluation for closed spinal dysraphism.[1]

Answers

1. The conus medullaris normally terminates at or above the inferior aspect of the L2 vertebral body. It has reached its mature adult level at term in most infants; however, the ascent of the conus may be delayed by up to 3 months in some cases.[1]
2. Spinal dysraphisms result from abnormalities in normal embryologic development occurring between gestational weeks 2 and 6.

REFERENCES

1. Tortori-Donati P, Rossi A, Biancheri R, et al. Magnetic resonance imaging of spinal dysraphism. *Top Magn Reson Imaging.* 2001;12(6):375–409.
2. Schwartz ES, Barkovich AJ. Congenital anomalies of the spine. In: Barkovich AJ, Raybaud C, eds. *Pediatric Neuroimaging.* 5th ed. Philadelphia, PA: Lippincott Williams & Wilkins; 2012:857–922.

CASE 2.16

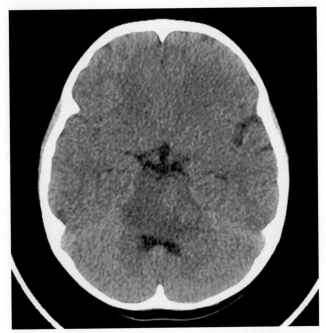

FIGURE 2.16A

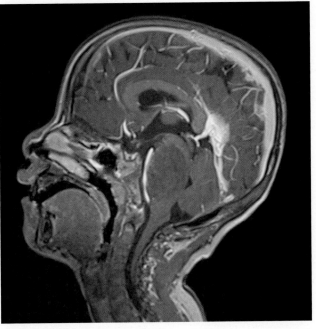

FIGURE 2.16B

FINDINGS Axial nonenhanced CT (**A**) demonstrates an ill-defined hypodense mass in the pons with mass effect on the fourth ventricle. Sagittal T1-weighted postcontrast MR image (**B**) demonstrates a T1-hypointense mass lesion centered in the pons, without significant contrast enhancement when compared to nonenhanced images (not shown). There is diffuse enlargement of the pons with anterior displacement of the basilar artery and posterior effacement of the fourth ventricle.

DIFFERENTIAL DIAGNOSIS Brainstem glioma, brainstem primitive neuroectodermal tumor (PNET), lymphoma, tumefactive demyelination, encephalitis

DIAGNOSIS Brainstem glioma

DISCUSSION Brainstem gliomas are the fourth most common posterior fossa mass occurring in children, following medulloblastoma, cerebellar astrocytoma, and ependymoma. Most brainstem gliomas arise in the pons, with the remainder in the midbrain and medulla. The majority of pontine gliomas are high-grade, infiltrative astrocytomas, as in this case.[1] The classic imaging appearance is that of an ill-defined mass that causes diffuse pontine enlargement with bowing of the ventral contour, the so-called "pregnant pons"

appearance. Enhancement following the administration of contrast material is variable, but is typically subtle or absent. Outcomes are poor, and treatment is palliative with corticosteroids and radiation therapy.

In contrast to pontine gliomas, gliomas arising elsewhere in the brainstem and posterior fossa are usually well circumscribed, histologically low grade, and have better outcomes.[2,3] These gliomas tend to be more heterogeneous in their imaging appearance, often demonstrating focally exophytic or cystic components and enhancement. Treatment depends on location, but is typically radiotherapy with or without chemotherapy. Aggressive surgical resection can be beneficial in selected cases, including dorsally exophytic tumors, cystic tumors, and enhancing tumors with well-defined margins. Surgery is typically avoided in midbrain gliomas due to their tendency for slow progression and proximity to the corticospinal tracts.

Questions for Further Thought

1. What is the typical clinical presentation of children with pontine glioma?
2. What imaging feature is helpful in differentiating brainstem gliomas from lymphomas and PNETs arising in the brainstem?

Reporting Responsibilities

- Describe the location and extent of involvement, including exophytic components and their relationship to the basilar artery.
- Assess for mass effect on the fourth ventricle and presence of hydrocephalus.

What the Treating Physician Needs to Know

- MR is the modality of choice to detect brain stem pathology, as beam hardening artifact decreases sensitivity of CT in the posterior fossa.
- Infiltrative pontine gliomas with typical imaging features are not routinely biopsied, and presumptive diagnosis is made on the basis of imaging alone. Atypical features should prompt consideration of alternative etiologies, as this can trigger biopsy and potentially alter prognosis and management.

Answers

1. Patients classically present with a short duration of cranial nerve or long tract signs. Symptoms are often mild relative to imaging findings because the infiltrative growth pattern leaves the underlying neural architecture relatively undisturbed.
2. Pronounced restricted diffusion is atypical for a brainstem glioma and can suggest a densely cellular tumor such as PNET or lymphoma.

REFERENCES

1. Lima MA. Brainstem gliomas: an overview. In: Hayat MA, ed. *Tumors of the Central Nervous System, Volume 2.* New York, NY: Springer; 2011:387–395.
2. Kwon JW, Kim IO, Cheon JE, et al. Paediatric brain-stem gliomas: MRI, FDG-PET and histological grading correlation. *Pediatr Radiol.* 2006;36(9):959–964.
3. Mauffrey C. Paediatric brainstem gliomas: prognostic factors and management. *J Clin Neurosci.* 2006;13(4):431–437.

Jason Nixon and Edward Weinberger

CASE 2.17

CLINICAL HISTORY *A 16-year-old male with lifelong history of dysarthria and impaired fine motor skills*

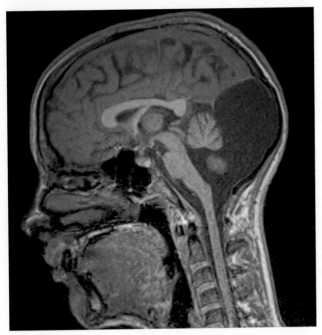

FIGURE 2.17A

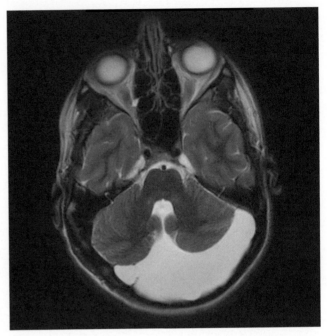

FIGURE 2.17B

FINDINGS Sagittal T1-weighted (**A**) and axial T2-weighted (**B**) MR images demonstrate a large posterior fossa, inferior vermian hypoplasia, and a large retrocerebellar cyst in communication with the fourth ventricle. Corpus callosum is intact.

DIFFERENTIAL DIAGNOSIS Dandy–Walker malformation (DWM), Dandy–Walker variant (DWV), Blake pouch cyst (BPC), mega cisterna magna (MCM), arachnoid cyst

DIAGNOSIS DWM

DISCUSSION DWM is the most severe manifestation of a spectrum of posterior fossa developmental abnormalities which are broadly termed the Dandy–Walker complex (DWC).[1] The complex further encompasses the DWV and MCM. Some authors also include the BPC.[2] DWM is classically defined by the triad of (1) an enlarged posterior fossa with lambdoid–torcular inversion, (2) a retrocerebellar cyst in communication with the fourth ventricle, and (3) vermian hypoplasia or aplasia. Although the definitions of DWV are varied, the term is most commonly used in cases with a normal-sized posterior fossa and inferior vermian hypoplasia. BPC is defined by the presence of a retrocerebellar cyst typically in continuity with the fourth ventricle, in the absence of vermian dysgenesis. Posterior fossa enlargement is variably present. MCM is enlargement of the subarachnoid space of the cisterna magna in the absence of either vermian dysgenesis or a retrocerebellar cyst. It is the least severe expression of the DWC, and is considered by most to be a normal variant.

Questions for Further Thought

1. What is the underlying pathophysiology of the DWC?
2. What imaging clue can help to distinguish between the cyst as seen in DWM or DWV, a BPC, and an arachnoid cyst?

Reporting Responsibilities

- Describe the spectrum of posterior fossa abnormalities.
- Describe associated supratentorial anomalies such as heterotopic gray matter, dysgenesis of the corpus callosum, or hydrocephalus.

What the Treating Physician Needs to Know

The spectrum of clinical abnormality associated with the DWC is broad, and depends largely on the degree of vermian hypoplasia and associated supratentorial as well as extracranial abnormalities. Clinical abnormalities can range from completely asymptomatic to profound psychomotor retardation.[1]

Answers

1. The DWC is believed to result from failure of normal development of the membranous roof of the fourth ventricle during fetal development. There is failure of perforation of the posterior membranous area, which consequently balloons out into a posterior fossa cyst. If the cyst is ultimately transient, the result is enlargement of the cisterna magna. If it persists, a BPC will result.[2] When the anterior membranous area is involved as well, there will be associated hypoplasia or aplasia of the vermis, resulting in the stigmata of DWV or DWM.

2. The status of the fourth ventricle choroid plexus can be helpful: It is absent in the cyst of DWM or DWV, displaced into the anterior roof of the BPC, and normally located in the arachnoid cyst.[3]

REFERENCES

1. Barkovich AJ, Kjos BO, Norman D, et al. Revised classification of posterior fossa cysts and cystlike malformations based on the results of multiplanar MR imaging. *AJR Am J Roentgenol.* 1989;153(6):1289–1300.

2. Tortori-Donati P, Fondelli MP, Rossi A, et al. Cystic malformations of the posterior cranial fossa originating from a defect of the posterior membranous area. Mega cisterna magna and persisting Blake's pouch: two separate entities. *Childs Nerv Syst.* 1996;12(6):303–308.

3. Nelson MD, Maher K, Gilles FH. A different approach to cysts of the posterior fossa. *Pediatr Radiol.* 2004;34(9):720–732.

Gisele E. Ishak

CASE 2.18

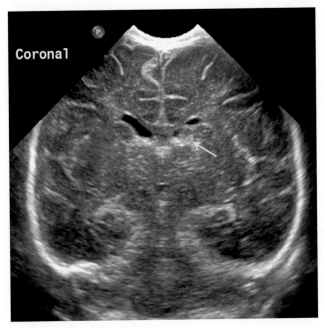

FIGURE 2.18A

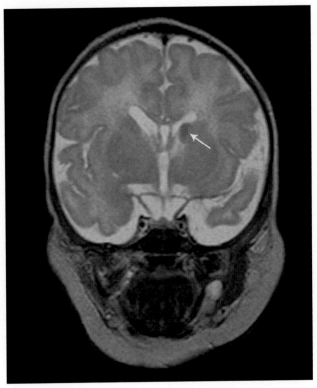

FIGURE 2.18B

FINDINGS Coronal image from a cranial ultrasound (**A**) shows a small echogenic focus in the left caudothalamic groove (*arrow*) consistent with grade I germinal matrix hemorrhage (GMH). There is no definite extension into the ventricles which are of normal size. Coronal T2-weighted MR image (**B**) shows a corresponding low T2 signal intensity focus (*arrow*) consistent with blood product.

DIFFERENTIAL DIAGNOSIS GMH, subependymal calcification

DIAGNOSIS GMH

DISCUSSION Preterm infants with hypoxic-ischemic injury are at increased risk for GMH. This is because the germinal matrix, which lines the walls of the lateral ventricles in fetal life and is the precursor of neurons and glial cells, is a highly vascularized and cellular region which is susceptible to ischemia and hemorrhage. The germinal matrix involutes by 34 weeks of gestation. The last portion to involute is located at the caudothalamic groove, where most GMH originates.[1]

GMH–intraventricular hemorrhage (GMH-IVH) grading is as follows:

Grade I: Subependymal hemorrhage with no intraventricular extension.

Grade II: Subependymal hemorrhage extending into the ventricles without ventricular enlargement.

Grade III: Subependymal hemorrhage extending into the ventricles with ventricular enlargement.

Grade IV: Subependymal hemorrhage, usually with ventricular extension, as well as periventricular parenchymal hemorrhagic infarction (hemorrhage into white matter surrounding lateral ventricles thought due to concurrent hemorrhage within an area of venous infarction rather than direct extension of IVH).

In addition to GMH, premature infants with hypoxic-ischemic injury are also at increased risk for periventricular leukomalacia (PVL), also referred to as white matter injury of prematurity. Previously thought to be related to ischemia in hypovascular watershed zones in the preterm brain, PVL is now believed to be related to vulnerability of oligodendrocyte precursors which disappear after 32 weeks of gestation, in concordance with the declining prevalence of PVL after 32 to 34 weeks of gestation. PVL is typically initially imaged as increased periventricular echogenicity by ultrasound (although ultrasound may not always pick up this finding) and increased T2 signal by MRI. Subsequent cavitation and periventricular cyst formation may be noted 3 to 6 weeks later. By 6 months of age, findings of end-stage PVL are usually noted, often with resolution of the cysts, progressive loss of volume with possible cystic encephalomalacia, ventriculomegaly, and thinning of the corpus callosum.[2,3]

Questions for Further Thought

1. What is the screening modality for GMH?
2. Is GMH-IVH common after 34 weeks of gestation?

Reporting Responsibilities

- Report grading of GMH and associated hydrocephalus.
- Report abnormal echogenicity/signal in the periventricular white matter that could be related to periventricular parenchymal hemorrhagic infarction or represent PVL.

What the Treating Physician Needs to Know

Premature infants may develop ventriculomegaly which may be due to communicating hydrocephalus (from obstruction of arachnoid granulations by blood in the subarachnoid CSF spaces) or noncommunicating hydrocephalus, such as due to the presence of blood clot in the cerebral aqueduct. Ventriculomegaly may also occur due to ex vacuo dilatation associated with end-stage PVL. Depending on the specific clinical situation, shunting may be warranted.

Answers

1. Intracranial ultrasound is an excellent screening modality for GMH and hydrocephalus. Ultrasound may also identify increased echogenicity in the periventricular white matter suggestive for PVL.[4]
2. GMH-IVH is not common after 34 weeks of gestation because the germinal matrix will have involuted by that time.

REFERENCES

1. Schwartz ES, Barkovich AJ. Brain and spine injuries in infancy and childhood. In: Barkovich AJ, Raybaud C, eds. *Pediatric Neuroimaging*. 5th ed. Philadelphia, PA: Lippincott Williams & Wilkins; 2012:240–366.
2. Huang BY, Castillo M. Hypoxic-ischemic brain injury: Imaging findings from birth to adulthood. *Radiographics*. 2008;28(2):417–439.
3. Argyropoulou MI. Brain lesions in preterm infants: Initial diagnosis and follow-up. *Pediatr Radiol*. 2010;40(6):811–818.
4. Chao CP, Zaleski CG, Patton AC. Neonatal hypoxic-ischemic encephalopathy: Multimodality imaging findings. *Radiographics*. 2006;26(suppl 1):S159–S172.

Gisele E. Ishak

CASE 2.19

CLINICAL HISTORY *A 6-month-old child with bilateral sensorineural hearing loss (Fig. 2.19A)*

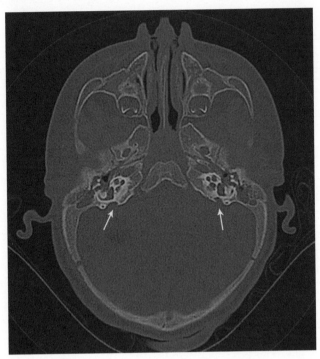

FIGURE **2.19A**

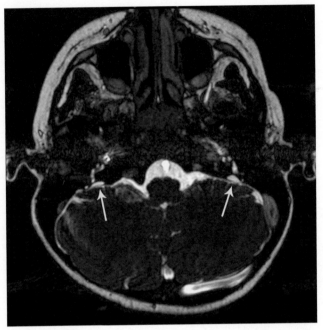

FIGURE **2.19B**

FINDINGS Axial thin-slice CT of the temporal bones (**A**) shows enlarged vestibular aqueducts bilaterally (*white arrows*). Axial CISS (constructive interference in steady state heavily T2-weighted MRI sequence) (**B**) in a different 5-year-old boy shows bilateral enlargement of the endolymphatic sacs (*white arrows*).

DIFFERENTIAL DIAGNOSIS Enlarged vestibular aqueduct or large endolymphatic sac anomaly

DIAGNOSIS Enlarged vestibular aqueduct or large endolymphatic sac anomaly

DISCUSSION Enlarged vestibular aqueduct or large endolymphatic sac anomaly is the most common congenital anomaly of the inner ear found by imaging in patients with childhood onset of sensorineural hearing loss (SNHL).[1] It is the radiologic marker for SNHL although the true etiology is thought to be caused by associated cochlear abnormalities which may not always be evident by imaging. This anomaly is a familial lesion with autosomal recessive inheritance. It is the result of arrest of inner ear develop-

ment at approximately the seventh week of fetal development. It is bilateral in 90% and is associated with cochlear dysplasia (75%) as well as vestibular or semicircular canal dysplasia (50%).[2] Hearing is typically normal at birth but deteriorates over the early years of life, leading to profound SNHL. Thin-section temporal bone CT shows enlarged bony vestibular aqueduct measuring greater than 1.5 mm at the mid aspect of the bony vestibular aqueduct, or measuring more than the diameter of the posterior semicircular canal. Thin-section, high-resolution T2-weighted imaging shows high T2 signal in an enlarged endolymphatic sac.[1]

Questions for Further Thought

1. What is one hypothesis of SNHL in large endolymphatic sac anomaly?
2. How does the endolymphatic sac appear normally on thin-section, high-resolution T2-weighted imaging?

Reporting Responsibilities

Report associated anomalies of the cochlea, vestibule, and semicircular canal.

What the Treating Physician Needs to Know

- Associated inner ear anomalies.
- Bilateral involvement, if present, because cochlear implantation is now used for bilateral disease associated with profound SNHL.

Answers

1. One hypothesis is that the cochlea is fragile and susceptible to injury from mild trauma, which is why avoidance of contact sports that may lead to head trauma is essential.

2. Normally, the endolymphatic canal is barely visible on thin-section, high-resolution T2-weighted imaging.

REFERENCES

1. Robson CD. Large vestibular aqueduct. In: Harnsberger HR, Glastonbury CM, Michel MA, Koch BL, eds. *Diagnostic Imaging: Head and Neck*. 2nd ed. Salt Lake City, UT: Amirsys; 2011;VI:4:14–17.

2. Atkin JS, Grimmer JF, Hedlund G, et al. Cochlear abnormalities associated with enlarged vestibular aqueduct anomaly. *Int J Pediatr Otorhinolaryngol*. 2009;73(12):1682–1685.

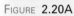

CASE 2.20

Robert Raines-Hepple and Edward Weinberger

CLINICAL HISTORY *A 2-year-old girl presents with leukocoria and unilateral impaired vision*

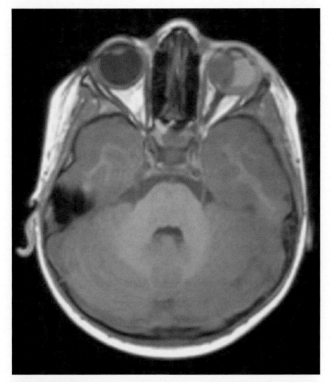

FIGURE 2.20A

FIGURE 2.20B

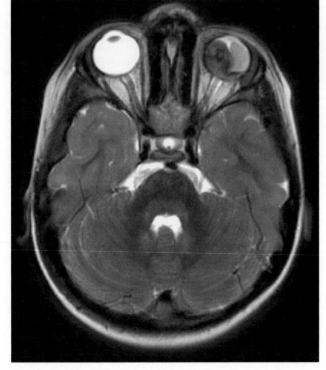

FIGURE 2.20C

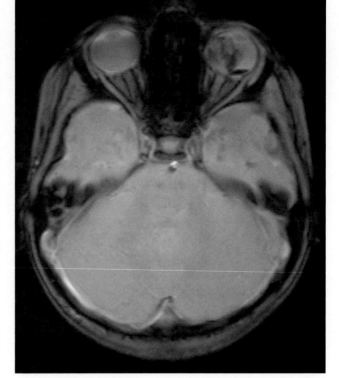

FIGURE 2.20D

FINDINGS T1-weighted precontrast (**A**), T1-weighted post-contrast (**B**), and T2-weighted precontrast (**C**) MR images demonstrate a heterogeneous, low T1 and T2 signal ocular mass in the medial aspect of the left globe with slight patchy enhancement. There is also hemorrhagic retinal detachment with a blood product—fluid level in the lateral portion of the left globe. Presumed presence of calcifications medially and dependent blood products laterally are suggested on GRE image (**D**) which demonstrates low signal. No extraocular extension, contralateral mass, pineal or suprasellar region mass was identified on remainder of examination.

DIFFERENTIAL DIAGNOSIS Retinoblastoma, persistent hyperplastic primary vitreous (PHPV), retinopathy of prematurity

DIAGNOSIS Retinoblastoma

DISCUSSION Retinoblastoma is the most common intraocular mass in children and manifests by age 5 years in 90% to 95% of cases. In utero, late childhood, and early adult presentations are rare. Retinoblastoma occurs in approximately 1/15,000 to 1/20,000 live births with minimal variation around the world, which leads to 7,000 to 8,000 new cases annually worldwide.[1,2]

Retinoblastoma has both noninherited and heritable forms. The noninheritable forms present as single-site tumors whereas the heritable forms are often bilateral or multifocal. The heritable form, related to loss of function of the tumor suppressor gene *RB1* on the long arm of chromosome 13, is autosomal dominant with 90% to 95% penetrance and is also associated with other intracranial tumors. Examples include pineoblastoma (the combination of bilateral retinoblastoma and pineoblastoma is called trilateral retinoblastoma) and rarely a suprasellar tumor, typically a PNET. Patients with the heritable form may also develop delayed second primary retinoblastomas and are at increased risk of developing other tumors, especially in those patients who have been treated with radiation. Osteosarcoma is the most common second tumor followed by rhabdomyosarcoma and other soft-tissue sarcomas.[1,3–7]

The most common presenting symptom of retinoblastoma is leukocoria, an abnormal light reflex on fundoscopic exam, seen in 56% to 75% of cases. Less common presenting symptoms include strabismus, visual disturbances, glaucoma, and pain. Periocular inflammation is an uncommon presentation that often leads to a delay in diagnosis due to mimicking orbital cellulitis.[3–6]

Ocular ultrasound demonstrates an intraocular mass, frequently with calcifications and retinal detachment. An array of characteristic patterns of growth and types of retinal detachment are well described in the ophthalmologic literature.[1,8] On CT, imaging findings include calcifications which occur in 95% of retinoblastoma, and occasionally enhancement (in 25% to 30%). On MR, retinoblastoma usually has heterogeneous, low T1 and T2 signal from calcification, and some enhancement. Retinoblastoma can be an aggressive tumor with spread through the sclera, along the optic nerve, intracranially through sphenoid bone invasion, or via lymphatic or hematogenous metastasis.[3–7]

Treatment has evolved from enucleation with radiation, to globe and frequently vision-salvaging procedures when possible with aggressive early local and systemic treatment. Examples include laser ablation and both intravenous and intra-arterial chemotherapy, often called chemoreduction. With these newer techniques, survival can exceed 95%. Since it is one of the most highly treatable cancers, disseminating the current standard of care around the world could decrease the annual death rate by up to 90%, from 3,000 to 4,000 children, to 400.[1,2]

In contradistinction to retinoblastoma, microphthalmia is characteristic of PHPV and calcifications are rare. Retinopathy of prematurity is typically seen in premature infants who received high-oxygen therapy. In this entity, calcification is rare, the orbit may or may not be small, and bilateral retinal detachment may occur.

Questions for Further Thought

1. What rare ocular malignancies could be considered in the differential diagnosis?
2. What is the differential diagnosis of leukocoria in the young child?

Reporting Responsibilities

- Describe invasion beyond the globe and evidence for multifocality within the same globe, as well as evidence for disease in the contralateral globe and if there is intracranial disease involving the pineal and suprasellar regions.
- A rare infiltrating form characterized by retinal thickening can be difficult to diagnose due to the absence of a discrete mass and rarity of calcifications.
- On studies ordered for suspected orbital cellulitis, look carefully for an intraocular mass.

What the Treating Physician Needs to Know

- Details relevant to the treating physician include tumor size, extraocular extension, intracranial extension, synchronous or metachronous primaries, and metastases.

- Intracranial masses tend to present approximately 2 years after the initial presentation of retinoblastoma.[5,6]

Answers

1. Additional malignant considerations include direct ocular metastases, such as neuroblastoma or sarcomas, and invasion of aggressive extraocular tumors including orbital metastases, rhabdomyosarcoma, and other sarcomas. Rare primary ocular malignancies include medulloepithelioma (which arises from the ciliary body) and ocular melanoma (also called choroidal or uveal melanoma).

2. Over half the patients with leukocoria have retinoblastoma. In addition to PHPV and retinopathy of prematurity, less common etiologies include *Toxocara* infection (non-calcified ocular mass associated with eosinophilia), Coats disease (retinal telangiectasia associated with hyperattenuating vitreous without calcification), and retinal astrocytoma (also known as astrocytic hamartoma and occurs in the setting of tuberous sclerosis complex (TSC) or neurofibromatosis type 1 (NF1)).[3,4]

REFERENCES

1. Houston SK, Murray TG, Wolfe SQ, et al. Current update on retinoblastoma. *Int Ophthalmol Clin.* 2011;51(1):77–91.

2. Shields CL, Shields JA. Retinoblastoma management: Advances in enucleation, intravenous chemoreduction, and intra-arterial chemotherapy. *Curr Opin Ophthalmol.* 2010;21(3):203–212.

3. Smirniotopoulos JG, Bargallo N, Mafee MF. Differential diagnosis of leukokoria: Radiologic-pathologic correlation. *Radiographics.* 1994;14(5):1059–1079.

4. Chung EM, Smirniotopoulos JG, Specht CS, et al. From the archives of the AFIP: Pediatric orbit tumors and tumorlike lesions: Nonosseous lesions of the extraocular orbit. *Radiographics.* 2007;27(6):1777–1799.

5. James SH, Halliday WC, Branson HM. Best cases from the AFIP: Trilateral retinoblastoma. *Radiographics.* 2010;30(3):833–837.

6. Provenzale JM, Gururangan S, Klintworth G. Trilateral retinoblastoma: Clinical and radiologic progression. *AJR Am J Roentgenol.* 2004;183(2):505–511.

7. Tateishi U, Hasegawa T, Miyakawa K, et al. CT and MRI features of recurrent tumors and second primary neoplasms in pediatric patients with retinoblastoma. *AJR Am J Roentgenol.* 2003;181(3):879–884.

8. Kaste SC, Jenkins JJ 3rd, Pratt CB, et al. Retinoblastoma: Sonographic findings with pathologic correlation in pediatric patients. *AJR Am J Roentgenol.* 2000;175(2):495–501.

Robert Raines-Hepple and Gisele E. Ishak

CLINICAL HISTORY *A 4-month-old girl presents with a right eyelid mass*

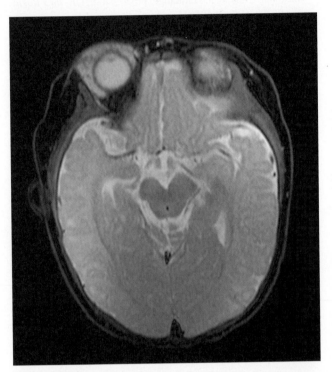

FIGURE 2.21A

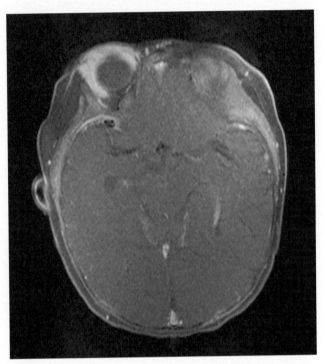

FIGURE 2.21B

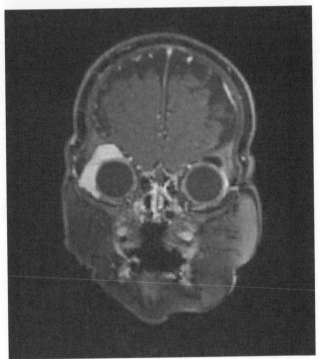

FIGURE 2.21C

FINDINGS Axial STIR MRI image (**A**) shows high signal lesion about the right eyelid and surrounding the anterolateral portions of the right globe. Axial (**B**) and coronal (**C**) post-contrast T1-weighted images with fat saturation demonstrate a nearly homogeneously enhancing extraocular orbital mass.

DIFFERENTIAL DIAGNOSIS Infantile hemangioma of the orbit, congenital hemangioma, vascular malformations (especially venous–lymphatic), rhabdomyosarcoma, nerve sheath tumors (neurofibroma, schwannoma), LCH, neuroblastoma metastasis, leukemia.

DIAGNOSIS Infantile hemangioma of the orbit

DISCUSSION Infantile hemangioma of the orbit is considered a true neoplasm with proliferative endothelium lining vascular channels. This lesion should be distinguished from developmental vascular malformations (which have variable components of arteries, veins, capillaries, or lymphatic vessels), as well as from malignancy such as rhabdomyosarcoma.[1,2]

Clinical presentation of infantile hemangioma of the orbit is usually within the first 6 months of life, and when superficial, consists of a reddish or bluish discolored lump that is often warm to the touch and occasionally pulsatile. This tumor represents 3% of all orbital lesions and 17% of vasculogenic orbital lesions. These lesions undergo characteristic growth phases with initial proliferation lasting up to 10 months, followed by a brief period of stabilization, then a long slow involution over up to 10 years. Involution proceeds from central to peripheral. One-third of infantile hemangiomas have additional lesions of the skin or viscera. Associated syndromes include Kasabach–Merritt, a consumptive thrombocytopenic coagulopathy, and PHACES, which is composed of posterior fossa anomalies, hemangiomas of the face, arterial abnormalities (including coarctation of the aorta), cerebral vascular anomalies, eye abnormalities, and sternal or ventral developmental anomalies. Congenital hemangioma of the orbit has a similar imaging appearance to infantile hemangioma of the orbit, but is formed at birth, and rather than a rapid proliferative phase, either involutes or may grow in proportion to growth of the child.[1-3]

Although first-line imaging of superficial orbital lesions may be ultrasound, MR is a better modality for tissue characterization and defining the extent of abnormality. On MR, infantile hemangioma of the orbit is iso- to slightly hyperintense on T1-weighted imaging relative to muscle and moderately hyperintense on T2-weighted imaging. Postcontrast imaging typically shows diffuse intense enhancement, and sometimes internal and peripheral flow voids as well as large feeding arteries. Additional findings on CT or MR include bony scalloping or orbital expansion, and well-circumscribed lobular margins. Calcifications are rare and indistinct margins are uncommon. As discussed above, infantile hemangioma of the orbit will have a time course showing growth and subsequent involution with progressive fatty infiltration and heterogeneity of enhancement.

Treatment of infantile hemangioma is generally conservative as most resolve completely. However, when vision is threatened, therapeutic options include surgery, systemic or intralesional corticosteroids, interferon, and laser therapy.[1-4]

DIFFERENTIAL DIAGNOSTIC CONSIDERATIONS

Rhabdomyosarcoma can be difficult to distinguish from infantile hemangiomas as they may have similar MRI features including homogeneous enhancement. However, rhabdomyosarcoma may have more heterogeneity as compared to hemangioma on T2-weighted imaging. Rarely, rhabdomyosarcomas may be sufficiently vascular to have internal flow voids. Aggressive or malignant features such as bony invasion, intracranial extension, and metastases are characteristic features of rhabdomyosarcoma in contrast to venous–lymphatic malformations and hemangiomas.[1,2,4,5]

Venous–lymphatic malformations are typically distinguished by the nonenhancing lymphatic component and irregular infiltrating margins that cross anatomic boundaries. Cystic components, internal hemorrhage, and the absence of flow voids or feeding vessels are characteristic.[1,2,4,5]

On dynamic MRI, infantile hemangiomas have initial diffuse enhancement as compared to nerve sheath tumors, where initial enhancement is typically more focal.[6]

Question for Further Thought

1. What is the difference between vascular tumors and vascular malformations?

Reporting Responsibilities
Describe the size, extent, and characteristics of the lesion including any identifiable vascular components.

What the Treating Physician Needs to Know
Extent of the lesion and whether there is involvement of any critical structures which could lead to compromised vision.

Answer

1. The terminology now in use was established by the International Society for the Study of Vascular Anomalies.[2] Vascular tumors are true neoplasms with proliferative endothelium lining vascular channels. Examples include infantile hemangiomas, the more rare congenital hemangiomas (both rapidly and noninvoluting subtypes), tufted angiomas, hemangioendothelioma and its many subtypes, and acquired dermatologic vascular tumors (pyogenic granuloma and rare acquired hemangioma variants) which are secondary to insults such as trauma, thermal injury, infection, insect bites, or retinoid treatment.

   Vascular malformations are congenital lesions with normal nonproliferative endothelium and are classified into slow-flow, fast-flow, and complex-combined vascular malformations. Slow-flow vascular malformations include capillary malformations (port-wine stain, telangiectasia, angiokeratoma), venous malformations (common sporadic, familial, glomangioma, Bean syndrome, Maffucci syndrome), and lymphatic malformations. Fast-flow vascular malformations involve an arterial component and include arterial malformations, arteriovenous fistula, and AVMs.

REFERENCES

1. Chung EM, Smirniotopoulos JG, Specht CS, et al. From the archives of the AFIP: Pediatric orbit tumors and tumorlike lesions: nonosseous lesions of the extraocular orbit. *Radiographics.* 2007;27(6):1777–1799.
2. Enjolras O, Wassef M, Chapot R. Introduction: ISSVA classification. In: Enjolras O, Wassef M, Chapot R, eds. *Color Atlas of Vascular Tumors and Vascular Malformations.* New York, NY: Cambridge University Press; 2007:1–11.
3. Jockin YM, Friedlander SF. Periorbital infantile hemangioma. *Int Ophthalmol Clin.* 2010;50(4):15–25.
4. Poon CS, Sze G, Johnson MH. Orbital lesions: Differentiating vascular and nonvascular etiologic factors. *AJR Am J Roentgenol.* 2008;190(4):956–965.
5. Shinder R, Al-Zubidi N, Esmaeli B. Survey of orbital tumors at a comprehensive cancer center in the United States. *Head Neck.* 2011;33(5):610–614.
6. Tanaka A, Mihara F, Yoshiura T, et al. Differentiation of cavernous hemangioma from schwannoma of the orbit: A dynamic MRI study. *AJR Am J Roentgenol.* 2004;183(6):1799–1804.

CLINICAL HISTORY *A 7-year-old boy who presents with bitemporal hemianopsia*

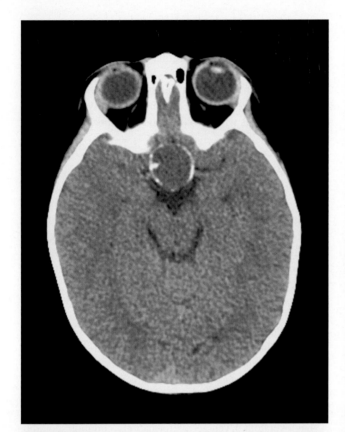

FIGURE 2.22A

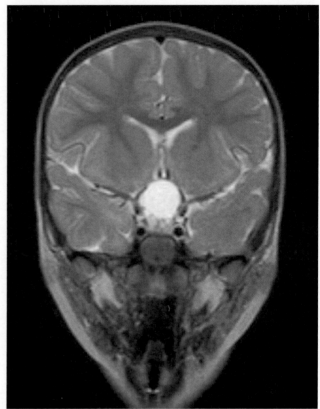

FIGURE 2.22B

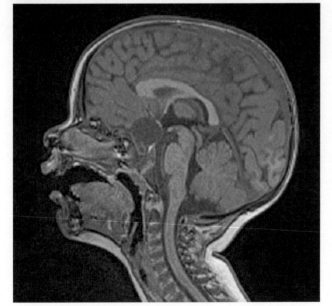

FIGURE 2.22C

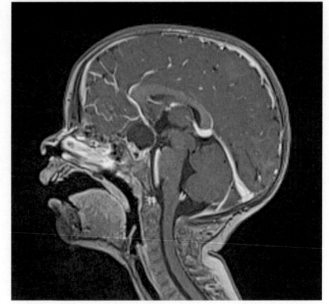

FIGURE 2.22D

FINDINGS Axial non-contrast CT (**A**) demonstrates a suprasellar cystic mass with rim calcifications that is also easily identified on coronal T2-weighted MRI (**B**). Sagittal T1-weighted precontrast imaging (**C**) and postcontrast imaging (**D**) show a small enhancing component at the inferior aspect of the cystic mass.

DIFFERENTIAL DIAGNOSIS Craniopharyngioma, germ cell tumor (GCT)/teratoma, astrocytoma, pituitary macroadenoma, chordoma[1,2]

DIAGNOSIS Craniopharyngioma

DISCUSSION Craniopharyngiomas are benign locally aggressive tumors that are presumed to arise from squamous epithelial remnants of Rathke pouch, also known as the craniopharyngeal duct, which is a precursor to the anterior pituitary. Another proposed etiology is ectopic embryonic cell rests of enamel organs.[3] Craniopharyngiomas represent 3% of childhood tumors and 50% of suprasellar tumors with a third to a half occurring in children under age 20.[3–5] Characteristic imaging findings include a predominantly cystic mass with some solid component, commonly with calcification and enhancement.[1–3,5] Craniopharyngiomas are usually suprasellar or both suprasellar and intrasellar in location. Rarely, a craniopharyngioma can be purely intrasellar in location. Outcomes are optimized with subtotal resection and external beam radiation treatment or stereotactic radiosurgery. Endocrine, neurologic, and vascular sequelae are minimized by avoiding gross total resection. Recurrence is common and can be difficult to treat due to involvement of or risk for damaging critical adjacent structures.[6–8]

Questions for Further Thought

1. What are typical presenting symptoms of patients with craniopharyngioma?
2. What are characteristic consequences of treatment?

Reporting Responsibilities

Location, size, shape, margins, composition, and involvement of critical structures pretreatment, and the identification of residual tumor and change in size or enhancement after treatment.

What the Treating Physician Needs to Know

- Location in order to determine the surgical approach: Prechiasmatic suprasellar, retrochiasmatic suprasellar, or limited to the sella.
- Extension of tumor into underlying bone and involvement of critical structures in the suprasellar region.

Answers

1. Typical presenting symptoms include headache, visual field deficits from compression of the optic chiasm and tracts, anterior pituitary dysfunction (hypopituitarism, especially growth hormone deficiency), and hypothalamic dysfunction (typically diabetes insipidus).
2. Consequences of treatment include endocrinopathies, visual disturbances, and new neurologic deficits. The most common endocrinopathies are diabetes insipidus, ACTH deficiency, anterior panhypopituitarism, and hypothyroidism. Vascular injury is rare and typically causes ischemic infarction.

REFERENCES

1. Johnsen DE, Woodruff WW, Allen IS, et al. MR imaging of the sellar and juxtasellar regions. *Radiographics.* 1991;11(5):727–758.
2. Eldevik OP, Blaivas M, Gabrielsen TO, et al. Craniopharyngioma: Radiologic and histologic findings and recurrence. *AJNR Am J Neuroradiol.* 1996;17(8):1427–1439.
3. Yousem DM, Grossman RI. Sella and central skull base. In: Yousem DM, Grossman RI, eds. *Neuroradiology: The Requisites.* 3rd ed. Philadelphia, PA: Mosby/Elsevier; 2010:356–384.
4. Bunin GR, Surawicz TS, Witman PA, et al. The descriptive epidemiology of craniopharyngioma. *J Neurosurg.* 1998;89(4): 547–551.
5. Raybaud C, Barkovich AJ. Intracranial, orbital, and neck masses of childhood. In: Barkovich AJ, Raybaud C, eds. *Pediatric Neuroimaging.* 5th ed. Philadelphia, PA: Lippincott Williams & Wilkins; 2012:637–807.
6. Sughrue ME, Yang I, Kane AJ, et al. Endocrinologic, neurologic, and visual morbidity after treatment for craniopharyngioma. *J Neurooncol.* 2011;101(3):463–476.
7. Barajas MA, Ramírez-Guzmán G, Rodríguez-Vázquez C, et al. Multimodal management of craniopharyngiomas: Neuroendoscopy, microsurgery, and radiosurgery. *J Neurosurg.* 2002; 97(5 Suppl):607–609.
8. Maira G, Anile C, Albanese A, et al. The role of transsphenoidal surgery in the treatment of craniopharyngiomas. *J Neurosurg.* 2004;100(3):445–451.

CASE 2.23

CLINICAL HISTORY *A 2-month-old boy born full term via an uneventful spontaneous vaginal delivery was noted to have an abnormal head shape shortly after birth*

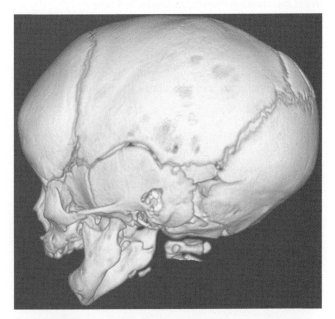

FIGURE **2.23A**

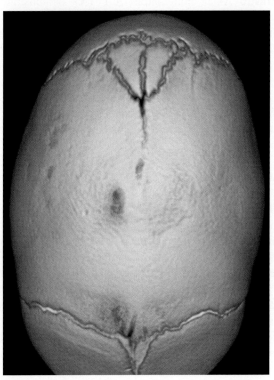

FIGURE **2.23B**

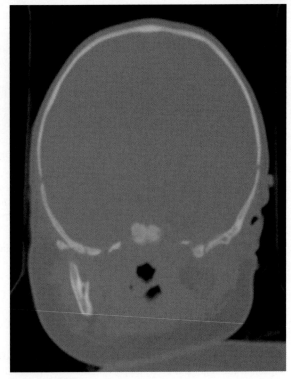

FIGURE **2.23C**

FINDINGS Selected images as viewed from the side (**A**) and the top (**B**) of a 3D surface-rendered CT reconstruction of the skull demonstrate an abnormal elongated shape of the skull (**A**) with associated premature closure of the sagittal suture (**B**). Coronal CT image of the head (**C**) optimized to evaluate the bones also shows bony fusion of the sagittal suture.

DIFFERENTIAL DIAGNOSIS Sagittal craniosynostosis with dolichocephaly

DIAGNOSIS Sagittal craniosynostosis with dolichocephaly

DISCUSSION Craniosynostosis is categorized as either primary (predominantly idiopathic premature closure and less frequently those associated with syndromes) or secondary, representing those cases with specific causes of premature sutural closure such as intrauterine compression of the skull, metabolic derangements, teratogens, or lack of brain growth.

The normal time course of sutural closure is variable among individuals with the metopic suture closing in the first 2 years of life, starting at or soon after 6 months of age. Normal closure of other sutures is generally in mid to late adulthood. The sagittal, coronal, and lambdoid sutures typically close by 40 years of age, but the squamosal, occipitomastoid, and sphenotemporal sutures may remain partly open through age 70 years.[1]

Primary craniosynostosis usually involves a single suture. Patients typically develop normally with normal intelligence and are operated on only for cosmetic reasons, if at all. Multisuture synostoses are typically inherited, syndromic, or secondary. Overall, approximately 15% of primary cases of craniosynostosis are syndromic. Of the rest, 75% to 80% are simple single suture synostoses and 20% to 25% are multisuture synostoses. Bilateral coronal synostosis is seen more frequently than would normally be expected in siblings, even in the absence of known familial inheritance or an associated syndrome. Inherited and syndromic forms of craniosynostosis have a strong association with genetic anomalies in fibroblast growth factor receptor (FGFR) and related genes.

Patterns of sutural closure are associated with specifically named abnormalities in head shape. Sagittal synostosis is the most common craniosynostosis and presents with an elongated, thin skull called dolichocephaly or scaphocephaly. There is often ridging of the fused suture. Metopic synostosis presents with a prominent wedge-shaped forehead called trigonocephaly. Unilateral coronal synostosis presents with a flattened oblique ipsilateral frontal region called anterior plagiocephaly. Unilateral lambdoid synostosis presents with a flattened oblique ipsilateral parieto-occipital region called posterior plagiocephaly. Posterior plagiocephaly should be distinguished from positional plagiocephaly, which is unilateral occipital flattening without associated synostosis, typically due to prolonged supine positioning.[1-5]

Bilateral coronal synostosis results in a short skull in AP dimension called brachycephaly. Turricephaly, oxycephaly, and acrocephaly are variably used terms for multisuture synostoses with characteristic head shapes and often secondary symptoms from microcephaly. Kleeblattschädel or cloverleaf skull is caused by a combination of sagittal, coronal, and lambdoid synostoses and is strongly associated with severe neurologic impairment. Proptosis and bulging temporal regions are common.[1-5]

Treatment, when indicated, is surgical and usually performed in the first 3 months of life. Options include strip craniectomies, suturectomies, extensive or total calvarial remodeling, and endoscopic suturectomy, followed by molding helmets. If orbitofrontal advancement is indicated, surgery is typically delayed until around age 1 year.[6,7]

Questions for Further Thought

1. What are the most common syndromes and secondary causes associated with craniosynostosis and their major associated features?
2. How do you distinguish posterior plagiocephaly from positional plagiocephaly?

Reporting Responsibilities

- Identify sutures which have closed prematurely.
- Identify restriction of brain growth or compression of critical structures.

What the Treating Physician Needs to Know

- The treating physician should be made aware of associated anomalies of the face or brain that could suggest a syndrome or chromosomal anomaly, for example: temporal bone anomalies, HPE or other midline anomalies, small skull base, Chiari I malformation, and encephalocele.

- In cases of multisuture synostosis, evaluate for signs of increased intracranial pressure such as dilated venous sinuses and accessory signs including small jugular foramina or enlarged foramina for emissary veins. CT or MR venography may be helpful.

Answers

1. Syndromes include the following:
   - Sagittal synostosis: Crouzon syndrome (maxillary hypoplasia and shallow orbits)
   - Coronal or all-suture synostosis, frequently with syndactyly: Apert (syndactyly of fingers and toes); Pfeiffer (broad thumbs and great toes, and mild soft tissue syndactyly); Carpenter (severe developmental delay, brachydactyly, syndactyly, and thumb duplication); Saethre–Chotzen (TWIST gene mutation, syndactyly, beaked nose, short stature)

   Secondary causes include the following:
   - Metabolic and endocrine derangements such as hyperthyroidism, hypophosphatasia, and rickets
   - Bony dysplasias such as mucopolysaccharidosis and thanatophoric dysplasia
   - Teratogens such as hydantoin

2. Posterior plagiocephaly from early unilateral closure of a lambdoid suture causes ipsilateral occipital flattening, relative posterior position of the ipsilateral ear, and contralateral frontal bossing. Positional plagiocephaly is occipital flattening with normal open sutures, which tends to have relative anterior position of the ipsilateral ear and ipsilateral frontal bossing.

REFERENCES

1. Flores-Sarnat L. New insights into craniosynostosis. *Semin Pediatr Neurol.* 2002;9(4):274–291.
2. Barkovich AJ, Raybaud CA. Congenital malformations of the brain and skull. In: Barkovich AJ, Raybaud C, eds. *Pediatric Neuroimaging.* 5th ed. Philadelphia, PA: Lippincott Williams & Wilkins; 2012:367–568.
3. Benson ML, Oliverio PJ, Yue NC, et al. Primary craniosynostosis: Imaging features. *AJR Am J Roentgenol.* 1996;166(3):697–703.
4. Glass RB, Fernbach SK, Norton KI, et al. The infant skull: A vault of information. *Radiographics.* 2004;24(2):507–522.
5. Khanna PC, Thapa MM, Iyer RS, et al. Pictorial essay: The many faces of craniosynostosis. *Indian J Radiol Imaging.* 2011; 21(1):49–56.
6. Mehta VA, Bettegowda C, Jallo GI, et al. The evolution of surgical management for craniosynostosis. *Neurosurg Focus.* 2010; 29(6):E5.
7. Hankinson TC, Fontana EJ, Anderson RC, et al. Surgical treatment of single-suture craniosynostosis: An argument for quantitative methods to evaluate cosmetic outcomes. *J Neurosurg Pediatr.* 2010;6(2):193–197.

CLINICAL HISTORY *A 16-year-old male with history of seizures* (*Fig. 2.24A*)

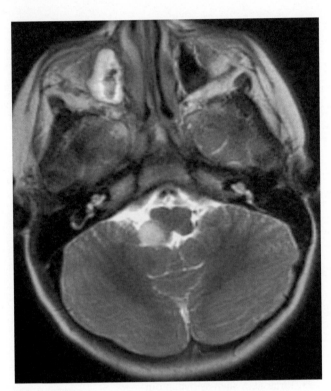

FIGURE **2.24A**

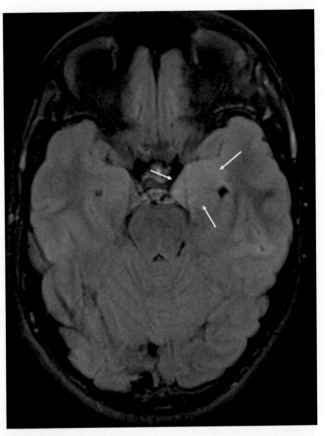

FIGURE **2.24B**

FINDINGS Axial T2-weighted (**A**) brain MRI image demonstrates a focal homogeneous T2-hyperintense mass arising from the right aspect of the dorsal medulla. Axial FLAIR (**B**) image in a different patient demonstrates a subtle FLAIR-hyperintense left medial temporal signal abnormality (*arrows*) with mass effect on the suprasellar cistern and an ill-defined loss of the gray–white interface in this area. Both lesions were T1 hypointense and neither demonstrated enhancement on postcontrast T1-weighted sequences (not shown).

DIFFERENTIAL DIAGNOSIS Low-grade glioma, anaplastic astrocytoma (Fig. 2.24A); low-grade glioma, cortical dysplasia, cerebritis, herpes encephalitis (Fig. 2.24**B**)

DIAGNOSIS Low-grade glioma

DISCUSSION Low-grade gliomas are more common in children than in adults. Appearance by MRI is typically that of a focal or diffuse nonenhancing white matter mass. On T1-weighted, T2-weighted, and FLAIR imaging, the mass usually appears homogeneous, with T1 hypointensity and T2/FLAIR hyperintensity that often appears ill-defined and may expand white matter and overlying cortex, with blurring of the gray–white interface. Hemorrhage, surrounding edema, calcification, and cystic degeneration are uncommon. The mass does not usually enhance or show restriction on diffusion imaging. Enhancement, if present, is usually mild. Often cortically based, the mass may be located in any part of supra- or infratentorial brain.

With the exception of the pontine glioma, most pediatric infratentorial gliomas are histologically low grade. Unfortunately, most brainstem gliomas arise in the pons, and these are usually high-grade infiltrative astrocytomas. Exophytic brainstem lesions, as in the presented case, tend to have a better prognosis. Pathologically, low-grade gliomas are WHO grade I (pilocytic) or grade II (fibrillary) astrocytomas.

DIFFERENTIAL DIAGNOSTIC CONSIDERATIONS

Anaplastic astrocytoma: As these are high-grade tumors, they typically appear infiltrative. Perfusion MRI has been used to differentiate anaplastic astrocytomas, which generally have increased vascularity, as compared to low-grade gliomas.[1,2]

Cortical dysplasia: This entity can often be indistinguishable from low-grade gliomas as they can appear similar on T2 and FLAIR sequences with an ill-defined blurring of the gray–white interface. Both low-grade glioma and cortical dysplasia may show stability in size with serial imaging but cortical dysplasia tends not to have mass effect.

Cerebritis: This is usually seen as an ill-defined area of signal abnormality that may enhance, may show restriction on diffusion imaging, and typically is seen in the setting of a constitutionally sick patient with neurologic findings.

Herpes encephalitis: This entity should be considered in the differential for low-grade gliomas if the abnormality is in the medial temporal lobe. Usually, there is a larger area of signal abnormality that may enhance.

Questions for Further Thought

1. What is a common clinical presentation in patients with low-grade glioma?
2. What is a common syndrome associated with low-grade gliomas in the pediatric population?

Reporting Responsibilities

Whether imaging findings are consistent with a low-grade neoplasm. Other differential possibilities. Any changes on serial imaging.

What the Treating Physician Needs to Know

Whether imaging findings are consistent with a low-grade neoplasm or is there a likely differential diagnosis. Any change in size and enhancement characteristics on serial imaging.

Answers

1. Seizures.
2. NF1.

REFERENCES

1. Hakyemez B, Erdogan C, Ercan I, et al. High-grade and low-grade gliomas: Differentiation by using perfusion MR imaging. *Clin Radiol.* 2005;60(4):493–502.
2. Knopp EA, Cha S, Johnson G, et al. Glial neoplasms: Dynamic contrast-enhanced T2*-weighted MR imaging. *Radiology.* 1999; 211(3):791–798.

Paritosh C. Khanna

CASE 2.25

CLINICAL HISTORY *A 10-month-old male with development of macrocephaly (head circumference greater than 95th percentile)*

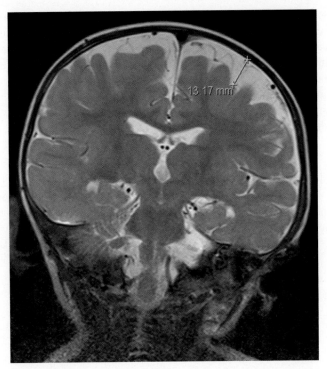

13.17 mm

FIGURE 2.25

FINDINGS Coronal T2-weighted MRI image of the brain shows bifrontal extra-axial space prominence that measures up to 13 mm on the left. The extra-axial spaces demonstrate vascular structures traversing them, suggesting that they represent the subarachnoid space. Underlying brain parenchyma appears normal. Myelination pattern was age appropriate.

DIFFERENTIAL DIAGNOSIS Benign macrocephaly of infancy, global cerebral atrophy, acquired extraventricular obstructive hydrocephalus, nonaccidental trauma

DIAGNOSIS Benign macrocephaly of infancy

DISCUSSION Benign macrocephaly of infancy is also known as external hydrocephalus, benign external hydrocephalus, or physiologic subarachnoid space enlargement. This entity is typically noted between ages of 3 and 8 months as patients present with a rapid increase in head circumference. A positive family history for this entity may be present. On imaging, prominent extra-axial spaces (over 4 to 5 mm in craniocortical dimension in the neonate) with traversing vessels, in the bifrontal or anterior interhemispheric regions,

is the main finding. Slight prominence of ventricles may also be seen. This entity is typically self-limited and usually resolves by age 2 years. A common theory for benign macrocephaly of infancy is that this is due to immature arachnoid villi, with CSF absorption by the arachnoid villi unable to keep up with CSF production.[1,2]

DIFFERENTIAL DIAGNOSTIC CONSIDERATIONS

Global cerebral atrophy: Paucity of white matter with enlarged ventricles, cisterns, sulci, and subarachnoid spaces.

Acquired extraventricular obstructive hydrocephalus: Prominent subarachnoid spaces secondary to arachnoid granulation obstruction from hemorrhage, exudate, or subarachnoid metastatic deposits.

Nonaccidental trauma: Enlarged subdural spaces with blood product of varying ages.

Questions for Further Thought

1. How is a subdural collection differentiated from a prominent subarachnoid space on MR?

2. How is volume loss or atrophy differentiated from benign macrocephaly of infancy?

Reporting Responsibilities

Whether there is enlargement of subarachnoid or subdural spaces and the MRI signal intensities of these spaces. Also note should be made of age appropriateness of myelination.

What the Treating Physician Needs to Know

Other conditions leading to prominent extra-axial fluid spaces, such as subdural hematomas from nonaccidental trauma.

Answers

1. With a subdural collection, blood vessels are typically noted to be flattened against the cortical surface. If the subdural collection is large, there may be flattening of the cortex. If proteinaceous or hemorrhagic, there may be T1 bright (hemorrhage, protein) and/or gradient dark (subacute or chronic blood product) signal.[3]

2. Findings suggestive of volume loss or atrophy include prominent ventricles, cisterns, and sulci in addition to enlarged subarachnoid spaces. There may also be white matter paucity, delayed myelination, or other underlying cause(s) identified within the parenchyma.

REFERENCES

1. Prassopoulos P, Cavouras D, Golfinopoulos S, et al. The size of the intra- and extraventricular cerebrospinal fluid compartments in children with idiopathic benign widening of the frontal subarachnoid space. *Neuroradiology.* 1995;37(5):418–421.

2. Zahl SM, Egge A, Helseth E, et al. Benign external hydrocephalus: A review, with emphasis on management. *Neurosurg Rev.* 2011;34:417–432.

3. Wilms G, Vanderschueren G, Demaerel PH, et al. CT and MR in infants with pericerebral collections and macrocephaly: Benign enlargement of the subarachnoid spaces versus subdural collections. *AJNR Am J Neuroradiol.* 1993;14(4):855–860.

CASE 2.26

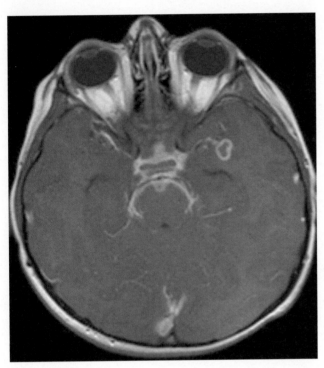

FIGURE **2.26A**

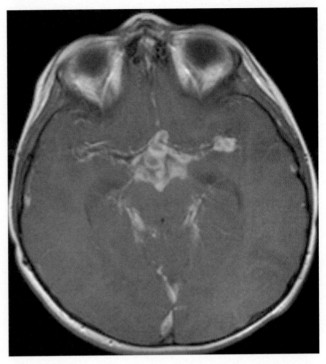

FIGURE **2.26B**

FINDINGS Consecutive axial contrast-enhanced T1-weighted MR images through the brain (**A** and **B**) demonstrate irregular contrast enhancement in the suprasellar and perimesencephalic cisterns. There were also several ring-enhancing areas, most conspicuous in the left medial temporal lobe, with mild parenchymal vasogenic edema on T2-weighted and FLAIR imaging (not shown).

DIFFERENTIAL DIAGNOSIS Tuberculous (TB) meningitis with tuberculoma, pyogenic meningitis with abscess, ring-enhancing temporal neoplasm with drop metastases, neurocysticercosis (NCC), neurosarcoid

DIAGNOSIS TB meningitis with tuberculoma

DISCUSSION Cranial tuberculosis is caused by the bacterium *Mycobacterium tuberculosis*. In the pediatric population, CNS involvement generally accompanies hematogenous spread from primary pulmonary tuberculosis. Dissemination can be widespread, including spine involvement (Pott disease) which may result in vertebral, and later, disc destruction. There may be associated epidural, prevertebral, and paravertebral (such as psoas) abscesses. Intracranial

TB infection manifests mainly as basilar meningitis with or without associated parenchymal lesions or tuberculomas. Tuberculomas may uncommonly present as extra-axial lesions, mimicking neoplastic masses.[1] Early MRI and CT may be normal. Non-contrast CT may demonstrate iso- to hyperdense exudate that appears to efface CSF spaces. Basilar meningitis is seen as enhancing thick, irregular exudate in the basal cisterns on contrast-enhanced CT or MRI, the latter being more sensitive. FLAIR sequence demonstrates hyperintense exudate within CSF spaces. Focal tuberculomas may be ring or solidly enhancing, solitary or multiple, with mild-to-moderate surrounding vasogenic edema, and may be diffusion restricted. Incidence of TB has increased in recent times due to immune compromise from HIV/AIDS. Imaging manifestations tend to be more florid in immunocompromised patients. Patients with TB meningitis may present with meningismus, seizures, neurologic deficits, and coma.[2]

DIFFERENTIAL DIAGNOSTIC CONSIDERATIONS

Pyogenic meningitis with abscess: Not generally localized to the basal cisterns. Pyogenic abscess can be indistinguishable, but the patient is generally more acutely sick.

Ring-enhancing temporal neoplasm with subarachnoid spread of leptomeningeal metastases: MRI would typically demonstrate mass effect, nodular tumor enhancement, and edema. Clinical presentation is useful in differentiating this entity from TB meningitis with tuberculoma.

NCC: Rarely causes meningitis; look for the central dot sign in the vesicular phase of the parenchymal form.

Neurosarcoid: Infrequent in the pediatric age group.

Questions for Further Thought

1. What potential complication of arteries may occur in patients with TB meningitis?
2. What are other complications of TB meningitis?

Reporting Responsibilities

Extent of involvement of cisterns and parenchyma, and complications such as hydrocephalus.

What the Treating Physician Needs to Know

Diagnosis, complications, and response to treatment.

Answers

1. The thick TB exudate in the basal cisterns can result in a vasculitis with resultant irregularity and narrowing of major arteries of the circle of Willis. This can potentially result in stroke.

2. Other complications include hydrocephalus, ventriculitis, and choroid plexitis.

REFERENCES

1. Khanna PC, Godinho S, Patkar DP, et al. MR spectroscopy-aided differentiation: "giant" extra-axial tuberculoma masquerading as meningioma. *AJNR Am J Neuroradiol.* 2006;27(7): 1438–1440.

2. Seth R, Sharma U. Diagnostic criteria for tuberculous meningitis. *Indian J Pediatr.* 2002;69(4):299–303.

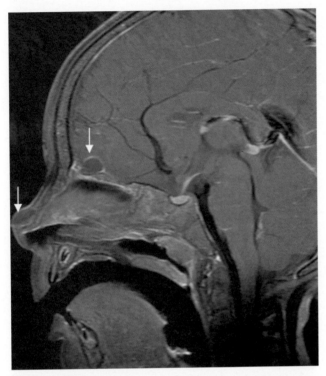

FIGURE **2.27A**

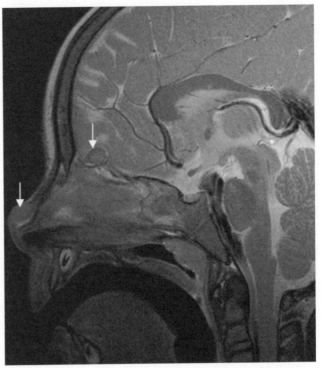

FIGURE **2.27B**

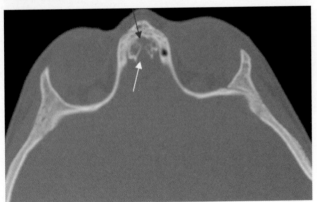

FIGURE **2.27C**

(**C**) demonstrates a "split" or "bifid" crista galli posteriorly (*white arrow*) and a large foramen cecum anteriorly (*black arrow*).

DIFFERENTIAL DIAGNOSIS Nasal and intracranial dermoids, nasofrontal cephalocele, nasal glioma, non-ossified midline anterior skull base structures

DIAGNOSIS Nasal and intracranial dermoids, presumably connected by a nasal dermal sinus (not identified on this examination)

DISCUSSION During normal embryonic development, a dural stalk herniates through the anterior neuropore through the region of the future foramen cecum into the nasofrontal region and then regresses spontaneously. Neuroectoderm may abnormally migrate along this stalk and persist resulting in a dermoid (fat, epithelium, keratin, skin appendages), epidermoid (desquamated epithelium), and/or nasal dermal sinus. Nasal dermoid, dermal sinus, and epidermoids are classified as type 1 anterior neuropore anomalies that result from failure of neuropore involution during the first month

FINDINGS Sagittal T1-weighted postcontrast fat-suppressed (**A**) and T2-weighted (**B**) MRI images demonstrate midline, well-circumscribed T1 fat-suppressed hypointense and T2-isointense masses at the nasal tip and in the midline of the anterior cranial fossa (*arrows*). Sagittal T1 non-fat-suppressed images (not shown) demonstrated hyperintense signal within these masses. Axial CT bone window image

of gestation. A minority of patients have an intracranial component. When present, the foramen cecum is usually enlarged, and the crista galli bifid—both indirect signs that are well visualized on CT with bone window. MR demonstrates one or more well-circumscribed lesions from the nasal tip to the crista galli apex that may either be hyperintense (dermoid) or hypointense (dermoid or epidermoid) on T1-weighted imaging. Care should be taken not to confuse this with fat that is normally present in the crista galli. The dermal sinus, even when present, may be difficult to visualize by MR and thin-section imaging may be helpful in this regard. As occurs with intracranial epidermoids, nasal epidermoids may also show diffusion restriction and this feature helps differentiate them from dermoids.[1,2]

DIFFERENTIAL DIAGNOSTIC CONSIDERATIONS

Nasofrontal cephalocele (type 2 anterior neuropore anomaly): Leptomeninges and/or brain tissue herniates through foramen cecum resulting in a large defect in cribriform plate.

Nasal glioma (type 3 anterior neuropore anomaly): Solid glial mass that appears separate from brain herniates through foramen cecum and resides within the nasal bridge, nasal cavity, or nasal septum.

Non-ossified midline anterior skull base structures: See Answer 2 for timing of ossification.

Questions for Further Thought

1. How do patients with nasal dermoid present?
2. What is an important caveat regarding timing of imaging?

Reporting Responsibilities

- Report presence of intracranial component and dermal sinus.
- Report any evidence of infection with contrast administration.

What the Treating Physician Needs to Know

Presence of intracranial component and dermal sinus. Any signs of infection such as meningitis.

Answers

1. Nasoglabellar mass, nasal pit with or without sebaceous discharge, craniofacial anomalies including broadening of nasal root and bridge, and rarely, meningitis.
2. The anterior skull base structures such as the crista galli, cribriform plate, and osseous structures around the foramen cecum ossify between 9 and 12 months of age. The foramen cecum normally completely closes by 5 years of age. In the young patient the lack of ossification can make it difficult to exclude abnormality by CT alone, and MRI is frequently necessary for complete evaluation of this region.

REFERENCES

1. Hedlund G. Congenital frontonasal masses: Developmental anatomy, malformations, and MR imaging. *Pediatr Radiol.* 2006; 36(7):647–662.
2. Huisman TA, Schneider JF, Kellenberger CJ, et al. Developmental nasal midline masses in children: neuroradiological evaluation. *Eur Radiol.* 2004;14(2):243–249.

CLINICAL HISTORY *An 11-year-old child with severe headache*

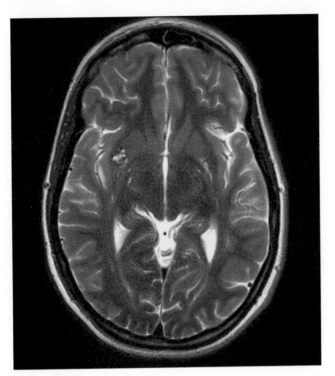

FIGURE 2.28A

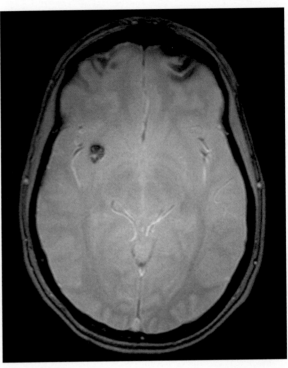

FIGURE 2.28B

FINDINGS Axial T2-weighted fast spin-echo (FSE) MRI image (**A**) demonstrates a cluster of punctate high-T2-signal foci surrounded by a rim of slightly low T2 signal centered in right putamen. Incidental note is made of some other tiny foci of high T2 signal about lateral aspects of anterior commissure, typical for normal perivascular spaces. T2-weighted GRE image (**B**) at the same level of **A** shows blooming (dark signal) of the lesion in right putamen, suggesting blood product.

DIFFERENTIAL DIAGNOSIS Cavernous malformation (cavernoma), hemorrhagic tumor, hematoma

DIAGNOSIS Cavernous malformation (cavernoma)

DISCUSSION The cerebral cavernous malformation (cavernoma) is composed of sinusoidal vascular channels lined by a layer of endothelium and separated by a collagen matrix devoid of elastin, smooth muscle, or other vascular wall elements, and without intervening brain parenchyma.[1,2] Intralesional hemorrhage is not uncommon, best diagnosed on

MRI where typically mixed-age blood products (methemoglobin and hemosiderin) lead to a "popcorn"-like appearance of both T2 hyper- and hypointensity.[2,3] Lesions are low-flow vascular malformations, and consequently do not typically require urgent management. However, rarely, significant acute hemorrhage occurs. Lesions are occult on conventional angiography, and MRI is typically diagnostic. Cavernous malformations may be either sporadic (usually a solitary lesion) or familial, with familial typically having multiple lesions. Evidence suggests the sporadic type is more likely associated with developmental venous anomalies (DVAs).[1]

Questions for Further Thought

1. What is the significance of the association with DVAs?
2. What is the significance of familial etiology?

Reporting Responsibilities

- Uncomplicated cavernous malformation does not represent an urgent or emergent finding. However, as with any new positive finding, direct communication with the referring physician is appreciated.

- It is important to evaluate for multiple lesions as this suggests a familial/hereditary form. A sequence with magnetic susceptibility sensitivity, such as a T2* GRE sequence or susceptibility-weighted imaging (SWI) should be performed as this will increase the sensitivity for lesion detection.

What the Treating Physician Needs to Know

- Lesions may be symptomatic; typical symptoms include seizures, headache, or focal neurologic deficit.
- Clinical course is not consistent. Lesions may enlarge, regress, or remain unchanged over many years. Patients with familial cavernous malformations may develop new lesions over time.

Answers

1. DVAs provide a pathway of normal venous drainage. If the choice is made to surgically resect a cavernous malformation in a patient who also has a DVA, care must be taken to preserve the venous drainage and avoid venous infarction.
2. If familial, the inheritance is autosomal dominant; imaging of possibly affected family members should be considered. Additionally, patients with familial cavernous malformations are more frequently symptomatic than those with sporadic lesions.

REFERENCES

1. Petersen TA, Morrison LA, Schrader RM, et al. Familial versus sporadic cavernous malformations: Differences in developmental venous anomaly association and lesion phenotype. *AJNR Am J Neuroradiol.* 2010;31(2):377–382.
2. Rivera PP, Willinsky RA, Porter PJ. Intracranial cavernous malformations. *Neuroimaging Clin N Am.* 2003;13(1):27–40.
3. de Souza JM, Domingues RC, Cruz LC Jr, et al. Susceptibility-weighted imaging for the evaluation of patients with familial cerebral cavernous malformations: A comparison with T2 weighted fast spin-echo and gradient-echo sequences. *AJNR Am J Neuroradiol.* 2008;29(1):154–158.

CLINICAL HISTORY *A 1-year-old child presents with macrocephaly and intractable epilepsy*

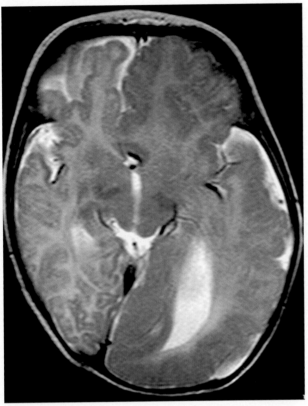

FIGURE 2.29A

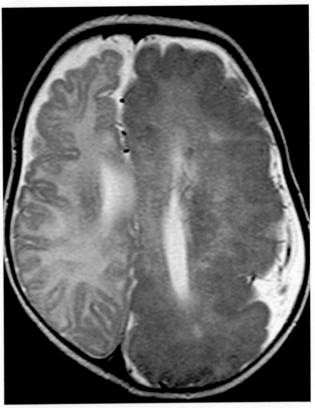

FIGURE 2.29B

FINDINGS Axial T2-weighted MRI images at the levels of midbrain (**A**) and centrum semiovale (**B**) show enlarged left cerebral hemisphere, thickened and abnormal cortex, dilation and straightening of the left lateral ventricle, and herniation of the cortex toward the right. The white matter in the left cerebral hemisphere is darker than the right, and on these T2-weighted images in a patient with incomplete myelination, this suggests accelerated myelination (as more immature white matter would have increased water content, resulting in increased, or less dark T2 signal). There is sharp definition between the cortex and white matter on the right, but blurring of this transition on the left, especially in the parietal lobe.

DIFFERENTIAL DIAGNOSIS Hemimegalencephaly, focal cortical dysplasia, pachygyria, gliomatosis cerebri, right cerebral infarct

DIAGNOSIS Hemimegalencephaly

DISCUSSION Hemimegalencephaly is a congenital disorder consisting of hamartomatous overgrowth of part or all of a cerebral hemisphere with abnormal neuronal migration. The etiology remains uncertain, and there is no known familial inheritance. There are three types of hemimegalencephaly.

The first is the isolated or sporadic form, affecting the cerebral hemisphere without associated systemic or posterior fossa involvement. The second type involves the ipsilateral brain stem or cerebellum (termed total hemimegalencephaly). The third type is a syndromic form where it is associated with other diseases including hypomelanosis of Ito, Klippel–Trenaunay–Weber syndrome, tuberous sclerosis (TS), NF1, Proteus syndrome, and epidermal nevus syndrome. Clinical presentation of hemimegalencephaly is often macrocephaly detected at birth with seizures typically beginning within the first year of life which eventually become intractable. Developmental delay and intellectual impairment are common.

On neuroimaging, the affected hemisphere is enlarged with a thickened abnormal cortex and dilation of the ipsilateral lateral ventricle with straightening of the frontal horn. There is often midline shift due to the enlarged hemisphere bulging across the midline. Ipsilateral cortical abnormalities such as polymicrogyria, pachygyria, or agyria and abnormal white matter myelination (generally hypermyelination) are often present. Blurring of the gray–white interface is common due to dysplastic neurons. Dystrophic calcification may be present. Contralateral cortical malformations can also occur.

A very important imaging feature is that hemimegalencephaly causes both cortical and ipsilateral ventricular enlargement. This finding is of key importance as this entity is often misdiagnosed as contralateral infarct, especially on CT. However, following infarct, it is the ventricle on the affected side that may enlarge and the cortex should be thinned. Histologically, there is no difference between focal cortical dysplasia and hemimegalencephaly. However, macroscopically, hemimegalencephaly typically involves much or all of a cerebral hemisphere with overgrowth, whereas focal cortical dysplasia is a much more limited entity.

Seizure control is the principal goal of therapy, but patients with hemimegalencephaly are often refractory to multiple antiepileptic medications. Anatomic or functional hemispherectomy is a mode of treatment offered to improve quality of life.

Question for Further Thought

1. What is the role of advanced neuroimaging techniques in hemimegalencephaly?

Reporting Responsibilities

Describe if there is unilateral, total, or syndromic hemimegalencephaly. Describe associated abnormalities of cortex and white matter. Describe any abnormalities, if present, in the contralateral hemisphere.

What the Treating Physician Needs to Know

Hemispherectomy is one treatment option that can help control intractable seizures, but this can only be undertaken if the contralateral hemisphere is normal. Careful scrutiny is required as the patient's epilepsy could continue if preoperative imaging and clinical assessment misses a contralateral cortical malformation.

Answer

1. Ictal 18F-fluorodeoxyglucose positron emission tomography ([18]FDG-PET) and MR perfusion have found hypermetabolism and hypervascularity within the involved hemisphere. Diffusion tensor imaging (DTI) can show completely disorganized axonal fibers that lack the normal perpendicular orientation to the lateral ventricles and hypermyelination. Advanced imaging techniques can also be very helpful in assessing for abnormality of the contralateral hemisphere which can appear morphologically normal.

REFERENCES

1. Barkovich AJ, Chuang SH. Unilateral megalencephaly: Correlation of MR imaging and pathologic characteristics. *AJNR Am J Neuroradiol.* 1990;11(3):523–531.
2. Sato N, Yagishita A, Oba H, et al. Hemimegalencephaly: A study of abnormalities occurring outside the involved hemisphere. *AJNR Am J Neuroradiol.* 2007;28(4):678–682.
3. Sasaki M, Hashimoto T, Furushima W, et al. Clinical aspects of hemimegalencephaly by means of a nationwide survey. *J Child Neurol.* 2005;20(4):337–341.
4. Hoffmann KT, Amthauer H, Liebig T, et al. MRI and 18F-fluorodeoxyglucose positron emission tomography in hemimegalencephaly. *Neuroradiology.* 2000;42(10):749–752.

CASE 2.30

CLINICAL HISTORY *A 5-year-old boy who presents with growth hormone deficiency and decreased visual acuity*

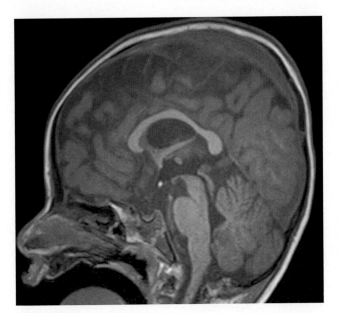

FIGURE **2.30A**

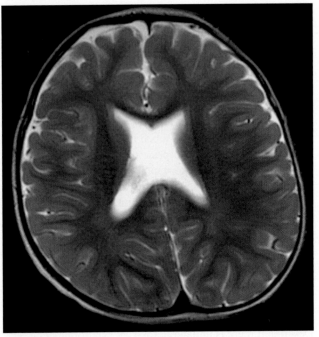

FIGURE **2.30B**

FINDINGS Sagittal T1-weighted MRI image (**A**) demonstrates an ectopic posterior pituitary gland. The normal "bright spot" of the posterior pituitary gland within the sella is lacking and is seen at the median eminence. The optic chiasm is also hypoplastic with small appearing anterior pituitary gland. Axial T2-weighted image (**B**) shows absence of the normal midline septum pellucidum between the lateral ventricles.

DIFFERENTIAL DIAGNOSIS SOD with ectopic posterior pituitary gland, isolated absence of the septum pellucidum, schizencephaly, lobar HPE

DIAGNOSIS SOD with ectopic posterior pituitary gland

DISCUSSION Originally described in a report by de Morsier in 1956, SOD entails absence of the septum pellucidum and hypoplasia of the optic nerves. In 1970, Hoyt described the pituitary dysfunction seen in up to two-thirds of patients with SOD (most often short stature due to decreased growth hormone and thyroid-stimulating hormone (TSH)). SOD is now considered as a heterogeneous disorder with maldevelopment of the midline prosencephalon including abnormality of the hypothalamic–pituitary axis, optic nerves, olfactory bulb, corpus callosum, and septum pellucidum, and sporadically associated with other malformations of cortical development. Schizencephaly or polymicrogyria are present in 30% to 40% of patients with SOD. Due to these numerous associations, some prefer the term SOD complex for this entity. SOD is also considered by some to be a milder form of lobar HPE. In patients with SOD but without schizencephaly, pituitary–hypothalamic dysfunction and visual symptoms such as nystagmus or diminished vision are commonly seen. In patients who also have schizencephaly or polymicrogyria, endocrine function is usually normal and seizures are often the presenting feature.

On neuroimaging of SOD, there is absence of the septum pellucidum resulting in a squared appearance of the frontal horns of the lateral ventricles with a flat roof. The fornices are low lying causing inferior pointing of the ventricles in the coronal plane. Optic nerve hypoplasia is not always perceptible on neuroimaging. Pituitary abnormalities may include a thin stalk, ectopic posterior pituitary, and a small anterior pituitary. The diagnosis is often established with a combination of fundoscopic exam demonstrating small optic discs, and neuroimaging showing absence of the septum pellucidum or other associated midline defects. Most clinicians make this diagnosis when two of the following three findings are present: optic nerve hypoplasia, absent septum pellucidum, and pituitary dysfunction.

Question for Further Thought

1. What syndrome is associated with olfactory nerve hypoplasia or aplasia and pituitary dysfunction?

Reporting Responsibilities

Isolated absence of the septum pellucidum is rare. Look for other congenital abnormalities such as schizencephaly, ectopic pituitary, optic nerve hypoplasia, encephalocele, HPE, and callosal dysgenesis/agenesis.

What the Treating Physician Needs to Know

Optic nerve hypoplasia may not be easily detected on neuroimaging. Ophthalmologic examination is crucial as this can detect optic disc atrophy and thereby help to confirm the imaging suspicion of SOD.

Answer

1. Kallmann syndrome (hypothalamic hypogonadism), a genetic syndrome typically associated with hyposmia or anosmia, and hypogonadism.

REFERENCES

1. Barkovich AJ, Fram EK, Norman D. Septo-optic dysplasia: MR imaging. *Radiology.* 1989;171(1):189–192.
2. Barkovich AJ, Raybaud CA. Congenital malformations of the brain and skull. In: Barkovich AJ, Raybaud C, eds. *Pediatric Neuroimaging.* 5th ed. Philadelphia, PA: Lippincott Williams & Wilkins; 2012:367–568.
3. Webb EA, Dattani MT. Septo-optic dysplasia. *Eur J Hum Genet.* 2010;18(4):393–397.

CASE 2.31

CLINICAL HISTORY *A 4-year-old child presents with lethargy, vomiting, and increasing headaches*

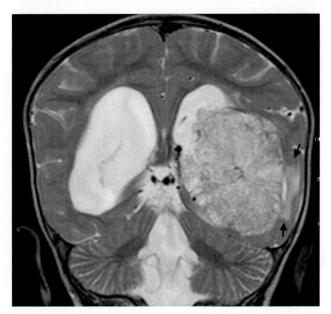

FIGURE **2.31A**

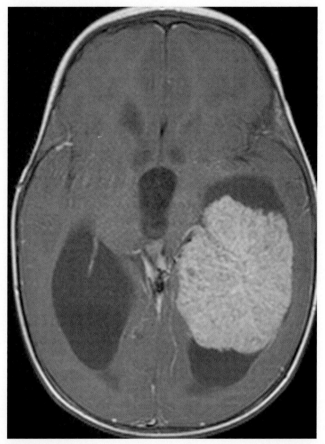

FIGURE **2.31B**

FINDINGS Coronal T2-weighted MRI image (**A**) demonstrates a large hyperintense mass in the left lateral ventricle with a microlobulated border with surrounding hydrocephalus. Some adjacent flow voids represent enlarged draining veins. Also note increased signal representing edema (*arrows*) in the adjacent white matter. Axial postcontrast T1-weighted image (**B**) demonstrates intense enhancement of the mass in trigone of left lateral ventricle with hydrocephalus.

DIFFERENTIAL DIAGNOSIS CPC, choroid plexus papilloma (CPP), villous hypertrophy of the choroid plexus

DIAGNOSIS CPC

DISCUSSION Choroid plexus tumors are uncommon neoplasms typically classified as CPP, which is a WHO grade I tumor, and CPC, which is a WHO grade III tumor. Recently, "atypical CPP" has been described which is categorized as a WHO grade II tumor.

Constituting less than 4% to 5% of pediatric supratentorial tumors, CPP and CPC are most often found within the first few years of life. CPC tends to occur slightly later than CPP and without the male predominance seen with CPP. Both tumors present with hydrocephalus, nausea, and vomiting. Neurologic deficits at presentation are more likely to be seen with CPC. CPPs have been associated with von Hippel–Lindau syndrome.

Choroid plexus tumors can arise anywhere from the epithelium of the choroid plexus, but there is a strong age–location relationship. They most frequently arise from the atrium of the lateral ventricle in children with left lateral ventricle more commonly involved than the right. While uncommon in adults, they usually tend to arise from the fourth ventricle or cerebellopontine angle.

On MRI, choroid plexus tumors appear as a large intensely enhancing intraventricular cauliflower-like mass, which is usually iso- to hypointense on T1-weighted imaging, and iso- to hyperintense to gray matter on T2-weighted imaging. The tumor is usually associated with hydrocephalus and may contain foci of calcification and hemorrhage. Hydrocephalus associated with these tumors is not fully understood. Theories include overproduction of CSF by the tumor itself as well as blockage of CSF drainage pathways by the tumor mass or hemorrhage. Given the propensity to spread in the CSF, contrast MRI of the spine is needed preoperatively to exclude drop metastases.

It is difficult with imaging to differentiate between CPC and CPP, and the final diagnosis is usually histologic.

Features favoring CPC are ependymal invasion into the brain parenchyma with surrounding vasogenic edema and CSF metastases. CPC tends to have a more heterogeneous appearance, often with areas of more cystic change or hemorrhage causing mixed signal on T1 and T2 imaging.

The distinction between CPP and CPC is important, as the prognosis is usually poor for CPC, with a 5-year survival rate ranging from approximately 26% to 40%, which is highly dependent on the success of surgical resection, with higher survival in cases of complete resection.

Question for Further Thought

1. What is villous hypertrophy of the choroid plexus?

Relevant Anatomy

Choroid plexus tumors generally arise in regions containing choroid plexus, including atria of lateral ventricles, third and fourth ventricles, and cerebellopontine angle (rare). These tumors can rarely be seen in a suprasellar or intraparenchymal location.

Reporting Responsibilities

Due to the hydrocephalus associated with these tumors, ensure there is no herniation or trapped ventricle. The entire neural axis should be imaged and assessed for metastatic spread.

What the Treating Physician Needs to Know

While the differentiation between CPP and CPC ultimately depends on histologic analysis, preoperative imaging diagnosis can help in surgical planning. Imaging the entire neural axis is recommended to assess for possibility of drop metastases.

Answer

1. Villous hypertrophy of the choroid plexus is diffuse, usually bilateral enlargement of the choroid plexus that typically presents with symptomatic hydrocephalus. Both villous hypertrophy and CPP are considered as points along a disease continuum.

REFERENCES

1. Wagle V, Melanson D, Ethier R, et al. Choroid plexus papilloma: Magnetic resonance, computed tomography, and angiographic observations. *Surg Neurol.* 1987;27(5):466–468.
2. Jeibmann A, Hasselblatt M, Gerss J, et al. Prognostic implications of atypical histologic features in choroid plexus papilloma. *J Neuropathol Exp Neurol.* 2006;65(11):1069–1073.

CASE 2.32

CLINICAL HISTORY *A 4-year-old child presents with intractable epilepsy*

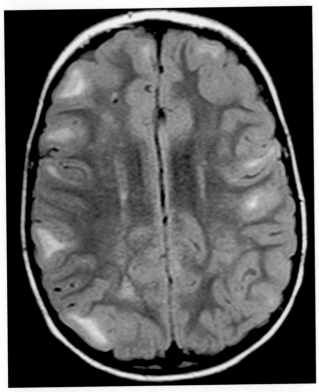

FIGURE **2.32A**

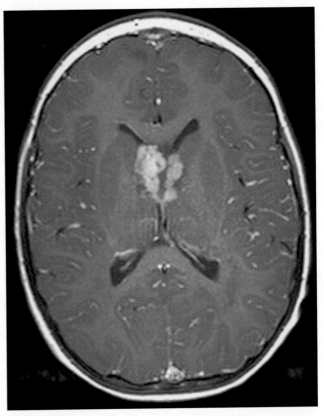

FIGURE **2.32B**

FINDINGS Axial FLAIR MRI image (**A**) shows multiple subcortical hyperintense foci in both cerebral hemispheres. Postcontrast axial T1-weighted image (**B**) shows enhancing masses in the region of foramina of Monro, right larger than left.

DIFFERENTIAL DIAGNOSIS Tuberous sclerosis complex (TSC), focal cortical dysplasia, neoplasm

DIAGNOSIS TSC

DISCUSSION TSC is an autosomal dominant neurocutaneous syndrome caused by a mutation of the *TSC1* (encodes for the protein hamartin) or *TSC2* (encodes for the protein tuberin) suppressor genes. Although a classical clinical triad of epilepsy, mental retardation, and adenoma sebaceum (facial angiofibromas) has been described, TSC can involve multiple organ systems. A combination of major and minor features (for example, subependymal nodules (SENs), cardiac rhabdomyoma, and renal angiomyolipoma are major features) is used to make a definitive diagnosis. About 50% of patients have mental retardation and 75% of patients with TSC have epilepsy. More than 95% of patients have neuroimaging abnormalities, which include cortical hamartomas (tubers) (the abnormalities described in **A**), SENs,

subependymal giant cell astrocytoma (SGCA) (the abnormalities described in **B**), and white matter abnormalities. Changes can be seen on ultrasound and CT, but MRI is the preferred imaging modality.

Cortical hamartomas (tubers) are usually multiple and supratentorial, though 10% to 15% of patients have infratentorial involvement. On CT, they are hypoattenuating and 50% eventually calcify. On MRI, the signal depends on the patient's age and degree of myelination. In neonates, tubers demonstrate T1 hyperintensity compared to the unmyelinated white matter and are hypointense on T2. As patients age, the lesions become iso- to hypointense on T1 and hyperintense on T2/FLAIR. A small portion (5%) will enhance with contrast, and this does not imply malignant degeneration.

SENs are nodular foci usually found along the walls of the lateral ventricles. They rarely calcify in the first year of life, but calcifications increase with increasing patient age and are easily seen on CT. SENs in infants demonstrate T1 hyperintensity and T2 hypointensity and can be confused with subependymal hemorrhages. Older children with myelin maturation show both T1 and T2 iso- or hypointensity. About half of these lesions demonstrate contrast enhancement, which does not have clinical significance.

SGCA is a WHO grade I tumor usually found near the foramen of Monro, seen in 10% to 15% of patients. MRI signal characteristics of SGCA are similar to SENs, and they demonstrate contrast enhancement. They are differentiated from SENs by location, size (>12 mm), and interval enlargement. Progressive interval enlargement rather than absolute size is the most important criteria to differentiate an SEN from SGCA at the foramen of Monro. Due to their location, they can cause ventricular obstruction, necessitating earlier intervention in these patients.

A range of white matter abnormalities can be seen on MRI in TSC. White matter abnormalities can range from hypomyelination to dysplastic, gliotic, or disorganized white matter usually appearing as fine lines extending radially from cortical tubers across the entire white matter.

Advanced neuroimaging techniques are being employed to determine which tuber is the most likely epileptogenic source, and hence can be resected to provide optimal cure from seizures. These techniques include DTI, PET, and magnetoencephalography (MEG).

Questions for Further Thought

1. What is the most important MRI sequence for evaluation of TSC in neonates and young infants?
2. How can one differentiate an SEN from subependymal heterotopia?

Reporting Responsibilities

- In patients with SGCA, follow-up imaging is obtained to assess for increase in size and possible development of obstructing hydrocephalus.

- Cortical hamartomas (tubers) and SENs may demonstrate enhancement, but the presence or absence of enhancement has no clinical significance.

What the Treating Physician Needs to Know

Oral rapamycin therapy is now used to induce regression of astrocytomas associated with TSC and offers an excellent alternative to resecting SGCA, thereby preventing operative morbidity.

Answers

1. In the neonate and young infant, the cortical tubers and SENs are hyperintense on T1-weighted imaging. A volumetric T1-weighted 3D gradient sequence is well suited for this evaluation.
2. Subependymal heterotopia will lack calcification and contrast enhancement and is isointense to gray matter on all sequences.

REFERENCES

1. Vezina G, Barkovich AJ. The Phakomatoses. In: Barkovich AJ, Raybaud C, eds. *Pediatric Neuroimaging.* 5th ed. Philadelphia, PA: Lippincott Williams & Wilkins; 2012:569–636.
2. Baskin HJ Jr. The pathogenesis and imaging of the tuberous sclerosis complex. *Pediatr Radiol.* 2008;38(9):936–952.
3. Kalantari BN, Salamon N. Neuroimaging of tuberous sclerosis: Spectrum of pathologic findings and frontiers in imaging. *AJR Am J Roentgenol.* 2008;190(5):W304–W309.
4. Osborn AG. Disorders of histogenesis: Neurocutaneous syndromes. In: Osborn AG, ed. *Diagnostic Neuroradiology.* St. Louis, MO: Mosby-Year Book, Inc.; 1994:72–116.

CLINICAL HISTORY *A 5-year-old boy presents with intractable epilepsy*

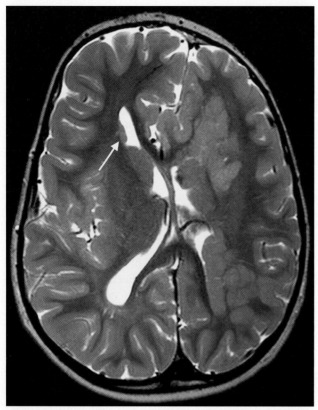

FIGURE **2.33A**

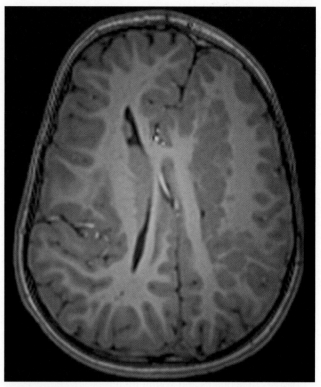

FIGURE **2.33B**

FINDINGS Axial T2-weighted MRI image (**A**) shows gray matter isointense nodular foci protruding into the left lateral ventricle as well as extending from the ventricular surface into the surrounding frontal and parietal white matter. The left cerebral hemisphere is smaller than the right, the overlying sulci are shallower, and there is no midline shift. There is also a small subependymal gray matter isointense focus abutting the frontal horn of the right lateral ventricle (*arrow*). Axial T1-weighted 3D gradient sequence image (**B**) at a slightly higher level shows gray matter isointense nodularity in the left periventricular white matter as well as a single small gray matter isointense focus abutting the frontal horn of the right lateral ventricle.

DIFFERENTIAL DIAGNOSIS Subependymal and focal subcortical heterotopia, hamartomas of TSC, subependymal hemorrhage, glioma

DIAGNOSIS Subependymal and focal subcortical heterotopia

DISCUSSION Gray matter heterotopias are malformations of cortical development that are thought to result from premature arrest of the migration of neurons from the germinal matrix to the developing cerebral cortex. Heterotopia refers to normal nerve cells located in an abnormal location. Three major subcategories are seen based on imaging: (1) subependymal heterotopia (SEH), (2) focal subcortical heterotopia, and (3) band heterotopia.

SEH: This is the most common type of heterotopia and is also referred to as periventricular heterotopia. SEH is often located at the trigone of the occipital or temporal horns of the lateral ventricles. Symptomatic patients usually present in the 10- to 20-year-old range with partial complex seizures and variable degrees of developmental delay. SEH can be an isolated abnormality but there is an association with Chiari II malformation, agenesis of the corpus callosum (ACC), and cephaloceles. Some cases are familial with a linkage to filamin-1 (*FLN1*) gene on chromosome Xq28. On imaging, SEH appears as nodular foci of varying sizes lining the ependymal surface and can be confused with the subependymal nodules (SENs) of TSC. SEH typically appears ovoid and smooth, parallel to the ventricular wall, follows signal intensity of gray matter on all sequences, and does not enhance. In contrast, the SENs of TSC usually have a more irregular shape with a long axis perpendicular to the ventricular wall, may enhance with contrast, and in older children are iso- or hypointense to mature white matter.

Focal subcortical heterotopia: These areas of gray matter heterotopia extend from the ventricular surface into the periventricular and subcortical white matter with irregular lobulation and without enhancement. They present in the first two decades with epilepsy, hemiplegia contralateral to the heterotopic tissue, intellectual impairment, and developmental delay. On imaging, focal subcortical heterotopia can appear masslike with associated effacement of the ventricle. Vessels and fluid can be found within these abnormal areas, often mimicking tumor, particularly on CT scan. The affected hemisphere, however, is typically small with a thin overlying cortex and shallow sulci, helping to differentiate focal subcortical heterotopia from a true mass lesion.

Band heterotopia: Subcortical band heterotopia (SBH) is also known as subcortical laminar heterotopia or double cortex syndrome. It may be classified as a form of incomplete lissencephaly. Over 90% of cases are found in females. The gene responsible for many cases is located on chromosome Xq22.3-23 (doublecortin gene (*DCX*)). The appearance is of a "double cortex" with a complete or partial band of normal-appearing heterotopic gray matter located between the ventricles and cortex with intervening normal-appearing white matter. Overlying cortex may be normal or have shallow cortical sulci. Diagnosis is usually simple on MRI, which shows the characteristic isointensity of the heterotopic band with respect to the cortex on all imaging sequences. When complete, findings are usually bilateral and symmetric. When partial, the frontal lobes are preferentially involved in females while the posterior lobes are involved more often in males. Increasing thickness of the band usually indicates increased symptomatology.

Question for Further Thought

1. What are the MR spectroscopy findings in heterotopia?

Relevant Anatomy

Neuronal migration is an orderly process occurring between gestational months 3 to 5. Neurons begin their journey at the ependymal surface of the germinal matrix, traveling along radial glial fibers, which guide them to their destination in one of the six cortical layers. Any disruption in this complex process may lead to areas of heterotopia.

Reporting Responsibilities

While periventricular and SEH can be isolated incidental imaging findings, they may be associated with other anomalies of cortical development; hence, a careful search should be made for these anomalies.

What the Treating Physician Needs to Know

In general, gray matter heterotopia is stable in both its imaging appearance and symptomatology, without tendency to progress. Epilepsy and varying degree of developmental delay are the two most common associated symptoms. Although appropriate surgery cannot reverse developmental disabilities, it may provide full or partial relief from seizures.

Answer

1. Studies of heterotopia with MR spectroscopy have shown conflicting results. Some studies have found similar levels of metabolites as normal brain tissue while others show an abnormal *N*-acetylaspartic acid (NAA)/creatine ratio. More research is needed before this becomes more incorporated into clinical practice.

REFERENCES

1. Barkovich AJ. Subcortical heterotopia: A distinct clinicoradiologic entity. *AJNR Am J Neuroradiol.* 1996;17(7):1315–1322.
2. Barkovich AJ. Morphologic characteristics of subcortical heterotopia: MR imaging study. *AJNR Am J Neuroradiol.* 2000; 21(2):290–295.
3. Widjaja E, Griffiths PD, Wilkinson ID. Proton MR spectroscopy of polymicrogyria and heterotopia. *AJNR Am J Neuroradiol.* 2003; 24(10):2077–2081.
4. Leite CC, Lucato LT, Sato JR, et al. Multivoxel proton MR spectroscopy in malformations of cortical development. *AJNR Am J Neuroradiol.* 2007;28(6):1071–1075.

CLINICAL HISTORY *A 14-year-old teenage boy presents to the emergency department with nasal mass and epistaxis*

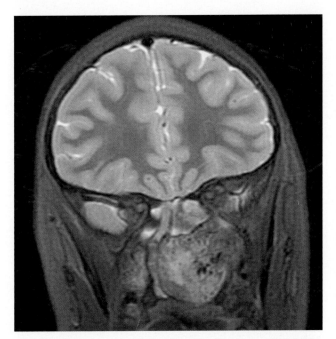

FIGURE **2.34A**

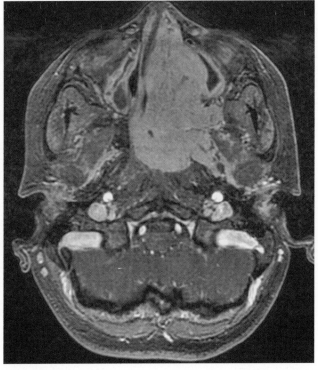

FIGURE **2.34B**

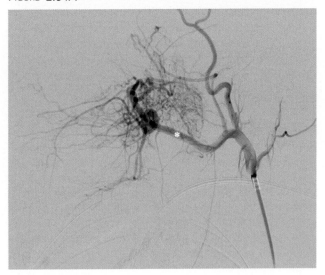

FIGURE **2.34C**

FINDINGS Coronal fat-suppressed T2-weighted MRI image (**A**) demonstrates a bulky mass in the left nasal/pterygopalatine region extending into the left infratemporal fossa with numerous hypointense flow voids representing tumor vessels. Bright signal in the ethmoid sinuses likely represents trapped fluid or secretions. Axial fat-suppressed postcontrast T1-weighted image (**B**) shows a large enhancing mass which originated in region of left sphenopalatine foramen with

extension into the nasal cavity, infratemporal fossa, and the nasopharynx. Angiographic injection of the left distal external carotid artery filmed in an oblique projection (**C**) shows intense tumor blush fed by branches of the internal maxillary artery (*asterisk*). Postembolization images (not shown) showed marked reduction in vascularity of the mass before surgery.

DIFFERENTIAL DIAGNOSIS Juvenile angiofibroma, rhabdomyosarcoma, angiomatous polyp, nasopharyngeal carcinoma, fibrous dysplasia, capillary hemangioma, solitary fibrous tumor, hemangiopericytoma

DIAGNOSIS Juvenile angiofibroma (also known as juvenile nasopharyngeal angiofibroma)

DISCUSSION Arising from the sphenopalatine foramen, this benign but aggressive highly vascular tumor classically presents in adolescent males with epistaxis or nasal stuffiness. This tumor has typically grown from the site of origin by the time of discovery. Lateral growth is commonly (90%) seen through the pterygopalatine fossa (PPF) and pterygomaxillary fissure into the infratemporal fossa causing anterior bowing of the posterior maxillary sinus antrum ("antral bowing" sign) originally described with lateral skull radiographs. Superior growth occurs into the sphenoid sinus or skull base, via the inferior orbital fissure into the orbit, or along the vidian canal or foramen rotundum into the middle cranial fossa. Medial growth occurs into the posterior nasal cavity and nasopharynx.

Full evaluation usually involves CT, MRI, and angiography. Maxillofacial CT best defines the osseous involvement of the posterior nasal cavity and skull base. Expansion of the PPF, sphenopalatine foramen, and nasal cavity is often seen, as well as bony remodeling of the maxillary antrum, if there is infratemporal fossa extension. Avid enhancement is seen with contrast on both CT and MR. The tumor is predominantly isointense on T1-weighted imaging and isointense to hyperintense on T2-weighted imaging. On both T1 and T2 imaging, multiple hypointense serpiginous structures are often seen representing tumor vessels. Postcontrast imaging with fat suppression is very helpful in defining tumor extent, particularly intracranial and intraorbital involvement.

Surgical resection is the primary mode of treatment. The majority of these tumors undergo preoperative embolization 1 to 2 days before craniofacial surgery. Preoperative embolization is especially useful in cases where newer image-guided, endoscopic, laser-assisted removal is being attempted in relatively localized tumors. Recurrence rates are as high as 20% due to the difficulty in complete resection. External radiation can be used for recurrence with fairly high success. Some centers use radiation as a primary treatment particularly in tumors with extensive or intracranial spread.

Questions for Further Thought

1. Would this diagnosis be likely in a female adolescent?
2. What syndrome has an increased incidence of juvenile angiofibroma?

Reporting Responsibilities

Detailed evaluation of the tumor spread is essential for operative planning and complete surgical resection. In a teenage male, an enhancing mass centered in the sphenopalatine foramen is an angiofibroma until proven otherwise.

What the Treating Physician Needs to Know

The diagnosis is often straightforward in a teenage male, but evaluation for skull base, sinus, and foraminal involvement is necessary for surgical planning. As the tumor extends laterally and/or intracranially, the staging designation, and therefore, the treatment plan, changes accordingly.

Answers

1. No, in a series of 150 patients examined at the Armed Forces Institute of Pathology, none were female. The tumor also has androgen receptors involved in its growth. Some suggest that genetic testing should be done in females with this diagnosis as genetic mosaicism can be found.
2. Familial adenomatous polyposis (FAP) syndrome. The same genetic mutations of the beta-catenin (β-catenin) pathway are seen in both FAP syndrome and juvenile angiofibroma.

REFERENCES

1. Hyams VJ. Tumors of the upper respiratory tract: vascular tumors. In: Hyams VJ, Batsakis JG, Micheals L, eds. *Atlas of Tumor Pathology, 2nd Series.* Washington, DC: Armed Forces Institute of Pathology; 1986:130–145.
2. Stokes SM, Castle JT. Nasopharyngeal angiofibroma of the nasal cavity. *Head Neck Pathol.* 2010;4(3):210–213.
3. Shaffer K, Haughton V, Farley G, et al. Pitfalls in the radiographic diagnosis of angiofibroma. *Radiology.* 1978;127(2):425–428.
4. Lee JT, Chen P, Safa A, et al. The role of radiation in the treatment of advanced juvenile angiofibroma. *Laryngoscope.* 2002;112(7 Pt 1):1213–1220.

Sumit Pruthi and Matthew D. Dobbs

CLINICAL HISTORY *A 7-year-old female with seizures*

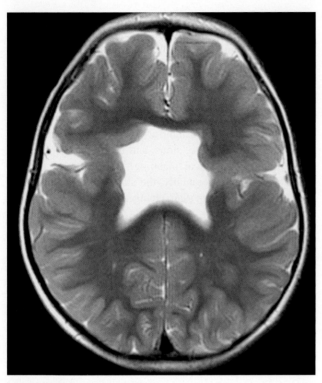

FIGURE **2.35A**

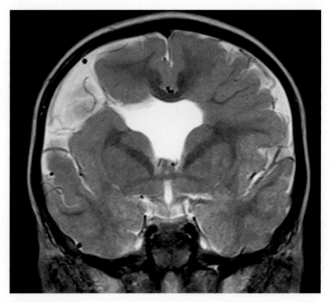

FIGURE **2.35B**

FINDINGS Axial T2-weighted MRI image (**A**) at the level of the lateral ventricles shows absence of the septum pellucidum. Corpus callosum is present. There are bilateral clefts lined by gray matter extending from the cortex to the ventricular surface. Notice the "dimple sign" bilaterally, which "points" toward the cleft. Coronal T2-weighted image (**B**) shows a small right-sided transcerebral cleft lined by gray matter and containing CSF which extends laterally from right lateral ventricle. Septum pellucidum is absent.

DIFFERENTIAL DIAGNOSIS Schizencephaly, transmantle heterotopia, porencephalic cyst, SOD

DIAGNOSIS Schizencephaly

DISCUSSION In schizencephaly, dysplastic gray matter lines an open (containing CSF) or closed transcerebral cleft extending from the pial surface to the ventricular ependyma (pial–ependymal seam), most often involving the frontal or parietal lobes in the parasylvian region. A "dimple" is often present at the ventricular surface in the closed-lip type "pointing" to the cleft. The dysplastic gray matter almost always consists of polymicrogyria. Polymicrogyria is also commonly seen along the adjacent cerebral cortex.

Most cases of schizencephaly appear to be sporadic. In utero vascular injury or infection during the early second trimester is the most favored etiology. Recent research has found a candidate gene for schizencephaly, the *EMX2* homeobox gene, but the true role of this gene is still debatable. Polymicrogyria and schizencephaly appear to be closely related. Some theories state that if injury is mild, polymicrogyria results. If injury is more severe, schizencephaly develops. Both entities are most often found in similar parasylvian regions unilaterally or bilaterally and both have associations with absence of the septum pellucidum.

Schizencephaly is categorized as closed (type I) or open lip (type II), with the gray matter apposed to one another with no intervening CSF in the closed type. In up to 40% of patients, the findings are bilateral, and often nearly symmetrical. There is an association with optic nerve hypoplasia (seen in about one-third of cases) and absence of the septum pellucidum. The term "SOD plus" is used when there are additional findings of schizencephaly, ACC, or other cortical malformation in addition to the typical findings of SOD.

Most patients with schizencephaly present with varying degrees of developmental delay, motor impairment, and seizures. Seizures often do not become apparent until the second decade of life but often become refractory. The clinical symptomatology depends upon the degree of anatomic defect and the amount of brain tissue involved. Bilateral clefts portend a worse clinical picture of intellectual impairment and earlier onset of epilepsy compared to unilateral presentation. Large clefts also tend to have increased clinical symptomatology. Anticonvulsant medicine is the first line of treatment in patients with schizencephaly. Refractory seizures can occasionally be treated with surgical excision of the cleft and surrounding dysplastic cortex.

Transmantle heterotopia can be confused with schizencephaly as it also has abnormal-appearing gray matter extending from the cortex toward the ventricle. It should not, however, reach all the way to the ependymal surface of the ventricle. The "dimple" of schizencephaly can be used to help differentiate these two entities. Porencephalic cyst can also be confused with open-lip schizencephaly as both can appear as fluid-filled spaces extending from the ventricles toward the cortex. However, as porencephalic cysts result from prior infection or infarction, they are typically lined by gliotic white matter rather than dysplastic gray matter as seen in schizencephaly.

Question for Further Thought

1. How does one differentiate open-lip schizencephaly from a porencephalic cyst?

Relevant Anatomy

Malformations of cortical development are broadly classified into three categories depending upon the timing of the insult in relationship to the cortical development. These include problems with (1) neuronal proliferation, (2) neuronal migration, and (3) late proliferation and cortical organization. Though classically classified as an abnormality of late proliferation and cortical organization, schizencephaly can result from an abnormality at any step in development.

Reporting Responsibilities

Assess the contralateral hemisphere for bilateral clefts (there can be open lip on one side with closed lip on the contralateral side), assess for presence/absence of septum pellucidum, and evaluate the optic nerves for hypoplasia. When unilateral, the contralateral hemisphere may have polymicrogyria or transmantle heterotopia.

What the Treating Physician Needs to Know

Unilateral or bilateral, open or closed lip, and any other associated malformations such as degree of polymicrogyria.

Answer

1. Gray matter will line the schizencephalic cleft. Gliotic white matter typically lines the porencephalic cyst.

REFERENCES

1. Barkovich AJ, Raybaud CA. Congenital malformations of the brain and skull. In: Barkovich AJ, Raybaud C, eds. *Pediatric Neuroimaging.* 5th ed. Philadelphia, PA: Lippincott Williams & Wilkins; 2012:367–568.
2. Oh KY, Kennedy AM, Frias AE Jr, et al. Fetal schizencephaly: Pre- and postnatal imaging with review of the clinical manifestations. *Radiographics.* 2005;25(3):647–657.
3. Raybaud C, Widjaja E. Development and dysgenesis of the cerebral cortex: Malformations of cortical development. *Neuroimaging Clin N Am.* 2011;21(3):483–543.

CLINICAL HISTORY *A 7-month-old boy who presents with seizures and mental retardation*

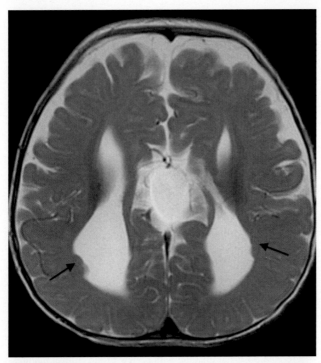

FIGURE 2.36A

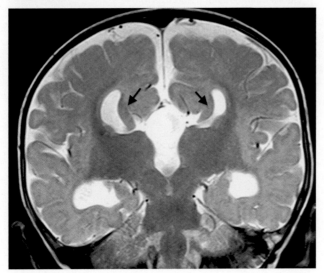

FIGURE 2.36C

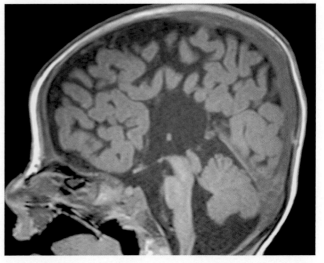

FIGURE 2.36B

FINDINGS Axial T2-weighted MRI image (**A**) demonstrates a high-riding third ventricle interposed between the lateral ventricles which themselves have a parallel configuration. Within the atria of both lateral ventricles are nodular projections that followed gray matter signal on all sequences representing areas of subependymal nodular heterotopia (*arrows*). Sagittal T1-weighted image (**B**) demonstrates complete absence of the corpus callosum with gyri extending to midline. Coronal T2-weighted image (**C**) shows a "Viking" or "longhorn" appearance of the upturned lateral ventricles bordered medially by Probst bundles (*arrows*), and a high-riding third ventricle. The hippocampi also have a more vertical appearance than usual.

DIFFERENTIAL DIAGNOSIS ACC, HPE, SOD, normal variant, callosotomy (postsurgical)

DIAGNOSIS ACC

DISCUSSION With an incidence of about 1:4,000, ACC is the most common abnormality seen with other brain anomalies. Since the corpus callosum may be partially (hypogenesis) or completely absent, the term dysgenesis is often used to describe the spectrum of callosal anomalies. When hypogenetic, the portions of the corpus callosum that form later in development, including the splenium and rostrum, are usually absent.

ACC is associated with numerous genetic mutations and syndromes, including fetal alcohol syndrome and Aicardi syndrome. It is often associated with other anomalies and malformations, the most common being encephaloceles, callosal lipomas, midline facial abnormalities, Chiari II malformation, malformations of cortical development, and DWM. Clinically, symptoms normally depend on the extent of associated anomalies rather than the absence of the callosum itself, and include seizures, mental retardation, developmental delay, and hypothalamic dysfunction. ACC may be present in isolation and without neurologic symptom.

Fetal MRI can depict absence of the corpus callosum as early as 20 to 21 weeks of gestation. Although the prognostic implications of prenatally detected ACC are not fully understood, fetal MRI can often help depict other associated anomalies thereby playing an important role in prenatal counseling and postnatal treatment planning. Postnatally, MRI is the preferred imaging modality to evaluate for ACC and associated anomalies. Sagittal views show absence of the corpus callosum, high-riding third ventricle, and radial orientation of the cingulate gyri extending up from the third ventricle. The lateral ventricles assume a classic parallel configuration and there may be colpocephaly (passive dilation of the trigones and occipital horns) due to lack of dense white matter fibers in the parietal white matter surrounding the occipital horns, which are lacking due to absence of the corpus callosum. Coronal images show the classic "Texas longhorn" or "Viking helmet" appearance of the anterior horns of lateral ventricles as well as vertical appearance of the hippocampi. The bundles of Probst are densely packed white matter bundles that extend parallel and medial to each lateral ventricle. They consist of white matter axons which attempted to cross the midline, but without a callosum, extended in an anterior and posterior direction. These axonal bundles indent the ventricles, thereby creating the upturned shape of the ventricles, which gives the "longhorn" appearance seen on coronal images. Lipomas, which are often associated with ACC, are typically found midline and can be large in size with rim calcification.

Question for Further Thought

1. What is Aicardi syndrome?

Relevant Anatomy

From anterior to posterior, the portions of the corpus callosum are the rostrum, genu, body, isthmus, and splenium. Embryologically, the order of development is genu, anterior body,

posterior body, isthmus, splenium, and rostrum. Knowing this order can help differentiate maldevelopment versus destruction. HPE is the only syndrome in which the posterior portions of the corpus callosum may be present without presence of the anterior portions of the corpus callosum, leading to an atypical pattern of callosal anomalies. Neonates have a normally thin corpus callosum due to lack of myelination. Hydrocephalus can also thin the corpus callosum which can mimic ACC if a careful search is not made. Radial orientation of the cingulate gyri extending up from the third ventricle with absence of cingulate sulcus helps differentiate ACC from an extremely thin unmyelinated corpus callosum.

Reporting Responsibilities

- Hypoplasia of the corpus callosum implies a fully formed, yet thinned appearance for the patient's age.
- Hypogenesis of the corpus callosum indicates an absence of a portion of the corpus callosum.

What the Treating Physician Needs to Know

More than half of patients with ACC will have other associated anomalies such as malformations of cortical development, midline facial anomalies, or posterior fossa abnormality such as Chiari II or DWM. The presence of these additional abnormalities generally governs the prognosis.

Answer

1. Aicardi syndrome is an X-linked dominant syndrome consisting of callosal dysgenesis, infantile spasms, and retinal lacunae. It is seen almost exclusively in females and presents with developmental delay and epilepsy. Interhemispheric cysts may also be present as well as choroid plexus papillomas, heterotopia, cortical dysplasia, microphthalmia, colobomas, and posterior fossa cysts.

REFERENCES

1. Barkovich AJ, Norman D. Absence of the septum pellucidum: A useful sign in the diagnosis of congenital brain malformations. *AJR Am J Roentgenol.* 1989;152(2):353–360.
2. Barkovich AJ, Raybaud CA. Congenital malformations of the brain and skull. In: Barkovich AJ, Raybaud C, eds. *Pediatric Neuroimaging.* 5th ed. Philadelphia, PA: Lippincott Williams & Wilkins; 2012:367–568.
3. Tang PH, Bartha AI, Norton ME, et al. Agenesis of the corpus callosum: An MR imaging analysis of associated abnormalities in the fetus. *AJNR Am J Neuroradiol.* 2009;30(2):257–263.

CASE 2.37

CLINICAL HISTORY *A 5-year-old child with headache, confusion, and tremulousness*

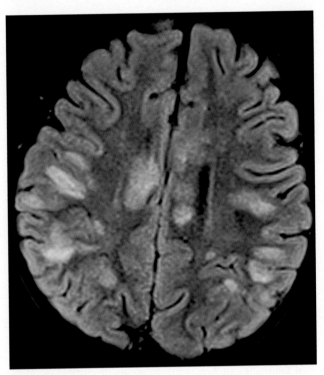

FIGURE **2.37A**

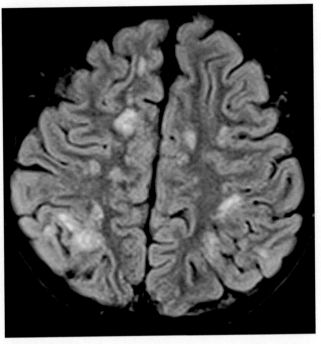

FIGURE **2.37B**

FINDINGS Axial FLAIR MRI images (**A** and **B**) demonstrate numerous regions of hyperintense signal abnormality of varying sizes predominantly within subcortical white matter and to a lesser extent periventricular white matter of bilateral frontal and parietal lobes.

DIFFERENTIAL DIAGNOSIS Acute disseminated encephalomyelitis (ADEM), multiple sclerosis (MS), viral encephalitis, vasculitis

DIAGNOSIS ADEM

DISCUSSION ADEM is generally a monophasic, focal or multifocal, perivascular inflammatory and demyelinating disorder, affecting brain and spinal cord, often presenting 7 to 14 days following a vaccination or an antecedent viral infection, and less likely other insults. A large number of infectious pathogens and a number of vaccinations have been associated with ADEM. That being said, in some cases, no definite history of prior infection or immunization is elicited. Measles, mumps, chickenpox, and rubella are some of the common viral pathogens associated with ADEM. The most common presenting signs/symptoms relate to motor deficits (including ataxia, paraparesis, etc.), brain stem dysfunction, and varying levels of altered consciousness. A seasonal distribution also has been observed, with most cases presenting in the winter and spring.

While ADEM and MS both involve autoimmune demyelination, they differ in many clinical, genetic, imaging, and histopathological aspects. Some authors consider MS and ADEM to constitute a spectrum, differing only in chronicity, severity, and clinical course, while others consider them discretely different diseases.

CT scan is relatively insensitive, and is often normal early on in the majority of cases of ADEM; MRI is a preferred imaging modality. On imaging, moderate to large areas of demyelination (hypodense on CT and hyperintense on fluid-sensitive MR sequences) can be seen involving the subcortical white matter of one or both hemispheres. The involvement is usually asymmetric. In approximately 50% of patients, there is involvement of the deep gray nuclei, with brain stem, spinal cord and cerebellar involvement seen in approximately 30% to 50% of the cases. Spinal cord lesions usually present as long segment confluent lesions. The lesions of ADEM show variable contrast enhancement and frequently lack associated restricted diffusion, a feature, which when present, is sometimes useful in differentiating ADEM from vasculitis. Lack of predominant periventricular white matter and corpus callosal involvement, and involvement of deep gray nuclei in ADEM, may help differentiate this entity from an initial episode of MS. Imaging findings in ADEM are not pathognomonic and the diagnosis is generally made after excluding other pathologies that can mimic ADEM. An important point to note is that imaging findings can lag behind clinical condition during both onset and resolution, leading to clinicoradiologic mismatch. Hence, a negative imaging study at presentation does not exclude the diagnosis. Similarly, worsening imaging appearance may be seen in the setting of resolving clinical infection. Follow-up imaging after treatment often reveals complete or partial resolution of lesions, confirming the true monophasic nature of the lesions.

Though primarily monophasic, relapses can happen in ADEM. If they happen during the course of treatment (corticosteroids), it is still considered as a monophasic event. If it happens during dose taper or after the completion of the therapy, it is considered multiphasic ADEM. That being said, if there is true passage of time in regard to the relapse (such as a 3-month interval between the first and second episodes), then a diagnosis of MS should be considered. This distinction is extremely crucial because it affects the diagnosis, management, and overall prognosis of the patient. Most patients with ADEM recover over a 4- to 6-week period, but residual neurologic deficit is not uncommon.

Question for Further Thought

1. What is acute hemorrhagic leukoencephalitis?

Reporting Responsibilities

Occasionally, there can be a delay between the onset of symptoms and the appearance of lesions on MR images; hence, a normal MRI does not exclude the diagnosis of ADEM. Similarly, clinical improvement may precede imaging changes and follow-up should be recommended to confirm the monophasic nature of the disease.

What the Treating Physician Needs to Know

- Clinical history of recent viral illness and/or vaccination is often helpful to confidently diagnose these lesions.
- Brain and spine MRI should both be obtained together to assess involvement of the entire neural axis.

Answer

1. Acute hemorrhagic leukoencephalitis is the most severe subform of ADEM characterized by an acute rapidly progressive fulminant inflammation of the white matter, first described by Hurst in 1941. It is also known as acute necrotizing encephalopathy, acute necrotizing hemorrhagic leukoencephalitis, Weston–Hurst syndrome, or Hurst disease. On neuroimaging, the lesions tend to be larger and associated with more edema and mass effect than those seen in ADEM, and frequently show hemorrhage, unlike ADEM. Though rare, it is unfortunately often fatal.

REFERENCES

1. Krupp LB, Banwell B, Tenembaum S, et al. Consensus definitions proposed for pediatric multiple sclerosis and related disorders. *Neurology.* 2007;68(16 Suppl 2):S7–S12.
2. Menge T, Hemmer B, Nessler S, et al. Acute disseminated encephalomyelitis: An update. *Arch Neurol.* 2005;62(11):1673–1680.

CLINICAL HISTORY *A 17-month-old child with seizures and increased head circumference*

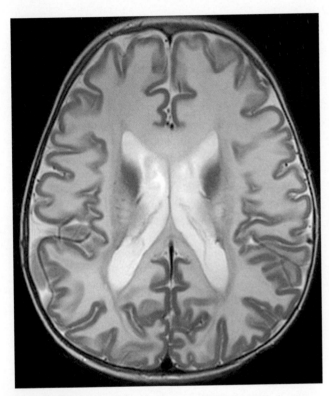

FIGURE **2.38A**

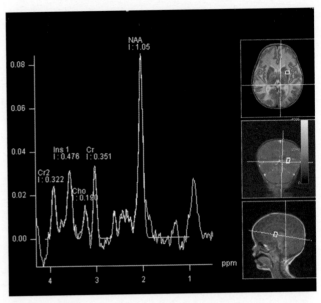

FIGURE **2.38B**

FINDINGS Axial T2-weighted image of the brain obtained at the level of centrum semiovale (**A**) reveals diffuse bilaterally symmetric increased signal intensity within entire white matter with involvement of subcortical U-fibers. Single-voxel ¹H MR spectroscopy with voxel placed over the left external capsule (**B**) shows a marked elevation of the NAA peak.

DIFFERENTIAL DIAGNOSIS MRI: Canavan disease, Alexander disease, metachromatic leukodystrophy, adrenoleukodystrophy, Pelizaeus–Merzbacher disease

MR SPECTROSCOPY Canavan disease

DIAGNOSIS Canavan disease

DISCUSSION Canavan disease, a spongiform degeneration of myelin, is an autosomal recessive childhood leukodystrophy caused by mutations in the gene for human aspartoacylase (ASPA), which leads to an abnormal accumulation of NAA in the brain, plasma, and urine. In the classic infantile form, patients typically present at 2 to 4 months of age with hypotonia, head lag, and macrocephaly, which progresses to developmental delay, optic atrophy, spasticity, and seizures, with death usually occurring within a few years of life. Increased head circumference, a clinical hallmark of the disease, may not be present at birth but head circumference increases rapidly after 6 months of life with obvious macrocephaly by 1 year of age. Atypical Canavan disease in juveniles, with mild manifestations, has been rarely reported.

Radiographically, spongiform changes or vacuolization of the white matter is easily evident on MRI as decreased T1 and increased T2 signal intensity within white matter. Although not always present and not uniform, there is generally diffuse and symmetric involvement of white matter with predominant involvement of the subcortical arcuate/U-fibers, especially early in the course of disease. This is in contrast to metachromatic leukodystrophy where subcortical white matter is relatively spared. In Canavan disease there is no lobar predominance, variable involvement of the basal ganglia and cerebellar white matter, and there is no associated abnormal contrast enhancement. This helps differentiate it further from adrenoleukodystrophy which tends to progress in an orderly manner from one portion of the brain to the next with an advancing edge of contrast enhancement.

With disease progression, there is eventual atrophy of the cortex.

Clinically, Canavan disease can be easily confused with Alexander disease and was historically differentiated on brain biopsy by demonstrating the presence of Rosenthal fibers in Alexander disease. MR spectroscopy is a very useful tool in differentiating these two entities as NAA is elevated in Canavan disease and usually normal or decreased in Alexander disease. In addition, extensive cerebral white matter abnormalities in Alexander disease usually present with a frontal preponderance.

Question for Further Thought

1. Which leukodystrophies are commonly associated with macrocephaly?

What the Treating Physician Needs to Know

There is considerable overlap in the imaging appearance of various leukodystrophies especially during late stages, and imaging distinction may not be possible. If there is a strong clinical suspicion for Canavan disease, MR spectroscopy should be obtained.

Answer

1. Of all the leukodystrophies, Alexander disease, Canavan disease, and megalencephalic leukoencephalopathy with subcortical cysts are most clearly associated with macrocephaly.

REFERENCES

1. Barkovich AJ, Patay Z. Metabolic, toxic, and inflammatory brain disorders. In: Barkovich AJ, Raybaud C, eds. *Pediatric Neuroimaging*. 5th ed. Philadelphia, PA: Lippincott Williams & Wilkins; 2012:81–239.
2. Cheon JE, Kim IO, Hwang YS, et al. Leukodystrophy in children: A pictorial review of MR imaging features. *Radiographics*. 2002;22(3):461–476.

CLINICAL HISTORY *A 23-month-old male with a dribbling urinary stream and dermal sinus tract on the back*

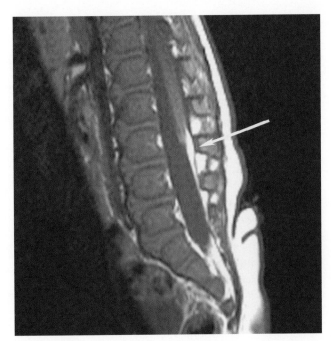

FIGURE **2.39A**

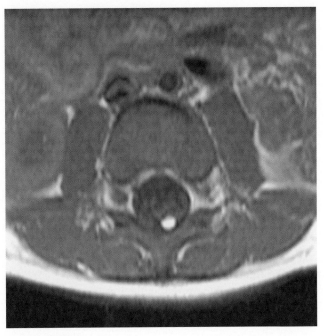

FIGURE **2.39B**

FINDINGS Sagittal (**A**) and axial (**B**) T1-weighted MRI images of the lumbar spine demonstrate a low-lying conus medullaris terminating at the L3-L4 vertebral body level. There is T1-hyperintense signal within the filum terminale with focal bulging of the filum at the L3-L4 level (*arrow*) consistent with a filar lipoma measuring up to 4 mm in maximal AP dimension.

DIFFERENTIAL DIAGNOSIS Filar lipoma, intradural lipoma, lipomyelomeningocele, lipomyelocele

DIAGNOSIS Filar lipoma (fatty infiltration of the filum terminale)

DISCUSSION Fatty infiltration of the filum terminale or filar lipoma is a closed spinal dysraphism characterized by a filum which is >2 mm in AP dimension and contains fat signal on MRI.[1] Fatty infiltration can cause stretching and tethering of the conus, resulting in neurologic symptoms of tethered cord which includes a constellation of progressive neurologic, gastrointestinal, urologic, and musculoskeletal symptoms. While filar lipoma is a common cause of cord tethering, cord tethering can also be seen as the presentation of several forms of closed spinal dysraphism.

Closed spinal dysraphisms are broadly classified on the basis of the presence or absence of a subcutaneous mass. Those with a subcutaneous fatty mass overlying the spinal defect include lipomyelocele and lipomyelomeningocele. Differentiating between these two entities depends on the location of the neural placode–lipoma interface with lipomyelomeningocele characterized by an interface located outside of the spinal canal. Other causes of closed spinal dysraphism with subcutaneous mass include meningocele and terminal myelocystocele resulting from cystic expansion of the caudal central canal. Closed spinal dysraphisms without subcutaneous mass include filar lipoma, intradural lipoma, diastematomyelia, caudal regression syndrome, and cystic intraspinal lesions such as neurenteric cyst. The dermal sinus tract mentioned above in the case history (which may not always be evident by MRI) represents an epithelial lined tract that connects neural tissue or meninges to the skin surface and is often associated with intraspinal dermoids, filar lipoma, and intradural lipoma. The dermal sinus tract may, of itself, be a cause of cord tethering. Recognition and surgical repair of these tracts is important to prevent complications of ascending infection including meningitis or abscess.

In cases of filar lipoma, the conus medullaris is often, but not always, low lying below the inferior endplate of L2.

Plain radiographs are often nonspecific although spina bifida occulta may be present. Scoliosis is seen in approximately 20% of cases of filar lipoma.[2] It is important to note that filar fat can be seen in normal patients without neurologic symptoms, estimated to occur in 3.7% of the population.[3] In these cases, the filum terminale is usually less than 2 mm in thickness. Conversely, the filum may be thickened without the presence of fat and some of these patients may have neurologic symptoms.

Questions for Further Thought

1. What clinical signs and symptoms alert clinicians to a possible tethered cord?
2. Are filar lipomas associated with other intraspinal lesions?

Reporting Responsibilities

- Report findings of closed spinal dysraphism, including whether the conus medullaris is low lying, as well as the presence or absence of associated subcutaneous mass.
- Report the level of the conus medullaris as well as any spinal cord abnormality.

What the Treating Physician Needs to Know

- Neurologic symptoms referable to a tethered cord can occur at any age and are not limited to the pediatric population.
- Incidental fat within the filum terminale can be seen in asymptomatic patients.[3]

Answers

1. Muscle stiffness or weakness, abnormal lower extremity reflexes, bladder dysfunction (dribbling stream), sensory changes, orthopedic deformities of the lower extremities (most commonly clubfoot), and back pain with exertion.
2. Filar lipomas can coexist with additional intraspinal lipomas, dermoids, or dermal sinus tract.

REFERENCES

1. Badve CA, Khanna PC, Phillips GS, et al. MRI of closed spinal dysraphisms. *Pediatr Radiol.* 2011;41(10):1308–1320.
2. Schwartz ES, Barkovich AJ. Congenital anomalies of the spine. In: Barkovich AJ, Raybaud C, eds. *Pediatric Neuroimaging.* 5th ed. Philadelphia, PA: Lippincott Williams & Wilkins; 2012:857–922.
3. Tortori-Donati P, Rossi A, Biancheri R, et al. Magnetic resonance imaging of spinal dysraphism. *Top Magn Reson Imaging.* 2001;12(6):375–409.

Stephen E. Darling and Gisele E. Ishak

CASE 2.40

CLINICAL HISTORY *A 12-month-old male with 2 days of vomiting and fever, now presenting with new onset seizure*

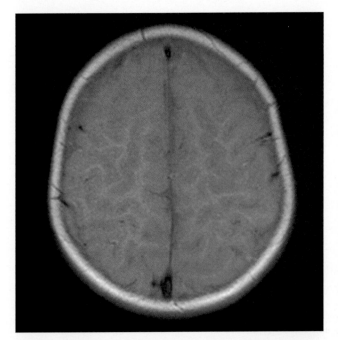

FIGURE 2.40A

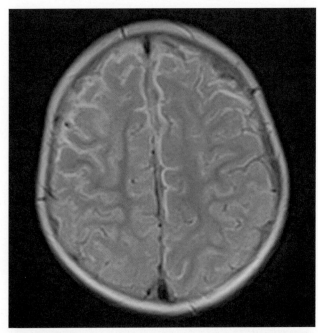

FIGURE 2.40B

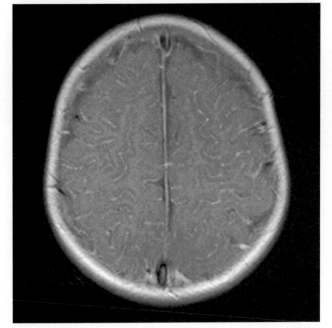

FIGURE 2.40C

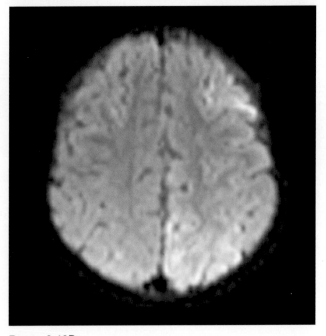

FIGURE 2.40D

FINDINGS Axial T1-weighted MRI image (**A**) shows no definite abnormality. Axial FLAIR (**B**) demonstrates diffuse subarachnoid signal abnormality with associated leptomeningeal contrast enhancement within the bilateral convexities as seen on axial T1-weighted postcontrast (**C**) imaging. In addition, there is abnormal high signal, indicating diffusion restriction, on DWI (**D**) within the left greater than right frontoparietal gyri at the vertex.

DIFFERENTIAL DIAGNOSIS Meningitis, leptomeningeal carcinomatosis, subarachnoid hemorrhage

DIAGNOSIS Meningitis

DISCUSSION The majority of cases of meningitis occur in children with diagnosis primarily being made on the basis of characteristic signs and symptoms as well as the results of lumbar puncture. Early CT and MRI examinations are often normal or may demonstrate small ventricles with effacement of sulci. Leptomeningeal enhancement may occasionally be seen on contrast-enhanced CT or MRI; however, meningeal enhancement is relatively rare and ultimately nonspecific.[1]

Ultrasound is sometimes used for evaluation of neonates with meningitis and can demonstrate subtle parenchymal echogenicity, echogenic sulci, extra-axial fluid collections, and ventricular dilation.[2] Imaging in meningitis is primarily reserved for the evaluation of children with a complicated clinical course and to assess for possible complications including venous thrombosis, venous or arterial infarcts secondary to infectious involvement of perivascular spaces, subdural empyema, ventriculitis (especially seen in neonatal meningitis), cerebritis, and abscess. Cerebritis most commonly occurs at the gray-white junction when infection travels through thrombosed venules into the cerebral parenchyma, and may progress to frank abscess over 1 to 2 weeks if incompletely treated. Surgical drainage is usually required for treatment once cerebritis liquefies into an encapsulated abscess.

If a patient with suspected meningitis has areas of restricted diffusion on MRI (as in the presented case), the possibility of concomitant cerebritis or infarct should be considered. Diffusion restriction may not always allow for this differentiation, but a watershed distribution would be more characteristic of infarct in a child with meningitis.[3]

Questions for Further Thought

1. Is there any role for imaging in the management of post-meningitic deafness?

2. What are the possible causes of diffuse subarachnoid FLAIR signal hyperintensity on MRI?

Reporting Responsibilities

• Report the presence or absence of possible complications of meningitis.
• Once cerebritis is identified, sequential imaging is important in management in order to determine response to antibiotic therapy.

What the Treating Physician Needs to Know

The diagnosis of meningitis is made primarily on clinical and laboratory data with imaging reserved for complicated or atypical cases.

Answers

1. Imaging is not useful in determining whether postmeningitic deafness is present; however, imaging can be useful in determining the potential success for cochlear implantation. Findings of calcification or ossification in the cochlea or of cochlear stenosis are poor prognostic signs for successful cochlear implantation.

2. Subarachnoid FLAIR signal abnormality can be seen with artifactual and pathologic processes, including subarachnoid hemorrhage, meningitis, and leptomeningeal carcinomatosis. Artifactual/nonpathologic causes of subarachnoid FLAIR signal abnormality include CSF or vascular pulsation, supplemental oxygen, and motion artifact.[4]

REFERENCES

1. Hedlund G, Bale JF Jr, Barkovich AJ. Infections of the developing and mature nervous system. In: Barkovich AJ, Raybaud C, eds. *Pediatric Neuroimaging.* 5th ed. Philadelphia, PA: Lippincott Williams & Wilkins; 2012:954–1050.

2. Soni JP, Gupta BD, Soni M, et al. Cranial ultrasonic assessment of infants with acute bacterial meningitis. *Indian Pediatr.* 1994;31(11):1337–1343.

3. Teixeira J, Zimmerman RA, Haselgrove JC, et al. Diffusion imaging in pediatric central nervous system infections. *Neuroradiology.* 2001;43(12):1031–1039.

4. Stuckey SL, Goh TD, Heffernan T, et al. Hyperintensity in the subarachnoid space on FLAIR MRI. *AJR Am J Roentgenol.* 2007;189(4):913–921.

CLINICAL HISTORY *A 10-year-old child with hearing loss*

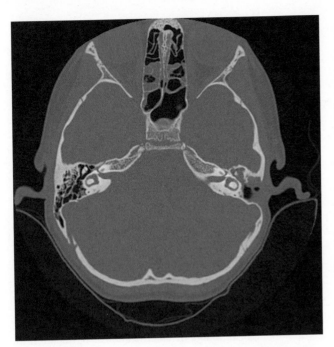

FIGURE **2.41A**

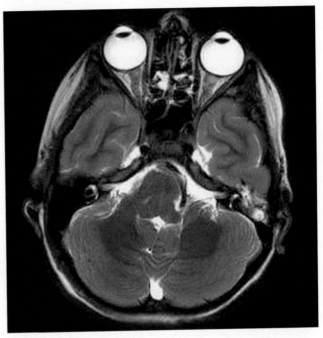

FIGURE **2.41B**

FINDINGS Non-contrast axial CT image (**A**) at the level of the internal auditory canals demonstrates opacification of the left middle ear with partial erosion of the malleus and incus. In addition, there is opacification of the left mastoid air cells with a large cortical defect of the lateral mastoid wall. Corresponding T2-weighted axial MR image (**B**) demonstrates T2 hyperintensity in and posterior to the left middle ear cavity, which did not enhance on postcontrast imaging.

DIFFERENTIAL DIAGNOSIS Cholesteatoma, rhabdomyosarcoma, LCH

DIAGNOSIS Cholesteatoma

DISCUSSION A cholesteatoma represents a collection of squamous epithelial cells that usually produce keratin debris and typically cause destruction of adjacent bones. Cholesteatomas can be classified as either congenital or acquired.

The congenital cholesteatoma represents an aberrant rest of squamous epithelial cells that can be located anywhere in the temporal bone. They are most commonly located in the middle ear (representing about 2% of all middle ear cholesteatomas) with less common locations being petrous apex and even intracranial extra-axial locations such as the cerebellopontine angle. The middle ear congenital cholesteatoma can cause conductive hearing loss, is usually small at time of presentation, and tends to cause bony destruction only late in the disease process.[1]

The much more common acquired cholesteatoma represents about 98% of middle ear cholesteatomas. These often present with conductive hearing loss but can also cause facial paralysis and vertigo. They are usually seen as a mass behind the tympanic membrane. Ossicular erosion is common. Additional local bony destruction can occur, including involvement of mastoid antrum, tegmen tympani, and facial nerve canal. The most common theories for origin of acquired cholesteatoma center on either tympanic membrane perforation or retraction pockets, with in-growths or relocation of squamous epithelial cells.[1,2]

The two major types of acquired cholesteatoma, classified on basis of site of origin, are the more common pars flaccida (attic) cholesteatoma, located at the upper one-third of the tympanic membrane, and the pars tensa cholesteatoma, involving the lower two-thirds of the tympanic membrane. The pars flaccida cholesteatoma is initially located lateral to the middle ear ossicles, which may be displaced medially, and typically extends into Prussak's space and causes erosion of the scutum. The pars tensa cholesteatoma is initially located medial to the ossicles.

On CT, the acquired cholesteatoma typically presents as a soft-tissue mass in the middle ear, often with ossicular erosion. Adjacent bone destruction may be present. On MRI, acquired cholesteatomas are usually hypo- to isointense on T1-weighted imaging and hyperintense on T2-weighted imaging compared to brain tissue. They do not enhance following gadolinium administration, although associated granulation tissue can enhance.[1,2]

The treatment of cholesteatoma is surgical resection. Diffusion imaging may be helpful in the postoperative patient where presence of diffusion restriction would suggest residual or recurrent disease rather than postsurgical change.[3]

DIFFERENTIAL DIAGNOSTIC CONSIDERATIONS

Rhabdomyosarcoma and LCH are both usually associated with bone destruction and variable enhancement. LCH may have evidence of disease elsewhere.

Questions for Further Thought

1. What other entity is associated with congenital cholesteatoma?
2. What are possible complications of cholesteatoma?

Reporting Responsibilities

Delineate extent of soft-tissue abnormality and bony change/destruction.

What the Treating Physician Needs to Know

- Extent of soft-tissue abnormality and bony destruction.
- Complications (see Answer 2 below).

Answers

1. External auditory canal dysplasia.
2. Fistulization into the semicircular canals; intracranial extension through the tegmen tympani; involvement of facial nerve canal.

REFERENCES

1. Baráth K, Huber AM, Stämpfli P, et al. Neuroradiology of cholesteatomas. *AJNR Am J Neuroradiol.* 2011;32(2):221–229.
2. Koch BL. Acquired cholesteatoma. In: Barkovich AJ, ed. *Diagnostic Imaging: Pediatric Neuroradiology.* Salt Lake City: Amirsys; 2007;II:1:34–37.
3. Aikele P, Kittner T, Offergeld C, et al. Diffusion-weighted MR imaging of cholesteatoma in pediatric and adult patients who have undergone middle ear surgery. *AJR Am J Roentgenol.* 2003;181(1):261–265.

Kalyan C. Tatineny and Edward Weinberger

CLINICAL HISTORY *A 21-month-old child with seizures (Figs. 2.42A and B)*

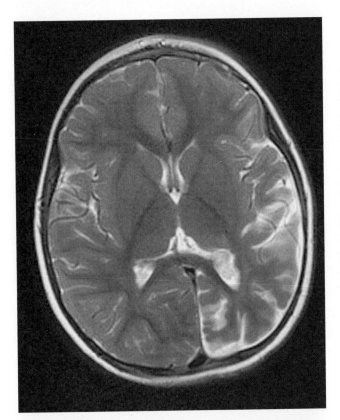

FIGURE **2.42A**

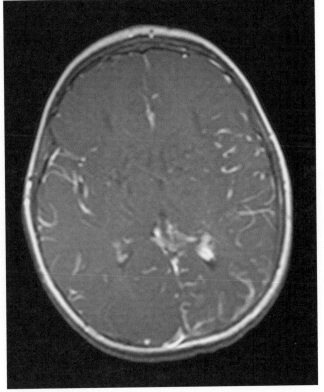

FIGURE **2.42B**

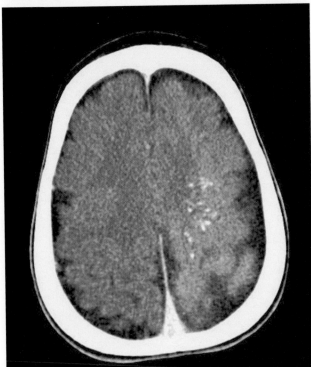

FIGURE **2.42C**

FINDINGS Axial T2-weighted MRI (**A**) shows left parieto-occipital volume loss with slight prominence of the left occipital horn and hypertrophy of the choroid plexus. Corresponding T1-postcontrast image (**B**) shows prominent leptomeningeal enhancement in the same region. Axial CT (**C**) in a different 6-month-old child demonstrates atrophy of the left frontal and parietal lobes, which contain multiple calcifications.

DIFFERENTIAL DIAGNOSIS Sturge–Weber syndrome, calcified infarct, cerebral AVM, infection

DIAGNOSIS Sturge–Weber syndrome

DISCUSSION Sturge–Weber syndrome, also known as encephalotrigeminal angiomatosis, is a neurocutaneous syndrome characterized by venous angiomas involving the face, choroid of the eye, and the leptomeninges, with most cases involving just one cerebral hemisphere.[1] This entity is caused by failure of cortical veins to develop properly, with lack of normal regression of an embryonic vascular plexus around cephalic portion of the neural tube resulting in some persistence of fetal venous anatomy and residual vascular tissue which forms the angiomas.[2] Cortical ischemic change can occur with various theories for this being that impairment of cortical venous drainage contributes to venous stasis and occlusion as well as a vascular steal phenomenon that may develop around the angiomas.

The most common clinical presentation is seizures within the first year of life. Other presentations include mental retardation, contralateral lower extremity paralysis, and contralateral lower extremity muscle hypotrophy. On physical exam, venous angiomas on the face usually present as a "port-wine stain" along the distribution of one of the branches of the trigeminal nerve, usually the V1 or V2 branch.[1]

The earliest intracranial manifestations of Sturge–Weber syndrome are best seen on MRI. Findings include prominent ipsilateral choroid plexus, prominent deep veins, and focal leptomeningeal enhancement, likely secondary to the delayed clearance of contrast in the areas of leptomeningeal angiomatous involvement[3] or breakdown of blood–brain barrier due to hypoxia and tissue scarring.[4] Later findings include parenchymal atrophy and calcification, secondary to the multiple episodes of ischemia that occur.[2] These later findings can be identified by CT. Plain radiograph of the skull may show subcortical calcifications in a gyriform or "tram track" configuration.[1]

Primary treatment of Sturge–Weber syndrome involves controlling the seizures. Treatment options if seizures cannot be controlled medically include vagal nerve stimulation that can help reduce seizure frequency[5] and focal cortical resection.[2] The "port-wine stain" can be treated by laser therapy.[2] In addition, an ophthalmologic evaluation is necessary as the choroid of the eye may also be involved.[2]

DIFFERENTIAL DIAGNOSTIC CONSIDERATIONS

While infection can present with leptomeningeal enhancement, there usually is no volume loss or prominence of either the vessels or choroid plexus in infection. Although volume loss may be seen in calcified infarct, choroid plexus prominence is not seen. Also, choroid plexus prominence is typically not seen in AVM.

Questions for Further Thought

1. What is the correlation between involvement of the branches of the trigeminal nerve and the brain?

2. What are some indications of poor outcome in Sturge–Weber syndrome?

Reporting Responsibilities

Location of the calcifications/leptomeningeal enhancement.

What the Treating Physician Needs to Know

If seizures need to be treated surgically, which areas of the brain are involved.

Answers

1. The trigeminal nerve distribution correlates with the area of ipsilateral brain which is affected: V1 distribution correlates with occipital lobe angiomas, V2 with parietal lobe, and V3 with frontal lobe.[1]

2. Indications of poor outcome include medically refractive seizures, increased seizure frequency and duration, progression of cortical atrophy or calcifications on subsequent examinations, decrease in cognitive abilities, and hemiparesis.

REFERENCES

1. Dähnert W. Brain disorders. In: Dähnert W, ed. *Radiology Review Manual*. 6th ed. Philadelphia, PA: Lippincott Williams & Wilkins; 2007:263–336.

2. Takeoka M, Riviello JJ Jr. Pediatric Sturge-Weber syndrome [Online exclusive]. *Medscape*. Retrieved December 3, 2011 from http://emedicine.medscape.com/article/1177523.

3. Lin DD, Barker PB, Kraut MA, et al. Early characteristics of Sturge-Weber syndrome shown by perfusion MR imaging and proton MR spectroscopic imaging. *AJNR Am J Neuroradiol*. 2003;24(9):1912–1915.

4. Evans AL, Widjaja E, Connolly DJ, et al. Cerebral perfusion abnormalities in children with Sturge-Weber syndrome shown by dynamic contrast bolus magnetic resonance perfusion imaging. *Pediatrics*. 2006;117(6):2119–2125.

5. Alexopoulos AV, Kotagal P, Loddenkemper T, et al. Long-term results with vagus nerve stimulation in children with pharmacoresistant epilepsy. *Seizure*. 2006;15(7):491–503.

CLINICAL HISTORY *A 6-week-old female (Fig. 2.43A) with suspected nonaccidental trauma*

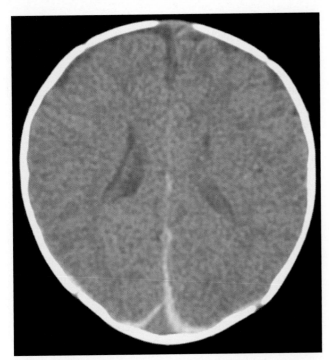

FIGURE **2.43A**

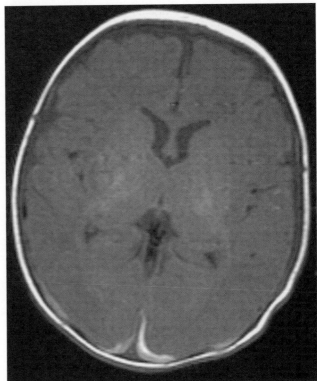

FIGURE **2.43B**

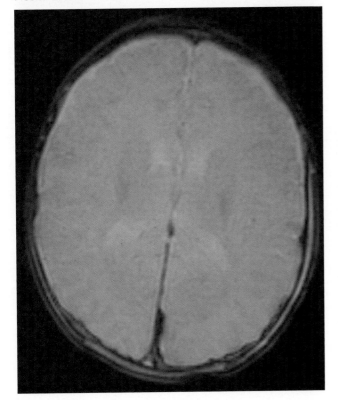

FIGURE **2.43C**

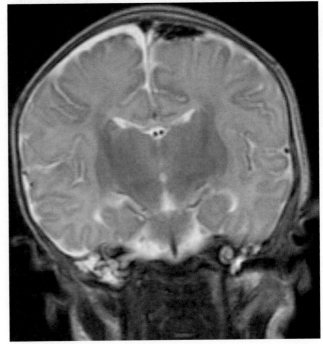

FIGURE **2.43D**

FINDINGS Axial CT (**A**) demonstrates hyperdense material layering along the dura adjacent to the posterior falx, and along right and left aspects of the superior sagittal sinus, consistent with acute subdural blood. In another 10-week-old patient, axial T1-weighted (**B**), axial GRE (**C**), and coronal T2-weighted (**D**) MR images show T1-hyperintense, T2-hypointense, and gradient-hypointense areas in the posterior subdural spaces, consistent with subacute subdural blood.

DIFFERENTIAL DIAGNOSIS Subdural hematoma, epidural hematoma, subdural hygroma, subdural empyema

DIAGNOSIS Subdural hematoma

DISCUSSION Subdural hematoma is blood between dura and arachnoid that, because of the location, typically appears crescentic when overlying the cerebral convexities and linear in the parafalcine region. Subdural hematoma can track across suture lines and may extend along the falx and tentorium. On axial CT, tentorial subdural hematoma is visualized as increased density of the tentorium cerebelli. Acute, subacute, and chronic subdural hematomas appear hyper-, iso-, and hypodense to brain parenchyma, respectively. Isodense hematomas can be subtle; a clue is the inward displacement of the gray–white interface. Blood of different ages, as seen in nonaccidental trauma, can have more than one density. On MRI, blood follows various stages of signal intensity on T1-weighted, T2-weighted, and gradient sequences. Subdural hematomas usually result from rupture of bridging veins with trauma (accidental, nonaccidental, birth trauma).[1] They may be seen in patients with minimal trauma who have enlarged extra-axial spaces as well as in patients with an underlying coagulopathy.[2] Subdural hematomas are often located diametrically opposite the site of head injury impact (contrecoup injury), may be holohemispheric, and can have mass effect on the underlying brain. They can be associated with parenchymal hemorrhagic contusions, shear injuries, subarachnoid and extradural hemorrhage, ischemic injury,

and edema. Subdural hematomas may be associated with calvarial fractures.

DIFFERENTIAL DIAGNOSTIC CONSIDERATIONS

Epidural hematoma: Typically biconvex configuration, usually occurs at the site of impact (coup injury), and often associated with calvarial fracture; should not cross sutures unless a fracture is present.

Subdural hygroma and empyema: CSF density/intensity. Empyemas show rim enhancement following contrast administration.

Questions for Further Thought

1. What is the characteristic appearance on CT of an active bleed into a preexisting subdural hematoma?
2. What are the imaging characteristics of subdural empyema?

Reporting Responsibilities

Extent and age of the subdural hematoma. Is there associated parenchymal injury? Is there blood of differing densities/intensities?

What the Treating Physician Needs to Know

Extent and age of injury. Are the findings concerning for nonaccidental trauma?

Answers

1. The "swirl" sign, with mixing of hyperdense (acute) and hypodense (less acute) blood products.
2. Peripheral enhancement of the subdural collection with restricted diffusion on MRI.

REFERENCES

1. Foerster BR, Petrou M, Lin D, et al. Neuroimaging evaluation of non-accidental head trauma with correlation to clinical outcomes: a review of 57 cases. *J Pediatr.* 2009;154(4):573–577.
2. Feldman KW, Bethel R, Shugerman RP, et al. The cause of infant and toddler subdural hemorrhage: A prospective study. *Pediatrics.* 2001;108(3):636–646.

CLINICAL HISTORY *A 15-year-old male with history of seizures (Fig. 2.44A)*

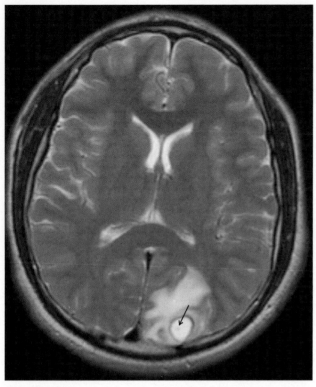

FIGURE **2.44A**

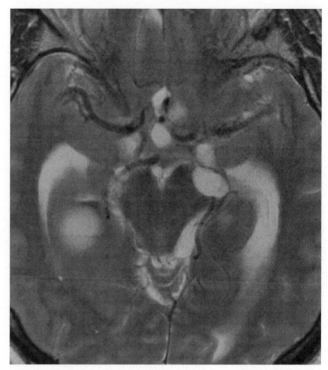

FIGURE **2.44B**

FINDINGS Axial T2-weighted MRI image (**A**) demonstrates a ring lesion in the left occipital lobe with a peripheral T2-hypointense rim and a central hypointense focus (*arrow*). There is surrounding vasogenic edema. Axial T2-weighted image (**B**) of a different patient, an 18-year-old male, demonstrates multiple CSF signal areas of varying sizes in the perimesencephalic and suprasellar cisterns. One of these has mass effect with scalloping of the left cerebral peduncle.

DIFFERENTIAL DIAGNOSIS NCC, other parasitic infestations, abscess, arachnoid cyst, neoplasm, large/giant perivascular spaces, tuberculoma

DIAGNOSIS NCC. The first case represents the colloidal vesicular phase (with surrounding vasogenic edema) of the parenchymal form and the second case represents the racemose form of NCC (see discussion below).

DISCUSSION NCC is an intracranial parasitic infestation caused by the larval stage of the tapeworm *Taenia solium* (undercooked pork). The larval stage may be found in the parenchyma (parenchymal and miliary form), basal cisterns and subarachnoid spaces (racemose form), or ventricles (intraventricular form) of the brain. When in the parenchyma, the larvae are commonly found at the gray–white interface. The parenchymal form has four phases: vesicular,

colloidal vesicular, granular nodular, and nodular calcified. The vesicular stage appears as a cyst with a central "dot," which is said to represent the larval scolex or head. The larva at this stage is viable and there is no surrounding edema. In the colloidal vesicular stage, the larva begins to degenerate, releasing toxic substances that incite vasogenic edema in the surrounding parenchyma. Patients present with seizures and headaches most commonly at this stage. A thickened, crenated cyst wall with resolving edema typifies the granular nodular phase. Variable rim enhancement can be seen in the first three phases. Dense calcification is noted in the fourth, nodular calcified phase. Widespread parenchymal infection termed miliary NCC may be encountered in endemic areas. The brain parenchyma of affected individuals is literally studded with larval forms. In the racemose form, multiple cysts of varying sizes are noted in the basal cisterns/subarachnoid spaces, some of which may demonstrate mass effect on the parenchyma. The intraventricular form usually occurs in the lateral or fourth ventricles and may lead to obstructive hydrocephalus.[1–3]

DIFFERENTIAL DIAGNOSTIC CONSIDERATIONS

Abscess: Rim enhancing, restricted, on diffusion.

Other parasitic infestations: In the calcified stage of NCC, differential diagnosis includes toxoplasmosis and other TORCH group of infections.

Arachnoid cyst: This may simulate the racemose form of NCC by demonstrating mass effect on parenchyma.

Neoplasm: With large cystic component, neoplasm may look similar to parenchymal NCC, particularly the colloidal–vesicular phase presented above as there is surrounding parenchymal edema. Cystic neoplasms, however, tend to have enhancing mural nodules or thick, irregular enhancing walls.

Large or giant perivascular spaces: These may sometimes look like the vesicular stage of NCC as there is no surrounding edema.

Tuberculoma: These are generally larger and rim enhancing.

Questions for Further Thought

1. What are potential complications of degenerating larval cysts in the racemose and intraventricular forms?
2. What are the imaging features of miliary NCC?

Reporting Responsibilities

Type and stage of NCC, edema, and mass effect if any.

What the Treating Physician Needs to Know

Response, if any, to medication. Complications (see Answer 1).

Answers

1. The inflammation may extend into the convexity subarachnoid spaces and potentially cause meningitis and/or vasculitis. The intraventricular form may also cause obstructive hydrocephalus.
2. Innumerable lesions in different phases (described above) within the brain parenchyma, sometimes referred to as the "starry-sky" appearance.

REFERENCES

1. Zee CS, Go JL, Kim PE, et al. Imaging of neurocysticercosis. *Neuroimaging Clin N Am.* 2000;10(2):391–407.
2. García HH, Del Brutto OH. Imaging findings in neurocysticercosis. *Acta Trop.* 2003;87(1):71–78.
3. Kimura-Hayama ET, Higuera JA, Corona-Cedillo R, et al. Neurocysticercosis: Radiologic-pathologic correlation. *Radiographics.* 2010;30(6):1705–1719.

Paritosh C. Khanna

CASE 2.45

CLINICAL HISTORY *A 2-year-old male with history of traumatic brain injury who presents with fever and seizures*

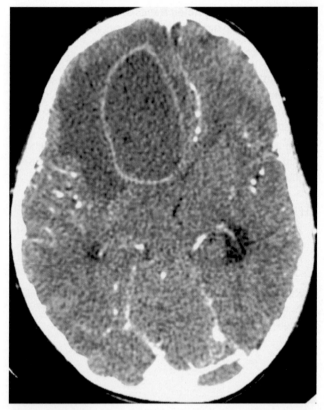

FIGURE **2.45A**

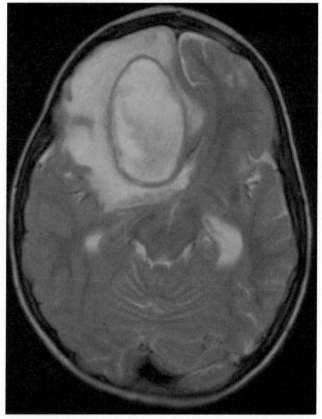

FIGURE **2.45B**

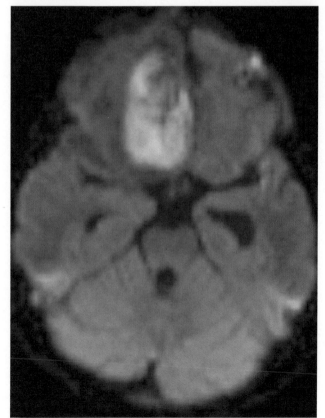

FIGURE **2.45C**

FINDINGS Contrast-enhanced axial CT head (**A**) demonstrates a slightly rim-enhancing lesion in the right inferior frontal lobe that is surrounded by hypoattenuating white matter with relative sparing of the gray matter, suggesting vasogenic edema. There is mass effect with right-to-left midline shift. Axial T2-weighted MRI image (**B**) demonstrates hyperintense lesion with a hypointense rim and surrounding hyperintense vasogenic edema with mass effect on the left frontal lobe. Axial DWI (**C**) demonstrates restricted diffusion (high signal) of the lesion (this was of low signal intensity on apparent diffusion coefficient (ADC) map, not shown).

DIFFERENTIAL DIAGNOSIS Brain abscess, neoplasm with necrotic center, tumefactive demyelination, tuberculoma, evolving hematoma/contusion, resolving/subacute infarct

DIAGNOSIS Brain abscess

DISCUSSION Intracranial abscesses are most commonly parenchymal, but can also be subdural or epidural in location (usually referred to as empyemas). They may result from hematogenous spread of infection, such as from septic emboli, or be secondary to head and neck infections (sinusitis or mastoiditis), trauma, and surgery. Contrast-enhanced

MRI is better than contrast-enhanced CT in evaluating abscesses. DWI helps differentiate abscess from other differentials, with abscess typically showing restricted diffusion. Spectroscopy is generally not needed but may be helpful in problem solving.[1] In the parenchyma, an abscess typically starts out as cerebritis which may only be evident as increased FLAIR signal (early cerebritis), and which may subsequently enhance and show restricted diffusion (late cerebritis). Subsequent necrosis and liquefaction of the center result in a rim-enhancing lesion which has restricted diffusion and is surrounded by vasogenic edema. The rim or capsule is low on T2-weighted MRI possibly from free radicals. In early stages, the capsule is thin-walled, regular, and may be thicker on its cortical aspect, postulated to be secondary to a higher blood supply to the cortex. Typically, in later stages, following treatment, the T2 hypointensity of the capsule decreases, the abscess no longer shows diffusion restriction, and eventually, rim enhancement is lost. Subdural and epidural abscesses/empyemas have similar peripheral enhancement and diffusion characteristics. Patients present with headaches, vomiting, seizures, and focal neurologic deficits. Surgical drainage is mandatory for larger abscesses with supportive antibiotic therapy. Antibiotics alone may be used for treatment of cerebritis and possibly for small abscesses.

DIFFERENTIAL DIAGNOSTIC CONSIDERATIONS

Neoplasm with necrotic center: Irregular enhancing walls; typically will not show restriction on diffusion.

Tumefactive demyelination: Restricted diffusion rare; typically, there is an incomplete rim of enhancement; no or minimal mass effect.

Tuberculoma: More chronic, indolent; fewer constitutional symptoms; may have history of TB elsewhere; diffusion restriction may be present.

Evolving hematoma/contusion: Has signal changes of blood products on T1 and T2 imaging; subacute blood products may restrict on diffusion imaging; appropriate antecedent history.

Resolving/subacute infarct: Enhancement when present is usually gyriform.

Questions for Further Thought

1. What are the phases of abscess evolution that might be seen at imaging?
2. What are the differences between pyogenic, TB, and fungal abscesses on DWI?

Reporting Responsibilities

Size and extent of abscess; mass effect and changes with therapy, if any.

What the Treating Physician Needs to Know

Diagnosis and response to treatment.[2]

Answers

1. Early and late cerebritis, early and late capsule phases.
2. Pyogenic: Frequently homogeneous diffusion restriction (bright on DWI and dark on ADC map).

   Fungal and TB: May or may not show restricted diffusion. If diffusion restriction is present, it usually is heterogeneous.[3]

REFERENCES

1. Kapsalaki EZ, Gotsis ED, Fountas KN. The role of proton magnetic resonance spectroscopy in the diagnosis and categorization of cerebral abscesses. *Neurosurg Focus.* 2008;24(6):E7.
2. Fanning NF, Laffan EE, Shroff MM. Serial diffusion-weighted MRI correlates with clinical course and treatment response in children with intracranial pus collections. *Pediatr Radiol.* 2006; 36(1):26–37.
3. Luthra G, Parihar A, Nath K, et al. Comparative evaluation of fungal, tubercular, and pyogenic brain abscesses with conventional and diffusion MR imaging and proton MR spectroscopy. *AJNR Am J Neuroradiol.* 2007;28(7):1332–1338.

Paritosh C. Khanna and Marguerite T. Parisi

CASE 2.46

CLINICAL HISTORY *A 1-year-old child, hospitalized with seizures following a motor vehicle accident, develops worsening mental status with coma (Figs. 2.46A and B)*

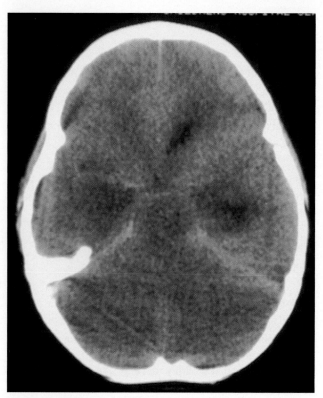

FIGURE 2.46A

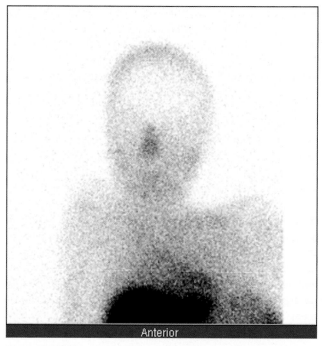

FIGURE 2.46B

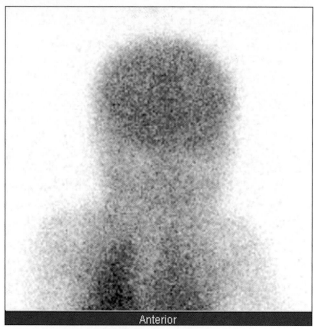

FIGURE 2.46C

FINDINGS Non-contrast CT (**A**) demonstrates severe cerebral edema and obliteration of the basilar cisterns. Static delayed anterior image obtained using technetium-99m hexamethylpropylene amine oxime (Tc-99m HMPAO) (**B**) demonstrates absence of radiotracer within the brain parenchyma. For comparison, in another patient, using the same radiopharmaceutical, normal uptake within brain parenchyma is demonstrated (**C**).

DIFFERENTIAL DIAGNOSIS CT: Global ischemic insult, diffuse cerebral edema. Nuclear medicine: Brain death

DIAGNOSIS Brain death

DISCUSSION Brain death is defined as the irreversible loss of function of the brain, including the brain stem.[1] It is essential, in view of the medicolegal implications of a diagnosis of brain death, that clinicians adhere to a uniform framework in making this determination. In 2010, the American Academy of Neurology issued new guidelines for determining brain death in adults.[2] While similar guidelines have not been issued for children, certain basic prerequisites apply.

First and foremost, the proximate cause of the patient's absence of clinical brain function must be known and be demonstrably irreversible. The three cardinal findings of brain death—coma or unresponsiveness, absence of brain stem reflexes, and apnea—must be present. Clinical neurologic testing is used to confirm absence of brain stem reflexes, including absent papillary and pain response, and may involve up to 25 different procedures. Apnea testing is then performed.[1,2]

Certain medical conditions may interfere with the clinical diagnosis of brain death. These include severe electrolyte or acid–base imbalance, endocrine disturbances, severe facial trauma, preexisting pupillary abnormalities, sleep apnea, or chronic pulmonary disease resulting in chronic carbon dioxide (CO_2) retention, hypothermia, poisoning, and drug intoxication (i.e., toxic levels of any of the following: sedative drugs, aminoglycosides, tricyclic antidepressants, anticholinergic agents, antiepileptic drugs, chemotherapeutic agents, or neuromuscular blocking agents). When any of the above conditions are present, the clinical diagnosis is not sufficient and ancillary, confirmatory testing becomes necessary in determining brain death.[1,2]

Conventional angiography, electroencephalogram (EEG), and nuclear medicine cerebral scintigraphy using the lipophilic class of agents are the preferred confirmatory tests when the clinical diagnosis of brain death is inconclusive. Cerebral scintigraphy is a simple, noninvasive method of determining the presence or absence of intracerebral perfusion, which does not require the withdrawal of medical therapy. It is particularly helpful when EEG is not possible due to severe head trauma, in cases of barbiturate, fentanyl, or pancuronium intoxication, hypothermia, hypovolemic shock, or when clinical examination is nondiagnostic.

There are two broad categories of radiotracers used for the determination of cerebral perfusion, cerebral blood flow (CBF), and lipophilic agents. The CBF agents are readily available and relatively inexpensive. These include technetium-99m pertechnetate (Tc-99mO$_4$) and technetium-99m diethylenetriaminepentaacetate (Tc-99m DTPA) which normally demonstrate activity in intracranial arteries and venous sinuses in the angiographic or flow phase. On the delayed static images, there is normally redistribution of radiotracer into the scalp soft tissues, calvarium, subarachnoid spaces that outline the hemispheres, as well as dural venous sinuses. These agents are excluded by a normal blood–brain barrier and do not enter the brain parenchyma.[3] Injection of an adequate bolus of radiotracer is essential for a diagnostic examination, and in the absence of distinct visualization of activity in the common carotid vessels in the neck, the radiotracer injection should be repeated.

The second category of radiotracers used for determination of cerebral perfusion is the lipophilic (brain-binding or brain-avid) agents including Tc-99m HMPAO and Tc-99m ethyl cysteinate dimer (Tc-99m EDC). These agents demonstrate a similar angiographic phase as the CBF agents, but with subsequent first-pass extraction by the brain parenchyma on delayed static images. These agents are taken up by the cerebral parenchyma in proportion to regional CBF (rCBF), and map brain perfusion in normal and pathologic states. Performance of the angiographic phase is optional when utilizing the lipophilic category of radiotracers.[4,5]

With the CBF agents (Tc-99mO$_4$ or Tc-99m DTPA), failure of visualization of radiotracer activity in the circle of Willis arteries on initial angiographic images (in the presence of an adequate bolus) and within dural venous sinuses on delayed planar images is consistent with brain death. There may be shunting of blood to the external carotid circulation resulting in the "hot nose" sign. Similarly, lack of first-pass uptake of lipophilic agents within the brain parenchyma is consistent with brain death (**B**). As a potential pitfall, it should be noted that the "hot nose" sign is a nonspecific finding which can be seen in brain death or those with occlusion of the internal carotid artery without brain death.

Questions for Further Thought

1. Which is the more sensitive radionuclide method in confirmation of a clinical suspicion of brain death?
2. Is ancillary testing always mandated for the determination of brain death and, if so, how many ancillary tests need to be performed?

Reporting Responsibilities

The technique (including the type of radionuclide agent used and documentation of adequacy of injection, if a CBF agent is utilized) as well as the presence or absence of intracerebral perfusion should be documented in the dictation. If nuclear cerebral scintigraphy confirms the clinical suspicion of brain death, the referring clinician should be immediately notified and the time of official interpretation documented for the medical record.

What the Treating Physician Needs to Know[1,2]

- When declaring a patient to be brain dead, the following must be known, demonstrated, and documented in the medical record:
  - The etiology and irreversibility of the underlying neurologic condition
  - Absence of brain stem reflexes
  - Absence of motor response to pain

- Absence of respiration with partial pressure of carbon dioxide (PCO_2) equal to or greater than 60 mm Hg
- Justification for confirmatory test (if performed) and result of such testing
- Repeat neurologic examination is NOT necessary but if performed, the interval is arbitrary. A 6-hour period is considered reasonable.
- The treating physician must, in accordance with federal and state law, contact an organ procurement organization.

Answers

1. Use of lipophilic group of agents is the more sensitive radionuclide method for confirmation of clinical diagnosis of brain death. This group of tracers allow for visualization of uptake within the cerebrum, cerebellum, and brain stem. Unlike the CBF agents which are highly dependent upon the adequacy of radiotracer bolus at time of injection, an angiographic phase is not mandatory when using lipophilic agents. Delayed images are usually definitive for the presence or absence of parenchymal uptake when using the lipophilic agents which also permit the performance of SPECT imaging to confirm absence of brain stem activity in difficult cases.

2. Ancillary/confirmatory testing is not mandatory for the determination of brain death and should be obtained only when clinical examination cannot be fully performed due to patient factors or if apnea testing is inconclusive.[2] When obtained, only one ancillary or confirmatory test is needed to confirm a clinical diagnosis of brain death.

REFERENCES

1. Practice parameters for determining brain death in adults (summary statement). The Quality Standards Subcommittee of the American Academy of Neurology. *Neurology.* 1995;45(5): 1012–1014.

2. Wijdicks EF, Varelas PN, Gronseth GS, et al. Evidence-based guideline update: determining brain death in adults: Report of the Quality Standards Subcommittee of the American Academy of Neurology. *Neurology.* 2010;74(23):1911–1918.

3. Mettler FA, Guiberteau MJ. Cerebrovascular system. In: Mettler FA, Guiberteau MJ, eds. *Essentials of Nuclear Medicine.* 5th ed. Philadelphia, PA: Saunders/Elsevier; 2006:53–57.

4. Society of Nuclear Medicine. *Society of Nuclear Medicine procedure guideline for brain death scintigraphy version 1.0.* Retrieved from http://www.snm.org/index.cfm?PageID=772 on 1/6/12.

5. American College of Radiology (ACR). ACR practice guideline for the performance of single photon emission computed tomography (SPECT) brain perfusion and brain death studies. Retrieved from http://www.acr.org/SecondaryMainMenuCategories/quality_safety/guidelines/nuc_med/ct_spect_brain_perfusion.aspx on 1/ 6/12.

CLINICAL HISTORY *A 2-year-old boy presents with developmental delay, sensorineural hearing loss (SNHL), and epilepsy (Figs. 2.47A and B)*

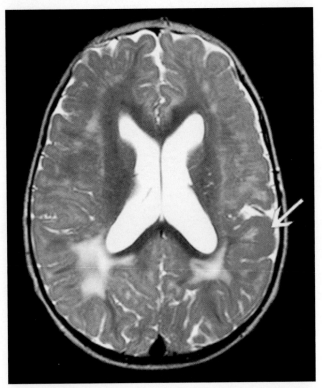

FIGURE **2.47A**

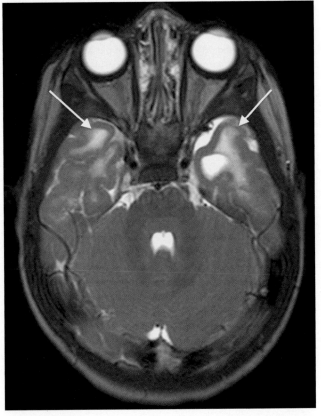

FIGURE **2.47B**

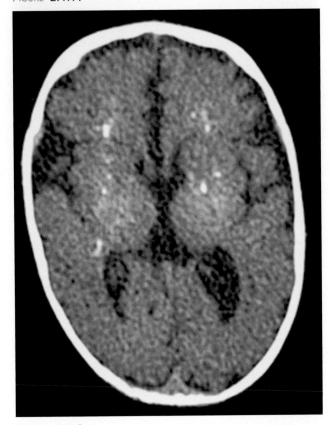

FIGURE **2.47C**

FINDINGS Axial T2-weighted MR images (**A** and **B**) show bilateral parietal white matter hyperintensity with ventriculomegaly. Also seen is diffuse subtle left-sided migrational abnormality (polymicrogyria), most pronounced in parietal region (*arrow,* **A**). Increased signal intensity in the anterior temporal lobes is also noted (*arrows,* **B**), a finding indicative of anterior temporal vacuolization/cyst formation. Axial non-contrast CT image (**C**) of another 2-year-old child shows fine punctate periventricular and basal ganglia calcifications.

DIFFERENTIAL DIAGNOSIS Congenital cytomegalovirus (CMV) infection, other TORCH infection such as toxoplasmosis, leukoencephalopathy with subcortical temporal cysts, and megalencephaly

DIAGNOSIS Congenital CMV infection

DISCUSSION Infecting 1% of all births, CMV is the most common intrauterine infection in the United States. Of infants infected with CMV, 10% to 20% come to clinical attention with signs and symptoms of hepatosplenomegaly, petechiae, hearing loss, seizures, microcephaly, intracranial calcifications, and chorioretinitis. CMV is a neurotropic DNA virus of the herpes family, transmitted by blood, urine, semen, cervical fluid, and breast milk, that hematogenously seeds the choroid plexus with replication in the ependymal cells.

Neuroimaging findings of congenital CMV depend on the fetal age at the time of infection. Common findings include intracranial calcification, migrational anomalies, volume loss, ventriculomegaly, and white matter disease. Infection at an earlier gestational age generally leads to poorer outcome. SNHL is common (up to 15% of infected patients), though temporal bone imaging studies (CT/MR) are usually normal. Microcephaly is present in up to 30% of patients, regardless of fetal age of infection.

Infection in the first half of the second trimester may result in multiple abnormalities including agyria-pachygyria, thinned cortex, abnormality of myelination, ventriculomegaly, periventricular calcification, and hypoplastic cerebellum. With infection in the late second trimester, findings may consist of polymicrogyria, ventricular dilation, and cerebellar hypoplasia (but typically less severe as compared to early second trimester infection). Perinatal infection may result in mild ventricular and sulcal prominence, and damaged periventricular and subcortical white matter with calcification or hemorrhage; the gyri are typically normal.

Cranial sonography of the newborn can show linear hyperechoic regions in the basal ganglia termed lenticulostriate vasculopathy. There can also be abnormal parenchymal hyperechogenicity, intraventricular septations, and sulcation abnormalities.

CT will show calcifications in 40% to 70% of patients. Common sites of calcification are periventricular regions, basal ganglia, and brain parenchyma. Calcifications are often thick in the periventricular region but tend to be punctate within the basal ganglia. Ventriculomegaly is the second most common finding after calcification. Imaging findings of calcifications with associated volume loss and hydrocephalus can also be seen in other TORCH infections, particularly congenital toxoplasmosis. However, the most important differentiating imaging feature of CMV is the presence of associated malformations of cortical development.

MRI has higher specificity than CT for showing subtle findings. MRI is very helpful in delineating the type and extent of migrational abnormality, white matter, and cerebellar involvement. Patients with agyria-pachygyria have worse neurologic outcome, and their presence implies earlier fetal infection.

White matter disease is common, and a distinct pattern of abnormal parietal or posterior white matter involvement with sparing of a small zone of subcortical and periventricular white matter is usually seen in asymptomatic patients with congenital CMV infection. Anterior temporal lobe cysts and vacuolization (hyperintense signal on fluid-sensitive sequences) can also be seen along with white matter involvement. Presence of anterior temporal lobe cysts and vacuolization with white matter disease strongly suggests congenital CMV infection as a combination of white matter disease along with anterior temporal lobe cysts has a very small differential of congenital CMV, vanishing white matter disease, and leukoencephalopathy with subcortical temporal cysts and megalencephaly. A combination of abnormal white matter disease and migration abnormalities also strongly suggests congenital CMV in asymptomatic patients.

Questions for Further Thought

1. Is periventricular calcification specific for CMV infection?
2. Does lack of calcification on CT exclude CMV infection?

Reporting Responsibilities

- White matter disease due to CMV is a static process. If there is progressive increase in disease, another explanation should be sought.
- Acquired postnatal CMV infection can occur in the setting of immunosuppression such as transplant and HIV patients. Findings include meningo-ventriculo-encephalitis.

What the Treating Physician Needs to Know

Early diagnosis can lead to antiviral treatment that can help minimize hearing loss.

Answers

1. No, periventricular calcification can be caused by other etiologies including other TORCH infections and anoxic/toxic brain injuries. However, if periventricular calcification is seen along with delayed myelination, cortical malformations, and cerebellar hypoplasia, CMV should be considered.
2. No. Up to 30% of patients will not have calcification.

REFERENCES

1. Fink KR, Thapa MM, Ishak GE, et al. Neuroimaging of pediatric central nervous system cytomegalovirus infection. *Radiographics.* 2010;30(7):1779–1796.
2. Van der Knaap MS, Vermeulen G, Barkhof F, et al. Pattern of white matter abnormalities at MR imaging: use of polymerase chain reaction testing of Guthrie cards to link pattern with congenital cytomegalovirus infection. *Radiology.* 2004;230(2):529–536.

CASE 2.48

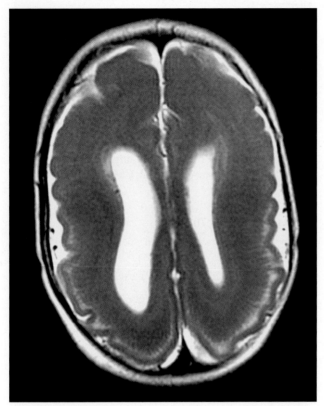

FIGURE **2.48A**

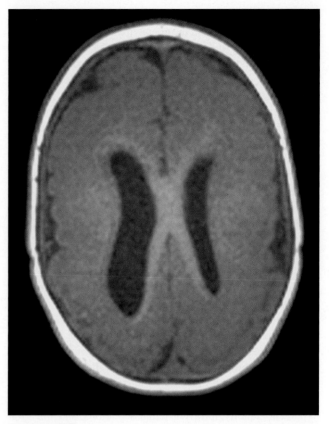

FIGURE **2.48B**

FINDINGS Axial T2-weighted MRI image (**A**) at the level of lateral ventricles shows agyria in the frontal lobes and pachygyria posteriorly. In the parietal lobes, a trilaminar appearance is seen with a thin outer cortex with very shallow sulci, an intermediate thin layer with T2 hyperintensity, and a thickened inner gray matter cortex. Axial T1-weighted gradient image (**B**) at the same level shows a smooth-appearing brain surface with diffuse abnormal thickened cortex.

DIFFERENTIAL DIAGNOSIS Lissencephaly, microcephaly with simplified gyral pattern, polymicrogyria

DIAGNOSIS Lissencephaly

DISCUSSION Lissencephaly (smooth brain), also referred to as "agyria-pachygyria" complex, is due to arrest of normal neuronal migration during the third and fourth months of gestation. On imaging, lissencephaly is characterized by a combination of complete or partial lack of gyri, and an excessively thick cortex. In agyria, there is complete

absence of gyri with a thickened cortex. In pachygyria, there are a few flat and broadened gyri, also with a thick cortex but not as thick as in agyria.

Clinical presentation of lissencephaly includes spasticity, global developmental delay, and intractable seizures. Genetic work has found many causes of lissencephaly. Up to seventy-five percent of cases are believed due to mutations in either the *LIS1* or *DCX/XLIS* genes. Acquired causes of lissencephaly include in utero CMV infection, radiation, and fetal alcohol syndrome. Consanguinity of parents can also result in lissencephaly.

Imaging of lissencephaly demonstrates a thickened cortex, a quintessential feature to diagnose this entity. A cell sparse zone, usually seen as an area of T2 prolongation, separates the outer cortex from a deeper cortical layer. This three-layer appearance on T2-weighted imaging is characteristic of lissencephaly. On imaging, complete lissencephaly appears as a brain with a smooth surface and lack of gyri. A figure-of-eight or hourglass appearance may be seen on axial images due to shallow and vertical sylvian fissures.

It is however important to note that if reviewing fetal MRI or prenatal ultrasound, the normal fetal brain has a smooth surface and an hourglass appearance up to 26 weeks of gestation. In incomplete lissencephaly, a gradient may be seen with areas of agyria, pachygyria, and even some intervening normal brain. Incomplete lissencephaly is much more common than the complete form.

Polymicrogyria, which refers to multiple small gyri, can often have a similar imaging appearance to pachygyria; distinction is aided with the use of high-resolution, thin-section imaging. In pachygyria, sulci that are present remain in normal anatomic locations, whereas in polymicrogyria the sulci may occur in nonanatomic locations. In addition, in polymicrogyria, the junction between the white and gray matter is irregular and bumpy with multiple indentations, whereas the junction of the thickened cortex with the underlying white matter is smooth with pachygyria.

Question for Further Thought

1. How can classic lissencephaly be differentiated from microcephaly with simplified gyral pattern?

Reporting Responsibilities

An area of polymicrogyria can resemble and is easily confused and reported as pachygyria. The difference can be difficult and may only be appreciated if high-resolution, thin-section imaging is obtained.

What the Treating Physician Needs to Know

The location of agyria in incomplete lissencephaly can suggest presence of a genetic mutation depending on involvement of the frontal (*DCX/XLIS* or *RELN* genes) or parieto-occipital (*LIS1* or *ARX* genes) lobes. Mothers of patients with DCX/XLIS X-linked lissencephaly usually have asymptomatic band heterotopia. Genetic testing and counseling of these mothers should be considered as future offspring could be affected.

Answer

1. The cortex will be always thickened in lissencephaly and is usually normal or thin in microcephaly with simplified gyral pattern.

REFERENCES

1. Barkovich AJ, Raybaud CA. Congenital malformations of the brain and skull. In: Barkovich AJ, Raybaud C, eds. *Pediatric Neuroimaging*. 5th ed. Philadelphia, PA: Lippincott Williams & Wilkins; 2012:367–568.

2. Ghai S, Fong KW, Toi A, et al. Prenatal US and MR imaging findings of lissencephaly: Review of fetal cerebral sulcal development. *Radiographics*. 2006;26(2):389–405.

3. Raybaud C, Widjaja E. Development and dysgenesis of the cerebral cortex: Malformations of cortical development. *Neuroimaging Clin N Am*. 2011;21(3):483–543.

Sumit Pruthi and Matthew D. Dobbs

CLINICAL HISTORY *A teenage male presents with paralysis of upward gaze*

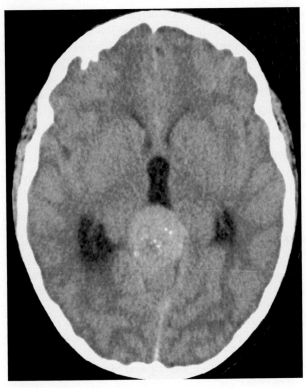

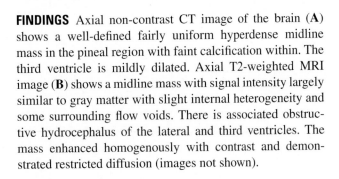

FIGURE **2.49A**

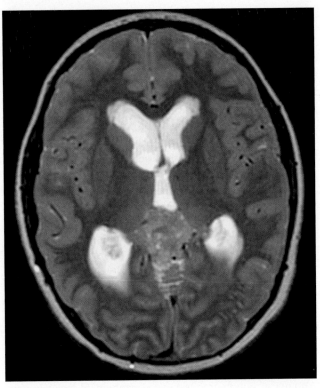

FIGURE **2.49B**

FINDINGS Axial non-contrast CT image of the brain (**A**) shows a well-defined fairly uniform hyperdense midline mass in the pineal region with faint calcification within. The third ventricle is mildly dilated. Axial T2-weighted MRI image (**B**) shows a midline mass with signal intensity largely similar to gray matter with slight internal heterogeneity and some surrounding flow voids. There is associated obstructive hydrocephalus of the lateral and third ventricles. The mass enhanced homogenously with contrast and demonstrated restricted diffusion (images not shown).

DIFFERENTIAL DIAGNOSIS Pineal germinoma, pineoblastoma, pineocytoma, astrocytoma, teratoma

DIAGNOSIS Pineal germinoma

DISCUSSION Primary CNS GCTs are broadly divided based on histology into germinomas and nongerminomatous GCTs (NGGCTs), with teratomas (mature and malignant), considered as separate entities. The NGGCTs include choriocarcinoma, yolk sac tumors, and embryonal carcinoma.

The vast majority of GCTs occur in the midline, in close association to the third ventricle. Germinomas constitute the majority of the GCTs with the most common location being the pineal region. The majority of germinomas occur in

10- to 30-year-old patients with a peak in the late teenage years, and a 10:1 male to female ratio in the pineal region. Thirty-five percent of germinomas occur in the suprasellar region, but in this area there is no sex predilection. Up to 10% of germinomas occur in the thalamus, basal ganglia and cerebral hemispheres.

Clinical features in germinomas are often related to tumor location and size. Hydrocephalus and paralysis of upward gaze (Parinaud syndrome) are the most common presenting complaints for pineal germinomas, even at a very early disease stage and small size of the tumor. Diabetes insipidus and endocrine abnormalities are seen with suprasellar germinomas.

On CT, germinomas usually are well-defined iso- to hyperdense masses with homogenous contrast enhancement. They often engulf the pineal gland calcifications. Classic teaching states that germinomas engulf the pineal gland calcifications, while pineocytoma/pineoblastoma "explodes" the calcification and has peripheral calcification, but exceptions to these rules are common. On both T1- and T2-weighted MRI imaging, germinomas typically demonstrate a hypo- to isointense well-defined lobulated mass lesion. Intense enhancement is usually seen with contrast administration. Due to their hypercellularity, diffusion restriction can be seen with DWI, which also accounts for the hyperdense appearance on CT and hypointense appearance on T2-weighted MRI.

The above-mentioned imaging characteristics are unable to reliably differentiate germinoma from NGGCT or from intrinsic pineal tumor as they often share similar imaging features. Hence, the diagnosis of specific pineal region tumor is often based on a combination of assessment of serum tumor markers (alpha-fetoprotein (AFP), beta-human chorionic gonadotropin (beta-HCG), and placental alkaline phosphatase), neuroimaging characteristics, and cytologic (CSF) and/or histologic assessments. Determination of type of tumor is important as the clinical behavior, treatment options, and prognosis of germinoma, NGGCT, and other intrinsic pineal region tumors are quite different.

CNS GCTs have a propensity to disseminate throughout the neural axis, even at early disease stages, and thus complete CNS staging is mandatory for all CNS GCTs. Radiation therapy is the first line of treatment with 5 year survival rates near 90%.

Questions for Further Thought

1. In a pediatric patient presenting with diabetes insipidus, what is the most likely differential diagnosis?
2. In a child with diabetes insipidus and a negative MR study, what should be recommended?

Relevant Anatomy

Astrocytomas and germinomas can appear similar, particularly in the suprasellar region, but germinomas usually have iso- to hypointense regions on T2-weighted imaging as well as extension along the pituitary infundibulum, as opposed to astrocytomas which usually are centered along the chiasm and are usually hyperintense. Patients with germinoma are also more likely to have diabetes insipidus compared to astrocytoma.

Reporting Responsibilities

It is difficult to differentiate, on imaging, pineal GCTs from pineal parenchymal tumors. On imaging, it is important to assess for CSF dissemination and acute hydrocephalus.

What the Treating Physician Needs to Know

- Is there hydrocephalus?
- Is there CSF dissemination?

Answers

1. LCH and germinoma.
2. Repeat MRI with contrast in 3 months. Symptoms occasionally precede imaging abnormalities of the hypothalamic stalk with germinoma. Lack of the normal bright signal of the posterior pituitary gland is an early finding of involvement.

REFERENCES

1. Smith AB, Rushing EJ, Smirniotopoulos JG. From the archives of the AFIP: Lesions of the pineal region: radiologic-pathologic correlation. *Radiographics.* 2010;30(7):2001–2020.
2. Raybaud C, Barkovich AJ. Intracranial, orbital, and neck masses of childhood. In: Barkovich AJ, Raybaud C, eds. *Pediatric Neuroimaging.* 5th ed. Philadelphia, PA: Lippincott Williams & Wilkins; 2012:637–807.

Sumit Pruthi and Matthew D. Dobbs

CLINICAL HISTORY *A 16-year-old female with uncontrolled hypertension who presents with sudden onset visual disturbance and headache*

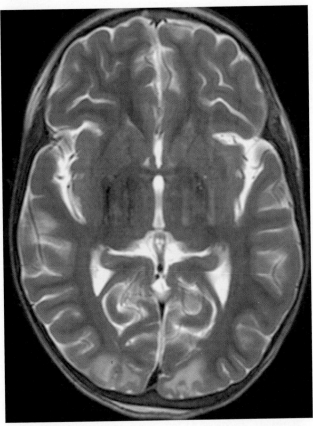

FIGURE **2.50A**

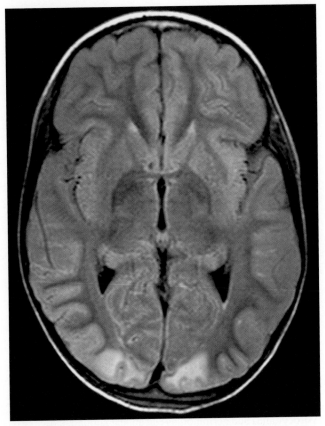

FIGURE **2.50B**

FINDINGS Axial MR T2-weighted (**A**) and FLAIR (**B**) images of the brain demonstrate bilateral, symmetric hyperintense signal within the occipital subcortical white matter.

DIFFERENTIAL DIAGNOSIS Posterior reversible encephalopathy syndrome (PRES), vertebrobasilar insufficiency or posterior stroke, encephalitis, reversible cerebral vasoconstriction syndrome, CNS vasculitis, status epilepticus

DIAGNOSIS PRES

DISCUSSION PRES is a clinicoradiologic entity which presents with headache, seizures, vomiting, and visual abnormalities in association with predominant posterior subcortical white matter vasogenic edema. These symptoms normally start abruptly, peaking within 24 hours. Symptoms usually resolve within 1 week. Resolution of imaging abnormalities lags behind clinical improvement.

There are numerous causes of PRES including pre-eclampsia/eclampsia, immune modulating drugs (cyclosporine and tacrolimus), renal failure, transplantation (solid organ and bone marrow), systemic lupus erythematosus, Wegener granulomatosis, scleroderma, shock, and sepsis. Most cases of PRES occur in the setting of uncontrolled hypertension or immunosuppression. The pathophysiology of PRES is still being investigated and debated. One principal theory is that hypertension leads to cerebrovascular dysregulation, subsequent hyperperfusion, endothelial injury, and vasogenic edema. The posterior circulation has a less developed sympathetic regulatory system explaining the preferential involvement. Other theories include systemic toxicity leading to endothelial dysfunction, with subsequent hypoperfusion and vasospasm.

CT is often negative and MRI is the preferred imaging modality. Abnormal signal is most often seen in the parieto-occipital lobes bilaterally in a somewhat symmetric manner, followed by superior frontal sulcus involvement. Other areas of the brain can be affected, but usually this is seen in conjunction with parieto-occipital abnormality. Subcortical white matter is normally involved, but there can also be involvement of cortex. Signal is low on T1-weighted and bright on T2-weighted/FLAIR imaging. Restricted diffusion, present in 10% to 20% of cases, suggests areas of cytotoxic rather than vasogenic edema, implying more severe injury. Patchy contrast enhancement can occasionally be seen. Intraparenchymal hemorrhage is seen in less than 15% on GRE or SWI. MR perfusion has shown significant posterior brain hypoperfusion with increased mean transit time and decreased cerebral blood volume in patients with PRES. Conventional angiography can demonstrate findings very similar to arteritis or vasospasm with areas of vasoconstriction and vasodilation. Follow-up MRI after appropriate therapy for the cause of PRES usually shows resolution unless the condition progresses to infarction or hemorrhage.

Question for Further Thought

1. What are the three common imaging patterns seen with PRES?

Relevant Anatomy

In PRES, signal abnormalities involving the occipital lobe typically spare the calcarine and paramedian occipital lobe, a feature which helps to distinguish this syndrome from bilateral infarctions of the posterior cerebral artery.

Reporting Responsibilities

Repeat imaging in 2 to 3 weeks will hopefully show resolution of abnormalities, strengthening a presumptive diagnosis of PRES.

What the Treating Physician Needs to Know

Clinical signs and symptoms of PRES are often nonspecific and imaging plays a very important role in diagnosis. The pattern of bilateral occipital edema is highly suggestive of PRES in the appropriate clinical setting. Early diagnosis and prompt treatment can prevent complications such as infarction and hemorrhage.

Answer

1. (a) Dominant parieto-occipital pattern; (b) superior frontal sulcus pattern; and (c) holohemispheric, watershed pattern.

REFERENCES

1. Bartynski WS. Posterior reversible encephalopathy syndrome, part 1: Fundamental imaging and clinical features. *AJNR Am J Neuroradiol.* 2008;29(6):1036–1042.

2. Bartynski WS. Posterior reversible encephalopathy syndrome, part 2: Controversies surrounding pathophysiology of vasogenic edema *AJNR Am J Neuroradiol.* 2008;29(6):1043–1049.

3. Bartynski WS, Boardman JF. Catheter angiography, MR angiography, and MR perfusion in posterior reversible encephalopathy syndrome. *AJNR Am J Neuroradiol.* 2008;29(3):447–455.

4. Bartynski WS, Boardman JF. Distinct imaging patterns and lesion distribution in posterior reversible encephalopathy syndrome. *AJNR Am J Neuroradiol.* 2007;28(7):1320–1327.

Sumit Pruthi and Matthew D. Dobbs

CLINICAL HISTORY *An 18-year-old girl with history of recurrent headaches who presents with a clinical episode of transient ischemic attack*

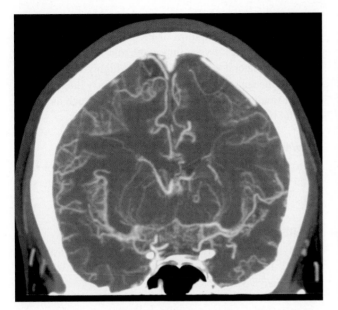

FIGURE **2.51A**

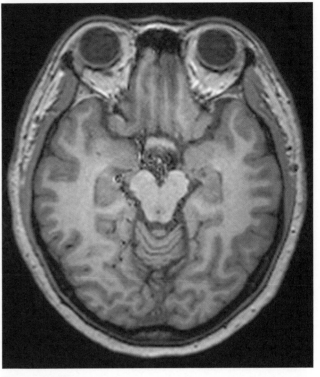

FIGURE **2.51B**

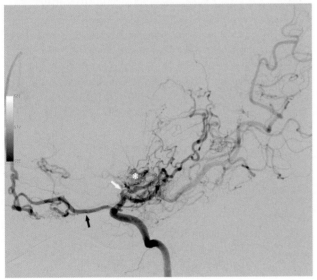

FIGURE **2.51C**

FINDINGS CT angiogram coronal reformat (**A**) at the level of the basal ganglia shows severe tapering of the distal supraclinoid internal carotid arteries and diminution of the middle cerebral arteries. There is marked hypertrophy of the lenticulostriate arteries within the basal ganglia as well as prominent meningeal collateral vessels. Axial image from a T1-weighted 3D gradient MRI sequence (**B**) shows numerous black serpentine flow voids coursing around the midbrain and interpeduncular cistern representing enlarged lenticulostriate arteries. Lateral angiographic projection of an internal carotid artery injection performed 3 months later (**C**) shows absence of the normal filling of the anterior and middle cerebral arteries. The supraclinoid internal carotid artery severely tapers (*white arrow*) and the lenticulostriate arteries constitute a "puff of smoke" on angiography (*asterisk*). Note the enlarged ophthalmic artery (*black arrow*) (first branch from the supraclinoid carotid) supplying an anterior frontal lobe meningeal collateral.

DIFFERENTIAL DIAGNOSIS Moyamoya disease or syndrome, vasculitis, carotid dissection, traumatic occlusion, atherosclerotic disease

DIAGNOSIS Moyamoya disease or syndrome

DISCUSSION Moyamoya is a slowly progressive vasculopathy that involves narrowing of the supraclinoid internal carotid arteries and proximal anterior and middle cerebral arteries, usually with sparing of the posterior circulation (until late in the disease process). Decreased blood flow spurs development of collateral vessels throughout the brain. Bimodal age peaks are at about age 5 years and patients in their mid-30s to mid-40s. Pediatric patients often present with transient ischemia, stroke, headache, or seizures while adults tend to present with subarachnoid or intraparenchymal hemorrhage. Seventy percent of cases are discovered within the first two decades of life. Originally described in Japanese patients, it has been observed in ethnicities around the world, but it is about 10 times more common in Japanese and Koreans. Female to male ratio is 2:1. It is the most frequent cause of stroke in Asian children.

Moyamoya disease, which is usually bilateral, is the term used for those patients with moyamoya vasculopathy with no associated risk factors. Patients with associated conditions are said to have moyamoya syndrome, which can be unilateral. Diseases classically associated with moyamoya syndrome are NF1, Down syndrome, sickle cell disease, and radiation therapy (particularly radiation for treatment of pituitary tumors, craniopharyngiomas, or optic pathway gliomas). Rare causes include glycogen storage disease Type 1a, TB meningitis, and chronic prothrombotic blood disorders.

Catheter angiography of the internal and external carotid arteries as well as the posterior circulation is the gold standard of imaging and preoperative planning, but CT or MR angiography is often the first imaging evaluation obtained as patients typically present with symptoms of ischemia or hemorrhage. Angiography demonstrates narrowing of the anterior cerebral circulation with dilation of lenticulostriate and thalamoperforator vessels. The dilated collateral network was originally described as "something hazy, like a puff of cigarette smoke" which translates into the Japanese word "moyamoya." In some patients, a radial appearance of dilated pial and medullary veins may also be seen.

CT imaging of patients with moyamoya is notable for cerebral infarctions most commonly in watershed vascular territories. On MRI, apart from the areas of infarction, dilated lenticulostriate vessels can be seen within the deep basal ganglia and thalamus as serpentine flow voids on T1- and T2-weighted sequences. The normal intravascular flow voids of the internal carotid, middle cerebral, and anterior cerebral arteries are diminished. On FLAIR and T1-weighted imaging with gadolinium, dilated leptomeningeal vessels are noted as bright vessels creeping along the cortical sulci and have been termed the "ivy sign." Advanced preoperative

imaging can include quantification of cerebral perfusion and cerebral reserves using modalities such as xenon CT, perfusion CT, PET, MR perfusion with acetazolamide or carbon dioxide challenge, and transcranial Doppler.

Most centers recommend early surgical revascularization for treatment. Moyamoya spares the external carotid system, allowing these vessels to be used for direct or indirect revascularization.

Question for Further Thought

1. What is the Suzuki grading system for moyamoya disease?

Reporting Responsibilities

- Look for signs of ongoing ischemia or new area of infarcts as well as imaging findings predictive of disease progression.
- In patients with unilateral disease, it is important to look for any abnormal vessels or signs of developing disease on the contralateral side.

What the Treating Physician Needs to Know

Without treatment, the majority of patients have symptomatic progression over a 5-year period. Following revascularization, the rate of progression significantly drops. Thus, early recognition and prompt treatment are crucial in order to alter the prognosis in this entity.

Answer

1. It is a grading system to assess severity of the disease at presentation. Severity of angiographic disease is assigned on a scale ranging from grade 1 to 6, with 6 being the most severe.

REFERENCES

1. Suzuki J, Takaku A. Cerebrovascular "moyamoya" disease. Disease showing abnormal net-like vessels in base of brain. *Arch Neurol.* 1969;20(3):288–299.
2. Fung LW, Thompson D, Ganesan V. Revascularisation surgery for paediatric moyamoya: A review of the literature. *Childs Nerv Syst.* 2005;21(5):358–364.
3. Scott RM, Smith ER. Moyamoya disease and moyamoya syndrome. *N Eng J Med.* 2009;360(12):1226–1237.
4. Yoon HK, Shin HJ, Chang YW. "Ivy sign" in childhood moyamoya disease: Depiction on FLAIR and contrast-enhanced T1-weighted MR images. *Radiology.* 2002;223(2):384–389.

CASE 2.52

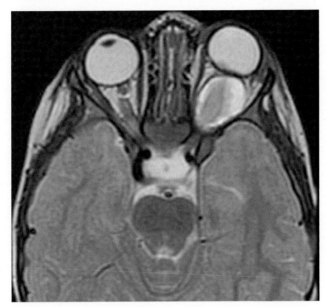

FIGURE 2.52A

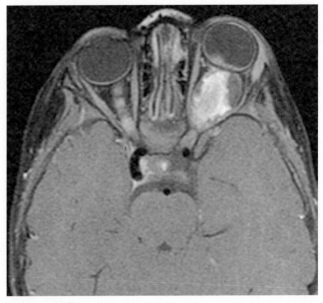

FIGURE 2.52B

FINDINGS Axial T2-weighted MRI image (**A**) demonstrates diffuse enlargement of the left optic nerve. There is associated diffuse enlargement of the surrounding CSF-containing optic nerve sheath. Axial postcontrast T1-weighted fat-suppressed MRI image (**B**) reveals significant enhancement of the enlarged left optic nerve.

DIFFERENTIAL DIAGNOSIS Optic pathway glioma (optic nerve glioma), orbital pseudotumor, meningioma, lymphoma

DIAGNOSIS Optic pathway glioma (optic nerve glioma)

DISCUSSION Optic pathway gliomas most often affect children less than 10 years of age, with a female predominance, and account for approximately 5% of pediatric brain tumors. There is a strong association with NF1 as 30% to 40% of patients with optic gliomas also have NF1. Children with optic gliomas often present with visual disturbances or hypothalamic dysfunction and/or hydrocephalus.

Pathologically, optic pathway gliomas are benign lesions with most classified as juvenile pilocytic astrocytomas (JPAs; WHO grade I). The majority of optic pathway gliomas in patients with NF1 remain stable over time, while the converse is true for optic pathway gliomas in patients without NF1. Therapy is only instituted if lesions progress rapidly and/or cause symptoms, predominantly visual decline.

Typical neuroimaging findings of optic pathway glioma include diffuse fusiform enlargement of the optic nerve without calcification that can often extend posteriorly toward the optic chiasm. The tumor can also arise from the optic chiasm and extend anteriorly or posteriorly along the optic pathway. Although intraconal orbital fat provides adequate tissue contrast on CT if only the optic nerve is involved, brain MRI is the preferred imaging modality to better evaluate for involvement posterior to the optic canal as well as for findings supportive of a diagnosis of NF1. MRI findings usually include T1 hypointensity, T2 hyperintensity, and variable contrast enhancement (ranging from none to intense). An important point to note is that imaging features and prognosis are different for optic gliomas with and without NF1. Features suggestive of optic glioma with NF1 include "kinked" or tortuous optic nerve, T2-hyperintense rim around the tumor reflecting perineural arachnoidal gliomatosis, bilaterality, tumor extension posterior to the chiasm along the optic tracts, and less intense to minimal contrast enhancement. Smooth fusiform enlargement is typically seen in children with NF1 versus more nodular and cystic enlargement in children without NF1. In the absence of NF1, these tumors are mainly located around the chiasm and on imaging are more likely to resemble the imaging features of pilocytic astrocytoma at other sites including presence of cystic and solid components with intense enhancement of the solid component. Optic glioma without NF1 also tends to have more intraneural as opposed to perineural spread, somewhat explaining the difference in prognosis.

DIFFERENTIAL DIAGNOSTIC CONSIDERATIONS

If there is isolated optic nerve involvement then the primary differential consideration is optic nerve sheath meningioma, with calcification in tramtrack-like manner and more peripheral as opposed to central enhancement favoring meningioma.

Orbital pseudotumor can affect any part of the orbit including muscles, tendons, fat, optic nerve, nerve sheath, and lacrimal gland, and would typically have more signs of surrounding inflammation with more fat stranding and edema.

Lymphoma is also in the differential and would likely have homogenous enhancement and possibly show restricted diffusion on DWI.

Question for Further Thought

1. What are pilomyxoid astrocytomas?

Relevant Anatomy

Pilocytic astrocytomas can also arise from the hypothalamus, which is in close proximity to the optic chiasm. In large tumors, it can be difficult to discern the site of origin. Hypothalamic involvement explains the endocrine abnormalities seen in many of these patients.

Reporting Responsibilities

If optic glioma is diagnosed, look for other supporting imaging features of NF1 as the prognosis of optic glioma differs depending on whether or not the patient has NF1.

What the Treating Physician Needs to Know

For young patients under the age of 5 years with NF1, annual ophthalmic exam rather than MRI is suggested to screen for asymptomatic optic pathway lesion. Once a lesion is identified, MRI at 3- to 12-month intervals, along with ophthalmic and endocrine evaluations, are recommended. Treatment is usually instituted if there is progressive worsening of visual symptoms or increase in size of the tumor.

Answer

1. Pilomyxoid astrocytomas are a relatively new subgroup of optic pathway gliomas that were once classified with pilocytic astrocytomas but are now considered as a distinct entity with more aggressive behavior and are classified as WHO grade II rather than WHO grade I tumors.

REFERENCES

1. Listernick R, Darling C, Greenwald M, et al. Optic pathway tumors in children: The effect of neurofibromatosis type 1 on clinical manifestations and natural history. *J Pediatr.* 1995; 127(5):718–722.

2. Kornreich L, Blaser S, Schwarz M, et al. Optic pathway glioma: Correlation of imaging findings with the presence of neurofibromatosis. *AJNR Am J Neuroradiol.* 2001;22(10):1963–1969.

3. Komotar RJ, Mocco J, Jones JE, et al. Pilomyxoid astrocytoma: Diagnosis, prognosis, and management. *Neurosurg Focus.* 2005; 18(6A):E7.

Sumit Pruthi and Matthew D. Dobbs

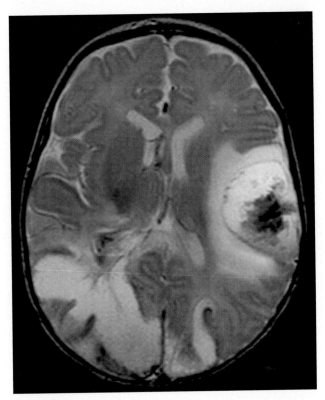

FIGURE 2.53A

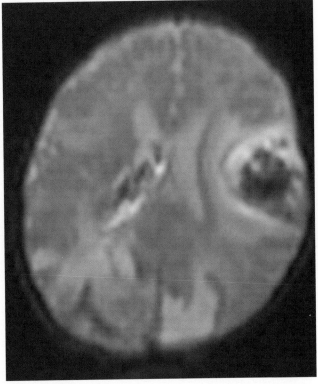

FIGURE 2.53B

FINDINGS Axial T2-weighted MRI image (**A**) shows a hyperintense lesion with central signal dropout (presumably blood product) in the left frontoparietal region with surrounding edema. There are additional areas of hyperintense signal abnormality in the white matter and cortex of bilateral parieto-occipital lobes. Blood is also present in the right lateral ventricle. Axial GRE sequence (**B**) shows blooming artifact (dark signal) in the right lateral ventricle and left frontal cortex indicating blood product. Abnormal increased signal is also present in bilateral parieto-occipital regions, better seen on the first image, with subtle hypointense signal surrounding the edge of these regions likely representing blood products.

DIFFERENTIAL DIAGNOSIS Neonatal herpes encephalitis, other TORCH infection, bacterial meningitis/encephalitis, ischemia/anoxic brain injury

DIAGNOSIS Neonatal herpes encephalitis

DISCUSSION Herpes simplex encephalitis (HSE) is the most common cause of sporadic, nonepidemic viral encephalitis in the United States. HSE occurs as two distinct entities. In children older than 3 months and in adults, it is usually caused by reactivation of prior latent infection from herpes simplex virus type 1 (HSV-1). In neonates and infants, herpes encephalitis is most often due to herpes simplex virus type 2 (HSV-2) acquired most commonly from the birth canal during delivery. A smaller percentage of cases can be transmitted in utero or postpartum. Only 20% to 25% of neonatal herpes encephalitis is due to HSV-1.

In neonatal HSE, symptoms usually begin at 2 to 4 weeks of life with fever, lethargy, bulging fontanelles, or seizures. Though neuroimaging plays a very important role in early diagnosis and timely initiation of therapy, a negative neuroimaging study does not rule out HSV encephalitis. Given the poor prognosis, treatment should be empirically initiated until the diagnosis is definitively excluded.

MRI is the most robust and sensitive imaging modality for the detection of HSE. DWI often shows restricted diffusion, and will be the first and most sensitive sequence to demonstrate an abnormality. Studies have shown that in neonatal herpes, areas initially showing restricted diffusion on DWI usually progress to areas of cystic encephalomalacia within a few weeks. Hypointense T1 and hyperintense T2 signal can be seen in affected areas. There can be patchy cortical and meningeal contrast enhancement.

In comparison to adult HSE, which typically and predominantly involves the temporal lobes, frontal lobes, and insular cortex bilaterally, the involvement is much more diffuse in neonatal HSE and quiet variable. All lobes can be affected and the cerebellum is involved in half of all cases. Basal ganglia, which are typically spared in adult HSE, are often involved with neonatal encephalitis. That being said, the imaging appearance of neonatal HSE can resemble adult onset HSV with typical involvement of the temporal lobes and limbic system with associated hemorrhage. Periventricular white matter involvement with restricted diffusion is also commonly seen in neonatal HSE. Infarction in a watershed distribution can also be seen, which could mimic a hypoxic injury. Brain tissue necrosis can be rapid with HSV-2 encephalitis and within 1 to 2 weeks significant cystic encephalomalacia can develop. Calcification of gyri or deeper brain parenchyma can be seen as a sequela of prior infection.

Questions for Further Thought

1. What is the prognosis of neonatal herpes encephalitis?
2. What is the most useful MRI sequence for detection of neonatal herpes encephalitis?

Relevant Anatomy

Imaging features suggest whether the infection occurred in utero or postnatally. In utero infection will have progressed to atrophy, scattered areas of calcification, ventricular enlargement, and cystic encephalomalacia. More recent infection will demonstrate restricted diffusion and lack the atrophic appearance.

Neonatal HSV infection has three patterns: (1) skin, eye, and mouth disease; (2) disseminated disease with or without CNS disease; and (3) encephalitis.

Reporting Responsibilities

Suspicion of herpes encephalitis is an urgent finding, and communication needs to be established quickly with the referring physician so antiviral medication and further testing can be initiated.

What the Treating Physician Needs to Know

There must be a high index of suspicion for neonatal herpes encephalitis, as treatment needs to be initiated before definitive diagnostic testing to decrease mortality. Only about 25% of mothers have herpetic genital rash at the time of delivery. Polymerase chain reaction (PCR) analysis of CSF is becoming the test of choice, but results can take several days to return. Intravenous acyclovir is the treatment of choice.

Answers

1. Mortality rate is approximately 50% without antiviral treatment. If disease is disseminated, mortality rate is about 85%. The earlier treatment is begun, the better the prognosis.
2. DWI. In one large series, in 20% of patients, only the DWI sequence demonstrated an abnormality at time of initial imaging.

REFERENCES

1. Vossough A, Zimmerman RA, Bilaniuk LT, et al. Imaging findings of neonatal herpes simplex virus type 2 encephalitis. *Neuroradiology.* 2008;50(4):355–366.
2. Kimberlin DW. Neonatal herpes simplex infection. *Clin Microbiol Rev.* 2004;17(1):1–13.

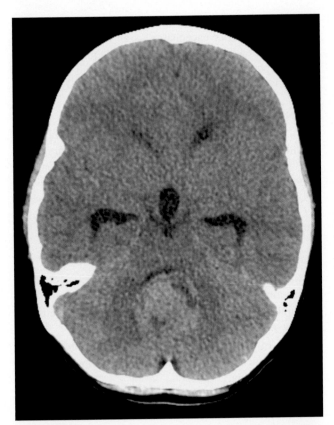

FIGURE 2.54A

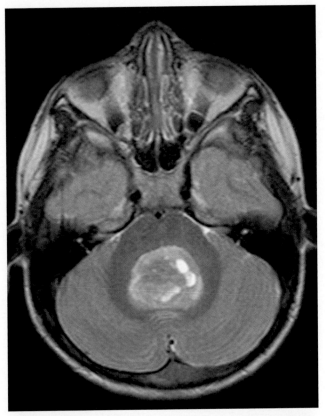

FIGURE 2.54B

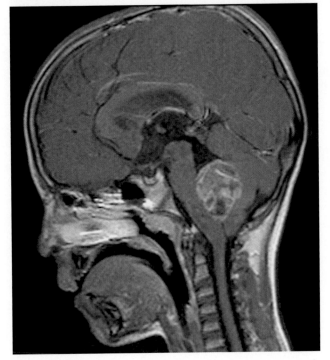

FIGURE 2.54C

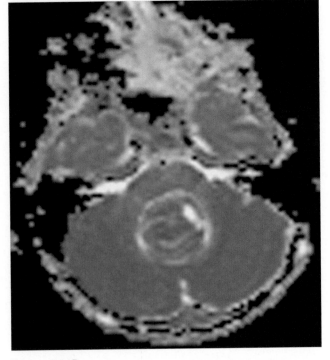

FIGURE 2.54D

FINDINGS (**A**) Nonenhanced CT demonstrates a hyperdense posterior fossa mass in the region of the fourth ventricle. Enlarged lateral and third ventricles indicate hydrocephalus. (**B**) Axial T2-weighted MRI demonstrates a heterogeneous hyperintense mass with internal cystic areas expanding the fourth ventricle. The mass heterogeneously enhances on sagittal T1-weighted postcontrast MRI (**C**). The mass has predominantly similar or decreased ADC values (darker) compared to adjacent parenchyma on ADC map (**D**).

DIFFERENTIAL DIAGNOSIS Medulloblastoma, ependymoma, atypical teratoid/rhabdoid tumor, exophytic brain stem glioma, pilocytic astrocytoma

DIAGNOSIS Medulloblastoma.

DISCUSSION Medulloblastoma is the second most common pediatric brain tumor after pilocytic astrocytoma, and the most common malignant brain tumor, with most cases presenting in children younger than 10 years of age. These WHO grade IV tumors arise from the roof of the fourth ventricle and often fill the ventricle, causing hydrocephalus. In older children and adults, these masses may arise laterally in the cerebellar hemispheres. Medulloblastomas are heterogeneous tumors with cystic areas, occasional calcifications, and rare hemorrhage.[1] Typical imaging features include hyperdensity on CT and relatively low ADC values (darker than adjacent brain parenchyma).[2] On diffusion-weighted MRI, medulloblastomas have significantly lower ADC values than those of JPA or ependymoma.[2] The imaging appearance and ADC values of medulloblastomas are similar to atypical teratoid/rhabdoid tumors, and these two entities can be indistinguishable by imaging. Up to one-third of patients may have leptomeningeal spread at the time of diagnosis, affecting the pial surfaces of the brain, the spinal cord, or both. Spread outside the CNS is rare. When it occurs, common metastatic sites are bone and lymph nodes.

Questions for Further Thought

1. How is this lesion differentiated from ependymoma?
2. What is the best way to determine if there has been subarachnoid spread of tumor?

Reporting Responsibilities

- Describe the lesion and determine if there is associated hydrocephalus
- Recommend/perform screening evaluation for spinal drop metastases.

What the Treating Physician Needs to Know

- Whether the child has hydrocephalus, a potentially life-threatening complication of this lesion.
- Whether there is evidence of leptomeningeal spread or drop metastases.

Answers

1. Ependymomas are soft tumors more likely to spread through fourth ventricular foramina into adjacent cisterns. In addition, ependymomas more commonly calcify.
2. Both MRI screening of the brain and spine and cytologic evaluation of CSF have been used to evaluate for drop metastases.

REFERENCES

1. Koeller KK, Rushing EJ. From the archives of the AFIP: Medulloblastoma: A comprehensive review with radiologic-pathologic correlation. *Radiographics.* 2003;23(6):1613–1637.
2. Rumboldt Z, Camacho DL, Lake D, et al. Apparent diffusion coefficients for differentiation of cerebellar tumors in children. *AJNR Am J Neuroradiol.* 2006;27(6):1362–1369.

CASE 2.55

CLINICAL HISTORY *A 7-year-old child with headache*

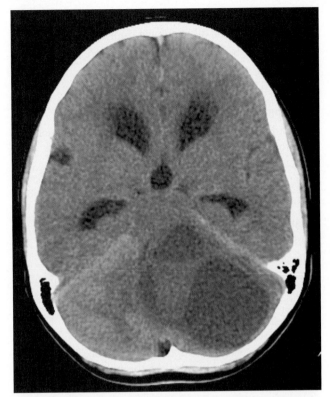

FIGURE 2.55A

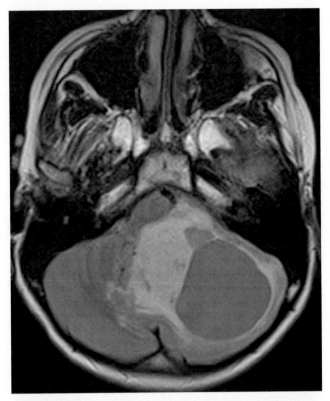

FIGURE 2.55B

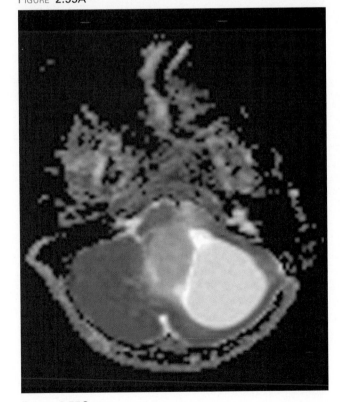

FIGURE 2.55C

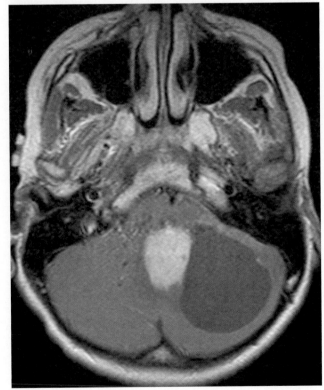

FIGURE 2.55D

FINDINGS Non-contrast CT (**A**) shows a mixed solid and cystic left cerebellar hemispheric mass lesion. The solid component is hypodense compared to adjacent cerebellum. Ventricles are markedly dilated, indicating hydrocephalus. On MRI FLAIR sequence (**B**), the solid component of the mass is hyperintense compared to the cerebellum. The cystic component is hyperintense compared to CSF, indicating proteinaceous fluid. On apparent diffusion coefficient (ADC) map, the solid portion of the mass exhibits higher (brighter) ADC values (**C**) than adjacent brain, and on T1-weighted postcontrast sequence (**D**), vividly enhances.

DIFFERENTIAL DIAGNOSIS Pilocytic astrocytoma, medulloblastoma, ependymoma, hemangioblastoma

DIAGNOSIS Pilocytic astrocytoma

DISCUSSION Pilocytic astrocytoma is the most common primary brain tumor in children, with peak incidence between the ages of 5 and 15 years.[1] This WHO grade I tumor has an excellent prognosis with greater than 90% 5-year survival rate. Pilocytic astrocytomas most commonly arise in the cerebellum, optic nerve/chiasm, or hypothalamic region, but can also occur elsewhere. Optic nerve and chiasm pilocytic astrocytomas are associated with NF1. Pilocytic astrocytomas most commonly manifest as a cyst with an enhancing mural nodule, although occasionally the cyst is absent. On CT, the solid component is typically hypodense to gray matter. Calcifications are uncommon and hemorrhage is rare. Hydrocephalus is common and ventricular size must be evaluated in any child with a posterior fossa mass. The solid component of a pilocytic astrocytoma is generally hypointense to gray matter on T1-weighted MRI, hyperintense on T2, and avidly enhances. The cystic component typically shows features of proteinaceous material, including increased T1 signal compared to CSF, and incomplete suppression on FLAIR sequence (brighter than CSF). Cyst walls may or may not enhance. On diffusion-weighted sequences, pilocytic astrocytomas have significantly higher ADC values than medulloblastomas and usually appear brighter than adjacent cerebellum.[2] CSF dissemination is rare, and does not necessarily worsen prognosis. Routine screening of the neural axis for drop metastases is typically not necessary. Gross total surgical resection can be curative, and radiation treatment is generally avoided.

Questions for Further Thought

1. How is this lesion differentiated from a medulloblastoma?
2. How does this lesion manifest in an adult?

Reporting Responsibilities

- Recognize and describe this lesion, which usually has a very favorable prognosis.
- Evaluate for hydrocephalus.

What the Treating Physician Needs to Know

- Whether the child has hydrocephalus, a potentially life-threatening complication of this lesion.
- Aggressive imaging features of this lesion do not portend a worse clinical prognosis. The prognosis of this lesion is favorable.

Answers

1. Medulloblastomas more commonly are midline, fill the fourth ventricle, and are hyperdense on CT, rather than hypodense.
2. Only 25% of pilocytic astrocytomas occur in adult patients. When they do, they are most commonly supratentorial.

REFERENCES

1. Koeller KK, Rushing EJ. From the archives of the AFIP: Pilocytic astrocytoma: Radiologic-pathologic correlation. *Radiographics.* 2004;24(6):1693–1708.
2. Rumboldt Z, Camacho DL, Lake D, et al. Apparent diffusion coefficients for differentiation of cerebellar tumors in children. *AJNR Am J Neuroradiol.* 2006;27(6):1362–1369.

CLINICAL HISTORY *A 2.5-year-old child with lethargy*

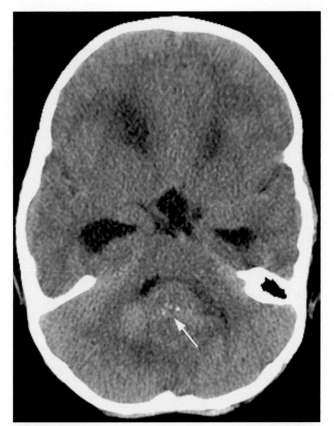

FIGURE **2.56A**

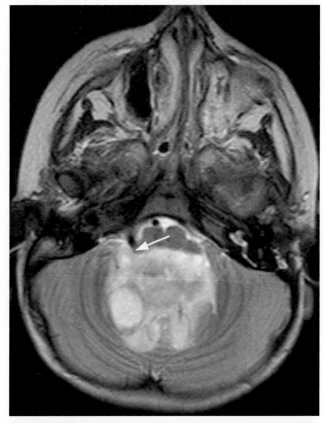

FIGURE **2.56B**

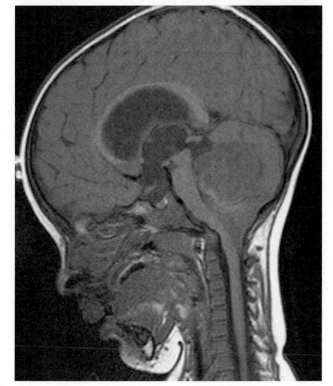

FIGURE **2.56C**

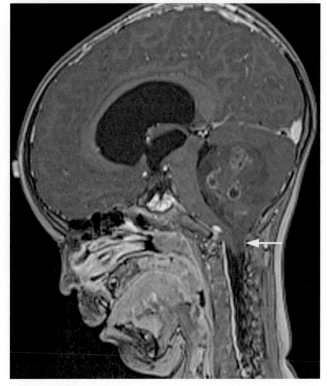

FIGURE **2.56D**

FINDINGS (**A**) Non-contrast CT demonstrates a mixed density posterior fossa mass with punctate calcifications (*arrow*). Enlargement of the temporal horns indicates hydrocephalus. (**B**) Axial T2-weighted MRI shows a heterogeneously hyperintense mass with extension through the right foramen of Luschka (*arrow*). Sagittal T1 pre- (**C**) and postcontrast (**D**) images show a T1-hypointense, heterogeneously enhancing mass, inferiorly extending out through the foramen of Magendie posterior to the cervicomedullary junction (*arrow, Fig. D*).

DIFFERENTIAL DIAGNOSIS Ependymoma, medulloblastoma, atypical teratoid/rhabdoid tumor

DIAGNOSIS Ependymoma

DISCUSSION Ependymoma is the third most common posterior fossa tumor in children, after pilocytic astrocytoma and medulloblastoma, with peak incidence between the ages of 1 and 5 years. Seventy percent of ependymomas are infratentorial and typically arise from the floor of the fourth ventricle. Seventy percent of supratentorial ependymomas are extraventricular.[1] Ependymomas are pliable tumors that fill and distend the fourth ventricle, frequently causing hydrocephalus. Other hallmarks of this lesion include extension through the foramina of Luschka and Magendie and the tendency to encase rather than compress adjacent structures. Ependymomas are heterogeneous by CT and MRI, with calcifications in up to 50% of cases. Cysts and hemorrhage may also be present. Ependymomas tend to be hypointense on T1-weighted and hyperintense on T2-weighted sequences. Heterogeneous enhancement is the norm. Although ependymomas typically manifest significantly higher ADC values than medulloblastoma and significantly lower values than JPA on diffusion-weighted images,[2] the ADC appearance is not sufficient for diagnosis. Intracranial ependymomas are WHO grade II or III (anaplastic) tumors. Subarachnoid spread can be detected with MRI of the neural axis or cytologic evaluation, and occurs more commonly at recurrence than at presentation. Younger children and those with WHO grade III (anaplastic) ependymomas are more likely to exhibit subarachnoid spread.

Questions for Further Thought

1. What other posterior fossa tumor can extend through fourth ventricular foramina?
2. How are intracranial ependymomas different from myxopapillary ependymomas?

Reporting Responsibilities

• Describe the lesion and determine if there is associated hydrocephalus
• Recommend/perform screening evaluation of the neural axis for drop metastases.

What the Treating Physician Needs to Know

• Whether the child has hydrocephalus, a potentially life-threatening complication of this lesion.
• Whether there is evidence of leptomeningeal spread or drop metastases.

Answers

1. Medulloblastomas can extend through foramina of Luschka or Magendie, but do so less frequently than ependymomas.
2. Myxopapillary ependymomas are WHO grade I tumors that occur almost exclusively in adults at the conus medullaris or filum terminale.

REFERENCES

1. Yuh EL, Barkovich AJ, Gupta N. Imaging of ependymomas: MRI and CT. *Childs Nerv Syst.* 2009;25(10):1203–1213.
2. Rumboldt Z, Camacho DL, Lake D, et al. Apparent diffusion coefficients for differentiation of cerebellar tumors in children. *AJNR Am J Neuroradiol.* 2006;27(6):1362–1369.

Kathleen Tozer Fink

CASE 2.57

CLINICAL HISTORY *A 2 year, 7-month-old child with developmental delay (Figs. 2.57A–C)*

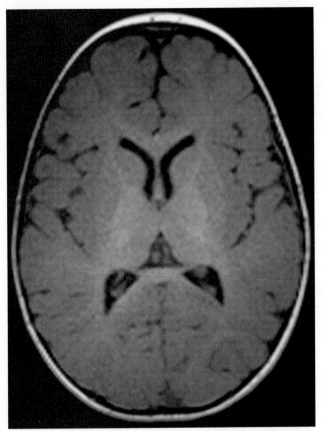

FIGURE 2.57A

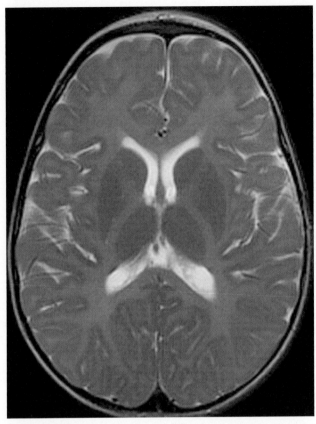

FIGURE 2.57B

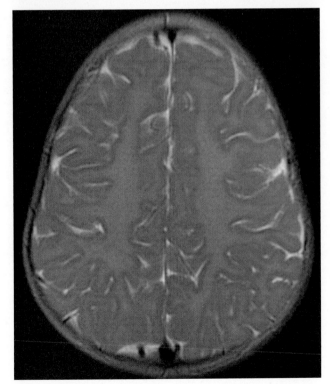

FIGURE 2.57C

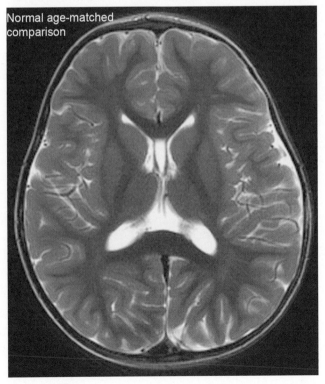

Normal age-matched comparison

FIGURE 2.57D

FINDINGS (**A**) T1-weighted gradient echo (MPRAGE) sequence demonstrates mild hyperintensity of the corpus callosum and internal capsule with respect to gray matter. T2-weighted images through the basal ganglia (**B**) and centrum semiovale (**C**) demonstrate persistent T2 hyperintensity of the white matter compared to gray matter. Extent of abnormality is more evident upon comparison to a normal age-matched control (**D**).

DIFFERENTIAL DIAGNOSIS Hypomyelination, cerebral edema

DIAGNOSIS Hypomyelination

DISCUSSION Cerebral myelination occurs in an orderly pattern during development, first manifesting as increasing T1 signal then as decreasing T2 signal. Myelination normally appears complete by 1 year on T1-weighted images, and by 2 to 3 years on T2-weighted sequences.[1] Before 10 months of age, T1-weighted sequences are best for assessing myelination. T2-weighted images are more helpful thereafter. Important milestones for assessing myelination on T1 include middle cerebellar peduncle at birth, anterior limb of internal capsule at 2 to 3 months, genu of the corpus callosum at 4 to 6 months, central white matter at 3 to 6 months, and peripheral frontal white matter at 7 to 11 months. Important T2 milestones include posterior limb of internal capsule at 40 gestational weeks, middle cerebellar peduncle by 2 months, anterior limb of internal capsule at 7 to 11 months, central frontal white matter at 11 to 16 months, and peripheral frontal white matter at 14 to 24 months. When assessing myelination, it is important to take into the consideration whether the child was born prematurely. There are many possible causes of delayed or reduced myelination, including primary hypomyelination syndromes, prematurity, and chronic debilitating conditions in infancy. Primary hypomyelination syndromes (such as Pelizaeus-Merzbacher disease) are often associated with chromosomal or genetic abnormalities resulting in delayed or defective myelin metabolism.

Question for Further Thought

1. How might DWI be used to evaluate demyelination?

Reporting Responsibilities

- For all children with imaging compatible with incomplete myelination, the radiologist should determine what milestones have been met and whether these are appropriate for the patient's age.
- In children with incomplete myelination that is delayed for chronologic age, correlation with prematurity (gestational age) is vital.

What the Treating Physician Needs to Know

- Whether degree of myelination is appropriate for age.
- Whether delayed/reduced myelination is global/symmetric, suggesting a primary hypomyelination or demyelination syndrome, or asymmetric and/or associated with secondary findings suggesting other etiologies of demyelination.

Answer

1. Diffusivity decreases as myelination progresses, with increasing fractional anisotropy values on DTI. This is because myelination facilitates diffusion along the direction of the axon tracts but restricts diffusion antiparallel to the tract direction.

REFERENCE

1. Jones BV. Hypomyelination. In: Barkovich AJ, ed. *Diagnostic Imaging: Pediatric Neuroradiology*. Salt Lake City: Amirsys; 2007;I:1:44–47.

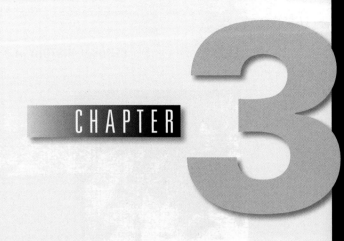

Gastrointestinal Imaging

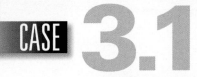

Grace S. Phillips

CLINICAL HISTORY *A 2.5-year-old boy with history of ingesting "callus eliminator"*

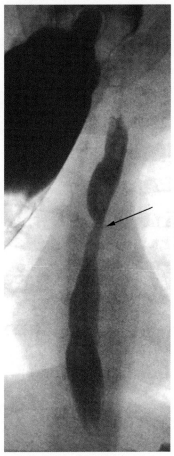

FIGURE **3.1A**

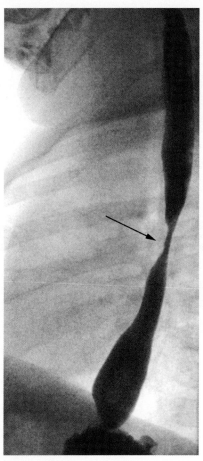

FIGURE **3.1B**

FINDINGS Frontal (**A**) and lateral (**B**) images from an upper gastrointestinal (UGI) series show smooth luminal narrowing of the mid-esophagus (*arrow*).

DIFFERENTIAL DIAGNOSIS Esophageal stricture, congenital esophageal stenosis; postsurgical (TEF repair), posttraumatic, or radiation-induced esophageal stricture

DIAGNOSIS Stricture of the mid-esophagus related to caustic ingestion

DISCUSSION Patients under the age of 5 are at greatest risk for accidental caustic ingestion. The most severe injuries are typically associated with ingestion of alkali substances such as household bleach and oven cleaner.[1] In the acute setting of caustic ingestion, the extent of esophageal injury is typically assessed clinically with esophagogastroduodenoscopy

(EGD). Stricture formation typically manifests between 1 and 3 months after caustic exposure.[2] UGI series is the study of choice for assessing stricture formation. Strictures related to caustic ingestion may be multifocal, and when most pronounced, may involve the entire esophagus.

Questions for Further Thought

1. What is the role of radiography in the acute setting of caustic ingestion?
2. Why are alkali agents associated with greater risk of injury compared to acid ingestion?

Reporting Responsibilities

In the acute setting, alert the physician if there is evidence of esophageal perforation, such as mediastinal air, pneumothorax, or pleural effusion. Esophageal perforation is considered a contraindication to EGD.

What the Treating Physician Needs to Know

- In the acute setting, alert the physician if there is evidence of esophageal perforation.
- Report the location, degree, and length of the stricture formation on UGI. Consider assessing with standardized barium tablet for quantifying severity of stricture.

Answers

1. Conventional radiography may be used to evaluate for evidence of esophageal perforation, which is considered a contraindication to EGD.
2. Alkali substances cause liquefactive necrosis, which is associated with a greater risk of penetrating injury, whereas acidic substances cause coagulative necrosis. In addition, alkali substances are often odorless and tasteless, and therefore greater quantities of these substances may be ingested. In contrast, acidic substances taste bitter, which is thought to deter ingestion of large quantities.[1,3]

REFERENCES

1. Dogan Y, Erkan T, Cokugras FC, et al. Caustic gastroesophageal lesions in childhood: An analysis of 473 cases. *Clin Pediatr (Phila)*. 2006;45(5):435–438.
2. Luedtke P, Levine MS, Rubesin SE, et al. Radiologic diagnosis of benign esophageal strictures: A pattern approach. *Radiographics*. 2003;23(4):897–909.
3. Kay M, Wyllie R. Caustic ingestions in children. *Curr Opin Pediatr*. 2009;21(5):651–654.

CASE 3.2

CLINICAL HISTORY *A 7-day-old infant with bilious emesis*

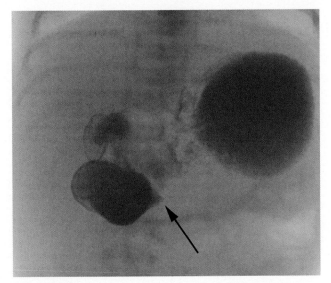

FIGURE **3.2A**

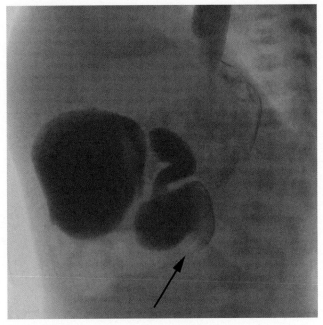

FIGURE **3.2B**

FINDINGS Frontal (**A**) and lateral (**B**) views from a UGI series show a beaked cutoff of the contrast column in the third portion of the duodenum (*arrow*). Lateral view shows a corkscrew configuration of the duodenum.

DIFFERENTIAL DIAGNOSIS Malrotation with midgut volvulus, duodenal obstruction related to annular pancreas, duodenal web, or duodenal atresia

DIAGNOSIS Malrotation with midgut volvulus

DISCUSSION Normal embryologic rotation and fixation of the bowel with respect to the mesenteric vessels occurs between the 4th and 10th weeks of gestational age. Disruption of this process results in abnormal rotation and fixation of the bowel, or "malrotation." Patients with malrotation are at risk for midgut volvulus and resultant ischemic injury to the small bowel, with potentially catastrophic results. Midgut volvulus may be visualized by ultrasound and computed tomography (CT).[1] However, the generally accepted method of evaluating for malrotation and midgut volvulus is the UGI series.[1] Normally, the duodenal–jejunal junction (DJJ), or ligament of Treitz, overlies the left pedicles of L1, at approximately the level of the pylorus or first portion of the duodenum. In malrotation, the DJJ is inferiorly displaced and typically more medial in position, often to the right of midline. Midgut volvulus should be suspected when there is associated obstruction in combination with an abnormally placed DJJ.

Questions for Further Thought

1. What situations can result in a false-positive UGI examination for malrotation?
2. Which syndromes are associated with malrotation?

Reporting Responsibilities

- Malrotation with midgut volvulus is a surgical emergency. Rapid communication of results is essential to ensure the best possible outcome for the patient.
- Malrotation without evidence of midgut volvulus is also considered an important finding that can have implications for patient management, and therefore, this result should also be communicated directly to the patient's physician.

What the Treating Physician Needs to Know

When malrotation is diagnosed, the referring physician needs to know whether or not there is evidence of midgut volvulus requiring emergent surgical management.

Answers

1. The DJJ may be displaced by a distended stomach, small or large bowel, and the presence of an enteric tube.[1] Documentation of the cecal position in equivocal cases of malrotation can help to assess the width of the mesenteric base, and thus, the potential for volvulus.[1]

2. Malrotation may be seen in the setting of gastroschisis, omphalocele, congenital diaphragmatic hernia (CDH), and heterotaxy syndrome, among others.[2]

REFERENCES

1. Lampl B, Levin TL, Berdon WE, et al. Malrotation and midgut volvulus: A historical review and current controversies in diagnosis and management. *Pediatr Radiol.* 2009;39(4):359–366.

2. Shew SB. Surgical concerns in malrotation and midgut volvulus. *Pediatr Radiol.* 2009;39(Suppl 2):S167–S171.

CASE 3.3

CLINICAL HISTORY *A 23-day-old former 35-week premature infant with bloody stools*

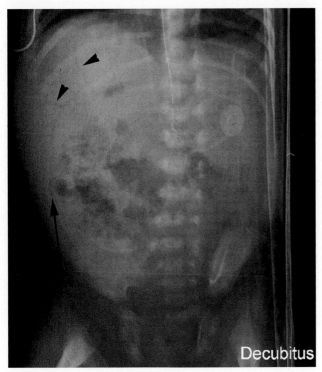

FIGURE **3.3A**

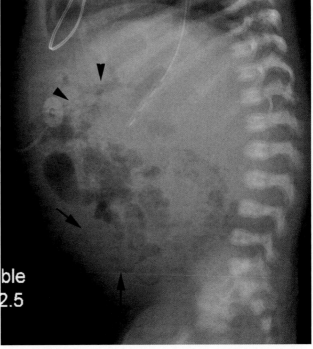

FIGURE **3.3B**

FINDINGS Left lateral decubitus (**A**) and cross-table lateral (**B**) views of the abdomen show bubbly lucencies (*arrows*) consistent with pneumatosis. Linear lucencies (*arrowheads*) projecting over the liver shadow on both views are consistent with portal venous gas.

DIFFERENTIAL DIAGNOSIS Necrotizing enterocolitis (NEC), occasionally portal venous gas may be related to injection of air through an umbilical venous catheter

DIAGNOSIS NEC

DISCUSSION Conventional radiography is the current standard for the initial diagnosis of NEC, as well as for assessing progression and detecting complications.[1] Plain film findings sometimes precede clinical symptoms of feeding intolerance, emesis, bloody stools, and diarrhea.[2] Radiographic patterns that suggest NEC include persistently dilated bowel loops, persistent asymmetric bowel dilatation, pneumatosis,

and portal venous gas.[1,2] Medical management includes antibiotics, nasogastric tube, and total parental nutrition (TPN). The presence of free intraperitoneal air and or fluid suggests bowel perforation, which necessitates surgical management.

Questions for Further Thought
1. Who is at risk for NEC?
2. What are common complications of NEC?

Reporting Responsibilities
- The clinician should be alerted to the possibility of NEC when suspicious plain film findings are detected so that prompt medical therapy may be initiated.
- The presence of free intraperitoneal air and/or fluid suggests bowel perforation, and therefore this critical finding should be rapidly communicated to the physician so that surgical consultation may be obtained.

What the Treating Physician Needs to Know

• Are there plain film findings consistent with NEC?

• Is there evidence of bowel perforation?

Answers

1. Preterm infants, particularly those <1500 g, are most at risk for NEC. However, 10% of patients with NEC are term infants. Typically, term infants with NEC have a concomitant illness such as congenital heart disease or birth asphyxia.[3]

2. Bowel perforation is a relatively common complication (12% to 31%), and is associated with increased mortality.

Long-term sequelae of NEC include stricture formation, which can be multiple, and short gut syndrome.[3]

REFERENCES

1. Epelman M, Daneman A, Navarro OM, et al. Necrotizing enterocolitis: Review of state-of-the-art imaging findings with pathologic correlation. *Radiographics.* 2007;27(2):285–305.

2. Daneman A, Woodward S, de Silva M. The radiology of neonatal necrotizing enterocolitis (NEC). A review of 47 cases and the literature. *Pediatr Radiol.* 1978;7(2):70–77.

3. Henry MC, Moss RL. Neonatal necrotizing enterocolitis. *Semin Pediatr Surg.* 2008;17(2):98–109.

Grace S. Phillips

CLINICAL HISTORY *A 2-month-old infant with persistent jaundice*

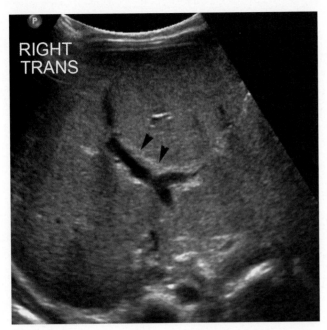

FIGURE **3.4A**

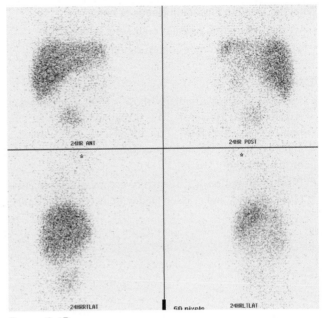

FIGURE **3.4B**

FINDINGS Transverse sonography of the liver (**A**) shows abnormal increased echogenicity anterior to the portal vein (triangle cord sign) (*arrowheads*). Hepatic scintigraphy (**B**) at 24 hours shows an absence of excretion of activity into bowel.

DIFFERENTIAL DIAGNOSIS Biliary atresia, neonatal hepatitis (NH), Alagille syndrome

DIAGNOSIS Biliary atresia

DISCUSSION Biliary atresia is a neonatal inflammatory cholangiopathy that obliterates bile ducts, most commonly the extrahepatic portions. Ultrasound may reveal an enlarged liver, and an absent or atretic gallbladder. The common bile duct (CBD) is typically not visualized. Detection of increased echogenicity at the porta hepatis (triangle cord sign) is a relatively specific but variably sensitive (49% to 73%) sign of biliary atresia.[1] Hepatic scintigraphy typically shows normal uptake of radiotracer and absent excretion into bowel. Magnetic resonance cholangiopancreatography (MRCP) may be considered for equivocal cases.[2] Diagnosis is typically confirmed by histology before or at the time of diverting portoenterostomy (Kasai procedure).

Questions for Further Thought

1. What pharmacologic agent helps to optimize hepatic scintigraphy in the setting of neonatal jaundice?
2. What finding at ultrasound may preclude portoenterostomy?

Reporting Responsibilities

Successful reestablishment of biliary drainage via Kasai procedure depends on prompt diagnosis. Therefore, prompt communication of abnormal sonographic or scintigraphic findings that suggest a diagnosis of biliary atresia is essential.

What the Treating Physician Needs to Know

- Bowel activity on hepatic scintigraphy excludes biliary atresia.
- Presence of a gallbladder on sonography does not exclude the diagnosis of biliary atresia. Approximately 25% of patients with biliary atresia have a gallbladder, which may be small or elongated.

Answers

1. Pretreatment with phenobarbital for 3 to 5 days before hepatobiliary imaging enhances biliary excretion of radiotracer and may increase the specificity of the test.[3]

2. The finding of a preduodenal portal vein typically precludes portoenterostomy. For this reason, Doppler evaluation of the hepatic vessels should be performed in patients with biliary atresia before portoenterostomy.

REFERENCES

1. Hartley JL, Davenport M, Kelly DA. Biliary atresia. *Lancet.* 2009;374(9702):1704–1713.
2. Anupindi SA. Pancreatic and biliary anomalies: Imaging in 2008. *Pediatr Radiol.* 2008;38(Suppl 2):S267–S271.
3. Balon HR, Fink-Bennett DM, Brill DR, et al. Procedure guideline for hepatobiliary scintigraphy. Society of Nuclear Medicine. *J Nucl Med.* 1997;38(10):1654–1657.

Deepa Reddy Biyyam

CASE 3.5

CLINICAL HISTORY *A 6-week-old infant presenting with progressive nonbilious projectile vomiting*

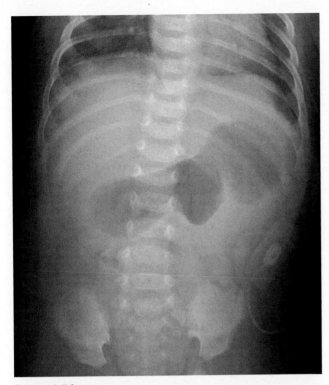

FIGURE **3.5A**

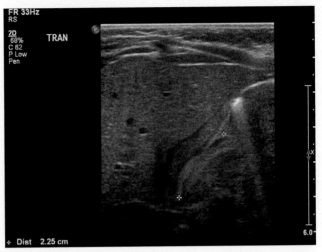

FIGURE **3.5B**

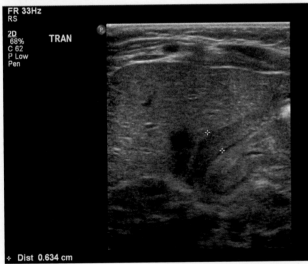

FIGURE **3.5C**

FINDINGS Plain radiograph (**A**) demonstrates a "caterpillar stomach", likely related to exaggerated gastric contractions. There is paucity of bowel gas distally.

Axial oblique and transverse ultrasound images through the pylorus, showing elongation of the pyloric channel (**B**) and thickening of the hypoechoic pyloric muscle (**C**).

DIFFERENTIAL DIAGNOSIS Infantile hypertrophic pyloric stenosis (IHPS), pylorospasm

DIAGNOSIS IHPS

DISCUSSION IHPS constitutes of idiopathic hypertrophy of the circular muscles of the pylorus, causing gastric outlet obstruction. The age at presentation is generally 2 to 12 weeks and these infants typically present with progressive projectile nonbilious vomiting. Ultrasound is the investigation of choice when IHPS is clinically suspected.[1] The measurements of pyloric muscle vary with authors; the commonly used measurements for diagnosis of hypertrophic pyloric stenosis are persistent pyloric muscle thickness >3 mm and pyloric channel length >16 mm.[1] Pylorospasm may mimic IHPS, however is typically transient. Prognosis of IHPS is excellent after pyloromyotomy.

Questions for Further Thought

1. What are the other common causes of nonbilious vomiting in an infant?
2. What is the study of choice in an infant presenting with bilious vomiting?

Reporting Responsibilities

In addition to appropriate measurements of the pyloric muscle thickness and the pyloric channel length, dynamic evaluation of gastric emptying by real-time ultrasound is important, especially in cases with borderline size measurements. Persistent pyloric muscle thickening with functional gastric outlet obstruction indicates IHPS.

What the Treating Physician Needs to Know

Patients presenting with bilious vomiting generally do not have IHPS. UGI series is the investigation of choice in these patients.[2] In a patient with malrotation, inversion of the normal relationship of the superior mesenteric artery (SMA) and superior mesenteric vein (SMV) may be observed at sonography; however, this may not be constant and UGI study is necessary to confirm the diagnosis.

Answers

1. Gastroesophageal reflux (GER; most common), pylorospasm, hiatal hernia, gastric bezoar, and preampullary duodenal stenosis are some of the common causes of nonbilious emesis in an infant.
2. Contrast UGI series. Malrotation with midgut volvulus which can manifest as bilious vomiting may lead to ischemia and necrosis of the small bowel. Hence, bilious vomiting should be considered as a radiologic emergency.

REFERENCES

1. Donnelly LF. Diagnostic Imaging. *Pediatrics.* 1st ed. Salt Lake City, Utah: Amirsys; 2005.
2. Hernanz-Schulman M. Infantile hypertrophic pyloric stenosis. *Radiology.* 2003;227:319–331.

CLINICAL HISTORY *A 3-month-old infant presenting with high output cardiac failure*

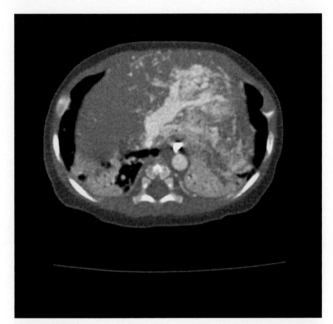

FIGURE **3.6A**

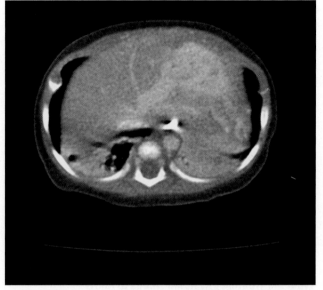

FIGURE **3.6B**

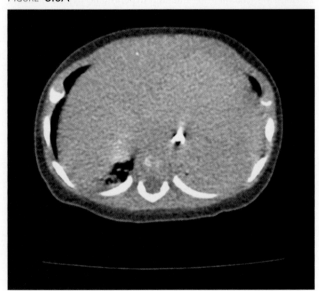

FIGURE **3.6C**

FINDINGS Multiphase contrast-enhanced CT images, demonstrating a hypervascular mass centered in the left lobe of the liver (**A**). Enlarged, early draining left hepatic vein is seen (**A**), indicating arteriovenous (AV) shunting. There is progressive centripetal fill-in of enhancement of the tumor in the delayed phase images (**B** and **C**). Imaging findings with the given history suggests infantile hemangioendothelioma.

DIFFERENTIAL DIAGNOSIS Infantile hemangioendothelioma, hepatoblastoma

DIAGNOSIS Infantile hemangioendothelioma

DISCUSSION Hepatic hemangioendothelioma or infantile hepatic hemangioma is the most common benign vascular tumor of the liver during infancy. They are typically high flow lesions, seen as a heterogeneous hypervascular mass with enlarged hepatic arteries and veins and tapering of the abdominal aorta below the origin of the celiac trunk. Three types are identified: focal, multifocal, and diffuse.[1] The serum alpha-fetoprotein (AFP) levels in these patients are generally normal. Even if elevated, they are much lower than that seen with hepatoblastoma.[1] Most of these lesions tend to involute spontaneously over few months to years. Follow-up is generally with ultrasound, to document resolution.

Questions for Further Thought

1. What are the complications that can occur with hemangioendotheliomas?
2. How are these lesions treated?

Reporting Responsibilities

- Describe the extent and enhancement characteristics of the mass.
- When detected on prenatal ultrasound, findings of fetal hydrops including anasarca, ascites, pleural effusion, and cardiomegaly should be looked for to comprehend prognosis.

What the Treating Physician Needs to Know

Biopsy of these masses is avoided due to risk of bleeding. Diagnosis is made on the basis of typical imaging findings and demonstration of resolution on follow-up imaging.

Answers

1. Congestive cardiac failure due to large AV shunting, consumptive coagulopathy (Kasabach–Merritt syndrome), and rarely hemoperitoneum due to rupture of tumor.
2. Most of them are asymptomatic and spontaneously involute; however, some may cause serious complications. Patients with focal or multifocal disease and symptoms related to tumor size or AV shunting are treated with steroids followed by alpha-interferon. Transcatheter embolization is performed to control cardiac failure when conservative measures have failed.[1]

REFERENCES

1. Chung EM, Cube R, Lewis RB, et al. Pediatric liver masses: Radiologic-pathologic correlation part 1. Benign tumors. *Radiographics*. 2010;30:801–826.
2. Donnelly LF. Diagnostic Imaging. *Pediatrics*. 1st ed. Salt Lake City, Utah: Amirsys; 2005.

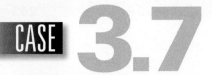

CASE **3.7**

Deepa Reddy Biyyam

CLINICAL HISTORY *A 16-month-old child presenting with a palpable abdominal mass*

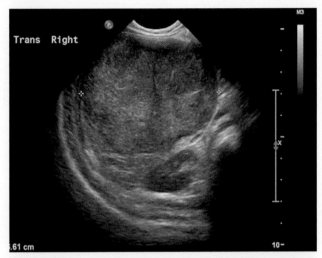

FIGURE **3.7A**

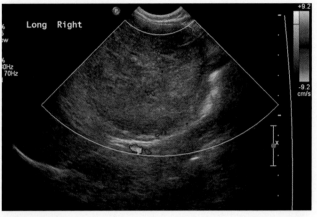

FIGURE **3.7B**

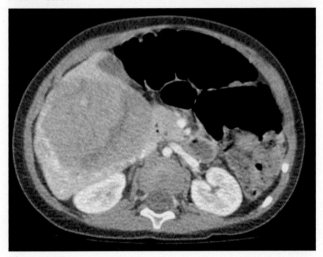

FIGURE **3.7C**

FINDINGS Gray scale (**A**) and color Doppler (**B**) ultrasound images through the liver demonstrating a well-circumscribed heterogeneous mass in the right lobe of the liver. Contrast-enhanced CT image (**C**) shows a large well-defined heterogeneous lesion in the segments 5 and 6 of the liver, predominantly hypodense compared to the normal adjacent liver parenchyma.

DIFFERENTIAL DIAGNOSIS Hepatoblastoma, metastatic neuroblastoma, hepatocellular carcinoma

DIAGNOSIS Hepatoblastoma

DISCUSSION Hepatoblastoma is a malignant embryonic hepatic tumor composed of epithelial cells and occasionally a mixture of epithelial and mesenchymal cells.[1] It is the most common primary liver tumor of childhood, mostly occurring in children under 3 years of age. AFP is elevated in >90 % cases.[1] They are usually single, well-defined masses with a pseudocapsule, may be multifocal. They can have a heterogeneous appearance due to hemorrhage or necrosis. They tend to displace rather than invade adjacent hepatic structures.[1] Neuroblastoma metastases are usually seen as multiple liver masses and an adrenal mass may be evident. Hepatocellular carcinoma is rare in children under 3 years of age.

Questions for Further Thought

1. Name few predisposing conditions associated with hepatoblastomas.
2. Which pediatric liver tumors are associated with elevated AFP levels?

Reporting Responsibilities

- Major role of imaging is to define the anatomic extent for preoperative planning as well as monitoring response to chemotherapy.
- Vascular invasion should be described if present.
- Metastasis to lung or abdominal lymph nodes should be described if present.

What the Treating Physician Needs to Know

In very large masses, it may be difficult to determine the organ of origin, whether arising in the liver, the kidney, or the adrenal gland.

Answers

1. Hemihypertrophy, Beckwith–Wiedemann syndrome, familial polyposis coli, Gardner syndrome, biliary atresia, and Wilms tumor.
2. Hepatoblastoma and hepatocellular carcinoma are associated with elevated AFP. Rarely hemangioendothelioma (<3% cases) can have elevated AFP, although the levels are much less than that typically seen with hepatoblastoma.

REFERENCE

1. Donnelly LF. Diagnostic Imaging. *Pediatrics.* 1st ed. Salt Lake City, Utah: Amirsys; 2005.

Deepa Reddy Biyyam

CASE 3.8

CLINICAL HISTORY *A 2-year-old child presenting with jaundice and palpable lump in the right upper quadrant*

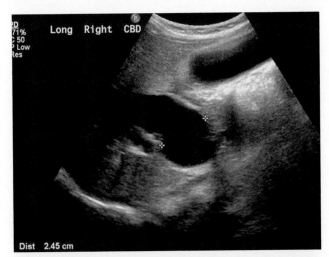

FIGURE **3.8A**

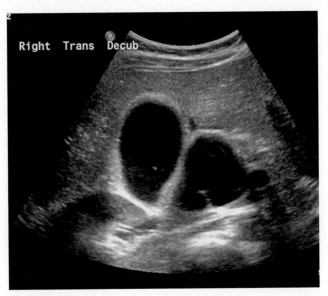

FIGURE **3.8B**

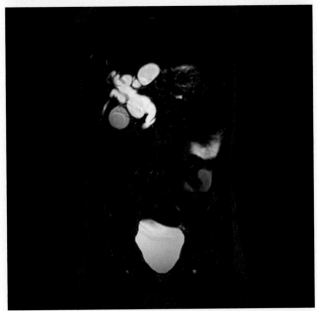

FIGURE **3.8C**

FINDINGS Longitudinal (**A**) and transverse (**B**) ultrasound images demonstrate a dilated CBD with sludge within. The gallbladder is seen separately. MRCP (**C**) demonstrates severe dilatation of the extra- and intrahepatic ducts. There is no obvious filling defect in the CBD.

DIFFERENTIAL DIAGNOSIS Choledochal cyst, choledocholithiasis causing obstruction, pancreatic cyst

DIAGNOSIS Choledochal cyst (type IVA)

DISCUSSION Choledochal cysts represent congenital cystic dilatation of the extrahepatic bile ducts, intrahepatic bile ducts, or both. They are classified into five major types as per Todani classification.[1] Type I, the most common type (accounting for 75% to 95% cases), consists of segmental or fusiform dilatation of the CBD. Type II represents a diverticulum arising from the wall of the CBD. Type III represents a choledochocele involving the intraduodenal portion of the CBD. Type IVA represents multiple cystic dilatations of both the intra- and extrahepatic ducts, whereas type IVB represents multiple cystic dilatations of only the extrahepatic ducts. Type V is characterized by dilatation of only the intrahepatic bile ducts, equivalent to Caroli disease. Infants may present with obstructive cholangiopathy, jaundice, acholic stool, hepatomegaly, or a palpable abdominal mass. Ultrasound is the best initial diagnostic test, although intestinal gas may obscure anatomic details. MRCP well demonstrates dilated fluid-filled bile ducts, and has replaced CT cholangiogram and percutaneous cholangiogram in the pediatric population. Biliary scintigrams may show accumulation of the radiotracer in the dilated ducts, confirming the diagnosis.[2]

Questions for Further Thought

1. What are the associated complications?
2. What is the treatment for choledochal cysts?

Reporting Responsibilities

- Describe the location of abnormality, that is, involvement of extrahepatic ducts, intrahepatic ducts, or both.
- Identify and describe any complications.

What the Treating Physician Needs to Know

Ultrasound is the best initial imaging modality of choice to evaluate the dilatation of the biliary tree. MRCP is helpful when diagnosis is uncertain as well as to see the relationship with the surrounding structures.

Answers

1. Complications include perforation, acute pancreatitis, biliary stone formation, ascending cholangitis with subsequent hepatic abscesses formation. Also, there is increased risk for cholangiocarcinomas.
2. Surgical excision of the cyst with reconstruction of continuity between the liver and gut.

REFERENCES

1. Todani T, Watanabe Y, Narusue M, et al. Congenital bile duct cysts: Classification, operative procedures, and review of thirty-seven cases including cancer arising from choledochal cyst. *Am J Surg.* 1977;134(2):263–269.
2. Kim OH, Chung HJ, Choi BG. Imaging of the choledochal cyst. *Radiographics.* 1995;15:69–88.

CLINICAL HISTORY *A 12-year-old child with epigastric pain and fever*

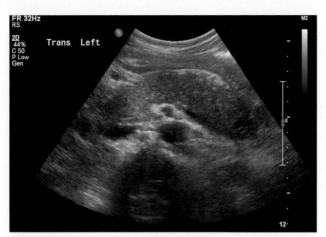

FIGURE **3.9A**

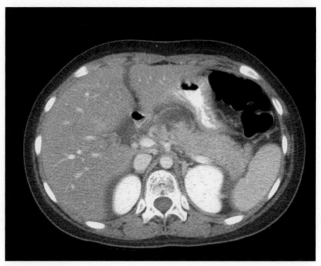

FIGURE **3.9B**

FINDINGS Abdominal ultrasound (**A**) demonstrates an enlarged and abnormally hypoechoic pancreas. Pancreatic duct dilatation is not evident. Coronal CT (**B**) demonstrates fluid attenuation infiltrating the pancreas with extensive fluid in the retroperitoneum.

DIFFERENTIAL DIAGNOSIS Acute edematous pancreatitis, necrotizing pancreatitis, ascites

DIAGNOSIS Edematous pancreatitis

DISCUSSION Pancreatitis in the pediatric population is recognized at a higher frequency than in the past[1] and may present clinically with abdominal pain, discomfort, or vomiting. Mild cases may be misdiagnosed as gastroenteritis or other nonspecific abdominal diagnoses. Laboratory evaluation reveals elevated amylase and lipase levels. The etiologies are numerous[2] and lead to acinar injury from inflammation or infection. This subsequently triggers the release of inflammatory mediators, which may be robust enough to lead to necrotizing pancreatitis or may affect multiple systems. Structural or anatomic causes of pancreatitis in the pediatric population may be safely evaluated and possibly treated by endoscopic retrograde cholangiopancreatography (ERCP)[3] and include gallstones, pancreas divisum (PD), papillary stenosis, sclerosing cholangitis, choledochocele, and trauma.

Medical causes include multisystem illness, viral or parasitic infection, bone marrow transplantation (BMT), autoimmune disorders, chemotherapy, and other drug toxicities. Many cases have no identifiable cause and are labeled idiopathic. Fatalities are generally limited to cases with multisystem causes or effects.

The role of imaging may be to diagnose the cause of abdominal symptoms, and if the diagnosis has been clearly made by the clinical presentation and by laboratory values, imaging may identify a structural cause of the pancreatitis or may identify complications, such as necrotizing pancreatitis, pseudocysts, or aneurysm. In children, ultrasound may be the initial imaging test performed, and may show diffuse pancreatic enlargement, altered echogenicity, or ductal dilatation. MRCP uses heavily T2-weighted sequences to optimally evaluate the ductal anatomy. Depending on the institution, the gland parenchyma and the adjacent vessels may be better evaluated by MR or by CT.

Questions for Further Thought

1. What is the standard clinical management for patients with pancreatitis?
2. Observation of the main pancreatic duct coursing anterior to the CBD should trigger what concern?

Reporting Responsibilities

- Define the extent of parenchymal involvement by edema, and search for areas of necrosis within the gland. The pancreatic duct may be disrupted in these cases.
- Report on the peripancreatic tissues, identifying pseudocyst formation (more common in older children and adolescents than in very young children) and vascular aneurysm.

What the Treating Physician Needs to Know

- Any diagnosable etiology, particularly cholelithiasis or congenital pancreatic anomaly, should be identified.
- Complications of pancreatitis, such as necrotized gland, pseudoaneurysm of an adjacent vessel, or pseudocyst formation must be conveyed to the referring physician urgently.

Answers

1. Pain control and pancreatic rest are the mainstays of therapy and have been for many years. Volume expansion with intravenous (IV) fluids early in treatment may reduce the likelihood of pancreatic necrosis. With severe courses, parenteral nutrition was historically initiated, although it is now recognized that jejunal feeds have fewer complications.[3]

2. It can be difficult to recognize a divisum pancreas, but the dorsal duct coursing anterior to the CBD before entering the ampulla will be a helpful observation.[4]

REFERENCES

1. Morinville VD, Barmada MM, Lowe ME. Increasing incidence of acute pancreatitis at an American pediatric tertiary care center: Is greater awareness among physicians responsible? *Pancreas.* 2010;39:5–8.

2. Lowe ME, Greer JB. Pancreatitis in children and adolescents. *Curr Gastroenterol Rep.* 2008;10:128–135.

3. Paris C, Bejjani J, Beaunoyer M, et al. Endoscopic retrograde cholangiopancreatography is useful and safe in children. *J Pediatr Surg.* 2010;45:938–942.

4. Shanbhogue AKP, Fasih N, Surabhi VR, et al. A clinical and radiologic review of uncommon types and causes of pancreatitis. *Radiographics.* 2009;29:1003–1026.

CLINICAL HISTORY *Four different 5-year-old patients with right lower quadrant pain and fever*

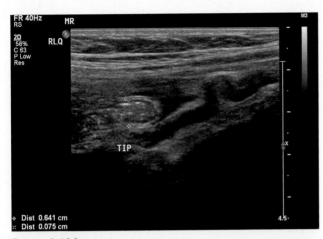

FIGURE **3.10A**

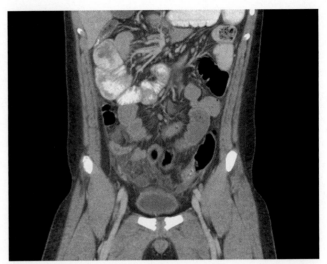

FIGURE **3.10B**

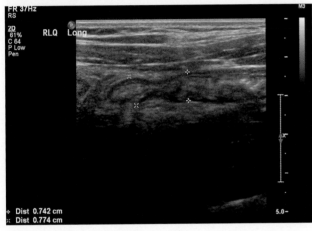

FIGURE **3.10C**

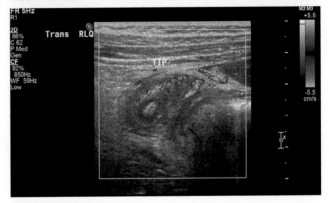

FIGURE **3.10D**

FINDINGS These images demonstrate a spectrum of abnormalities that might be found when imaging the abdomen for right lower quadrant pain and suspected appendicitis. Abdominal ultrasound (**A**) demonstrates a borderline enlarged (between 6.5 and 7.5 mm) appendiceal tip, without wall thickening and a small amount of periappendiceal fluid. In the second patient, coronal CT (**B**) shows a thickened appendix in the right lower quadrant with substantial fat stranding in the surrounding mesentery. A third patient undergoing limited abdominal ultrasound (**C**) shows an abnormally thickened appendix (7.7 mm) and no surrounding inflammation. Finally, a fourth patient's ultrasound (**D**) shows a blind-ending tubular structure with surrounding echogenic and hyperemic mesenteric fat.

DIFFERENTIAL DIAGNOSIS Appendicitis, inflammatory bowel disease, mesenteric adenitis

DIAGNOSIS (A) Early appendicitis; (B) Acute appendicitis; (C) Normal appendix in a cystic fibrosis (CF) patient; (D) Perforated appendicitis.

DISCUSSION Appendicitis in children is the most common surgical cause of abdominal pain in children presenting to the emergency department.[1] It is uncommon in children less than 4 years of age and very uncommon in the toddler age group. Because of the rarity of appendicitis in this age group and the difficulty in diagnosis, perforation of the appendix is quite common in these younger patients. Although appendicitis has a higher incidence in adolescents, perforation occurs much less frequently (10% to 15% in teenagers, compared with 80% to 100% in toddlers and preschoolers). Abdominal pain is a common complaint in older children and classically begins in the periumbilical region and then gradually migrates to the right lower quadrant over a period of hours to days. Fever, anorexia, and vomiting may be present. Laboratory evaluation may reveal leukocytosis, and inflammation in the right lower quadrant may render the urinalysis abnormal due to distal ureteral irritation.[1,2]

Since the clinical presentation may not be definitive, imaging plays an important role in assisting the pediatric surgeon in management decisions. Other processes mimicking appendicitis include mesenteric adenitis, inflammatory bowel disease, pyelonephritis, ovarian torsion, omental infarction, or infected urachal remnant, all entities identifiable by abdominal imaging.

At institutions with pediatric-trained ultrasound technologists, ultrasound is an effective way to accurately diagnose appendicitis. In experienced hands, the appendix can be identified in greater than 80% of asymptomatic patients, and the normal appendix characteristically measures 6.4 mm or less without compression.[3] In patients with CF, the expected diameter is higher due to mucoid secretions in the lumen and may measure as much as 14.5 mm (mean diameter is approximately 8 mm in these patients).[4] Secondary signs of inflammation include appendiceal wall thickening (greater than 2 mm), hyperemia based on increased flow detected with color Doppler, periappendiceal fluid, and mesenteric fat inflammation manifested by increased echogenicity. If ultrasound cannot identify the appendix, further imaging with CT may be pursued. Normal appendices measure less than 7 mm by CT.[5]

Questions for Further Thought

1. What is the importance of reporting the presence of a fecalith in a case of acute appendicitis?
2. What is the importance of diagnosing perforation as a complication of appendicitis?

Reporting Responsibilities

- It is critical to articulate whether the entirety of the appendix is visualized. The diameter of the appendix should be reported, as well as its contents, if apparent. Air and fecal material can distend a non-inflamed appendix. Secondary signs of inflammation including wall thickening, periappendiceal fluid, and mesenteric or omental echogenicity must be described.

- Alternative diagnoses to explain symptoms, most commonly mesenteric adenitis, which manifests as numerous prominent lymph nodes in the right lower quadrant, should be described.

What the Treating Physician Needs to Know

- Emphasize whether the entire appendix is visualized and if the entirety of its diameter is within normal limits or abnormally dilated.
- Convey signs of likely or definite perforation, such as hyperemia of the mesentery surrounding the inflamed appendix or obviously fluid collection.

Answers

1. Inflamed appendices with a fecalith are more likely to perforate in pediatric patients than in cases of acute appendicitis without a fecalith.
2. Perforated appendicitis can be managed nonoperatively and requires a longer hospital stay. If abscess develops, percutaneous drainage may be required.

REFERENCES

1. Bundy DG, Byerley JS, Liles EA, et al. Does this child have appendicitis? *JAMA.* 2007;298:438–451.
2. Morrow SE, Newman KD. Current management of appendicitis. *Semin Pediatr Surg.* 2007;16(1):34–40.
3. Wiersma F, Sramek A, Holscher HC. Ultrasound features of the normal appendix and surrounding area in children. *Radiology.* 2005;235:1018–1022.
4. Lardenoye SW, Puylaert JB, Smit MJ, et al. Appendix in children with cystic fibrosis: US features. *Radiology.* 2004; 232:187–189.
5. Victoria T, Mahboubi S. Normal appendiceal diameter in children: Does choice of CT oral contrast make a difference? *Emerg Radiol.* 2010;17:397–401.

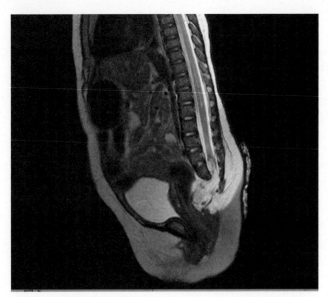

Teresa Chapman

CASE 3.11

CLINICAL HISTORY *Newborn with imperforate anus on clinical examination*

FIGURE **3.11A**

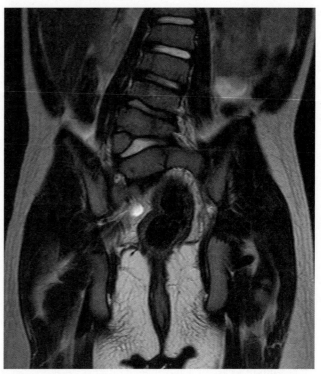

FIGURE **3.11B**

FINDINGS Sagittal T2-weighted MRI (**A**) through the lower spine shows a low-lying cord terminating imperceptibly in a neural placode and fatty material that protrudes anterior to the expected location of the sacrum. The sacrum is hypoplastic. Abnormal fatty tissue is also present dorsal to the lower spine posterior elements. The urinary bladder is in the expected location, although the bladder base and anus are not distinct from one another.

DIFFERENTIAL DIAGNOSIS Currarino triad, presacral teratoma

DIAGNOSIS Anorectal malformation (ARM) as part of the Currarino triad

DISCUSSION ARM is a relatively common congenital anomaly, affecting 1 out of 2,000 to 5,000 infants.[1,2] The term ARM encompasses a wide spectrum of defects, including the simpler low malformations as well as complex cloacal anomalies. The level of the lesion influences the surgical outcome and quality of life. Worldwide, an accepted classification system identifies the lesion as "high" (those without a perineal fistula) or "low" (those with a perineal opening).

Males with a bladder neck fistula and females with a high confluence cloaca (a common cavity into which the intestinal, urinary, and genital tracts open) have a significantly poorer prognosis than patients with a lower urogenital communication. Hypoplastic voluntary sphincter muscles, particularly the infralevator component, explain the poorer prognosis. Of note, the presence of severe sacral anomalies is associated with hypoplastic sphincters.

A considerable number of these patients (30% to 70%) have associated defects involving other organ systems, mostly commonly the urologic system. Importantly, the mortality of patients with high anomalies is higher than that of low anomaly patients, owing to the more severe associated anomalies. The mortality attributable to repair of the ARM itself is very low.[1]

Upon recognition of the malformation, it is critical to determine whether a colostomy or urinary diversion is necessary to prevent sepsis or metabolic acidosis. Early complications such as stricture and prolapse following colostomy and complications such as peritonitis or dehiscence following a traditional anterior-approach anal pull-through repair are seen much less in recent years, thanks to the development of the posterior sagittal anorectoplasty (PSARP). The most common complication following PSARP is constipation due to disordered motility.[1]

Questions for Further Thought

1. What is the Currarino triad?
2. In an adolescent female presenting with abdominal pain and a history of cloacal malformation, what imaging study is a reasonable initial approach?

Reporting Responsibilities

- At the time of diagnosis, radiography, fluoroscopy, and MR may all contribute to defining the anatomic anomalies. Vertebral anomalies and sacral hypoplasia should be well described. Cystography and voiding cystogram may be used to detect associated vesicoureteral reflux and may be elucidate fistula formation between the bladder base or urethra and rectum or vagina.
- Following anorectoplasty (see Fig. 3.11B), pelvic MR should define the sphincter symmetry, presence of perirectal fibrosis, and the position of the pull-through rectum (a central position is the expected postoperative finding). However, postoperative findings and manometric studies cannot accurately predict sphincter function since continence of multifactorial. Also note a hemivertebra in the lower lumbar spine and secondary right convex curve.[3]

What the Treating Physician Needs to Know

ARMs are often associated with other system anomalies, and the appropriate consultations should be acquired, including assessment of the patient by a cardiologist.

Answers

1. The Currarino triad is also known as the ASP triad, including ARM, sacrococcygeal osseous defect, and presacral mass. This is a rare syndrome that typically is autosomal dominant. The presacral mass is most commonly a teratoma or an anterior sacral meningocele, but may also be a dermoid cyst, hamartoma, duplication cyst, or a combination of these abnormalities.[4]
2. Mullerian anomalies are frequent in females with ARM, and obstruction of the Mullerian structures may result in menstrual blood collections that can lead to pain. Pelvic ultrasound is therefore the appropriate first imaging study in this scenario.

REFERENCES

1. Rintala RJ, Pakarinen MP. Imperforate anus: Long- and short-term outcome. *Semin Pediatr Surg.* 2008;17:79–89.
2. Al-Hozaim O, Al-Maary J, Al Qahtani A, Zamakhshary M. Laparoscopic-assisted anorectal pull-through for anorectal malformations: a systematic review and the need for standardization of outcome reporting. *J Pediatr Surg.* 2010;45(7):1500–1504.
3. Wong KK, Khong PL, Lin SC, et al. Post-operative magnetic resonance evaluation of children after laparoscopic anorectoplasty for imperforate anus. *Int J Colorectal Dis.* 2005;20:33–37.
4. Kocaoglu M, Frush DP. Pediatric presacral masses. *Radiographics.* 2006;26:833–857.

CASE 3.12

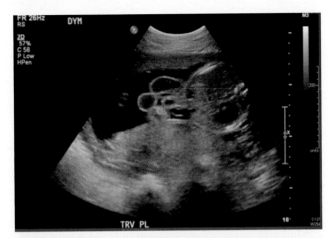

FIGURE **3.12A**

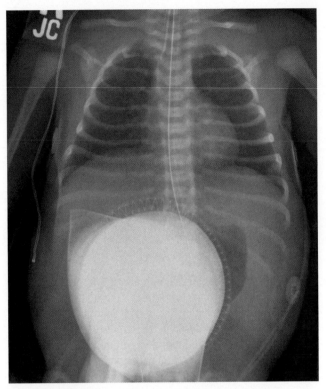

FIGURE **3.12B**

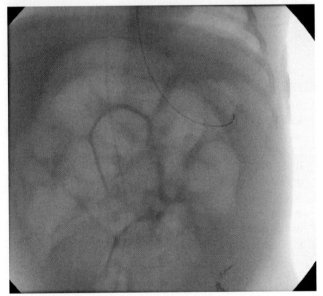

FIGURE **3.12C**

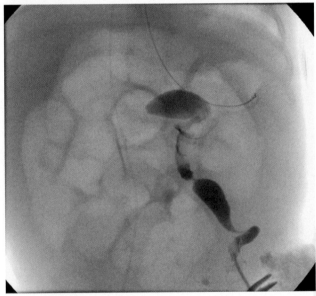

FIGURE **3.12D**

FINDINGS Third trimester fetal ultrasound (**A**) demonstrates an anterior fetal wall defect with few loops of abnormally dilated bowel in the amniotic cavity. Postnatal radiograph (**B**) demonstrates the appearance of a surgical silo containing the prenatally extra-abdominal loops of bowel. A scout abdominal radiograph (**C**) of the same patient several weeks into life shows abnormal dilatation of several featureless loops of bowel. Injection of water-soluble contrast through a left-sided stoma (**D**) opacifies a segment of bowel with narrowing and tapered margins, consistent with a bowel stenosis and resultant obstruction.

DIFFERENTIAL DIAGNOSIS Gastroschisis, omphalocele, limb-body wall complex

DIAGNOSIS Gastroschisis

DISCUSSION Resulting from a small defect in the abdominal wall to the right of the umbilical cord, gastroschisis leads to uncovered herniation of the bowel into the amniotic cavity in fetal life. The inflammation of the bowel by this exposure may lead to a complicated postnatal course, with bowel dysfunction and recurrent bowel stenoses. The etiology of gastroschisis may relate to a vasoconstrictive insult upon the omphalomesenteric artery causing focal ischemia of the paramedian abdominal wall, a theory supported by the higher incidence of this disorder in neonates born to young mothers who are more likely to be exposed to tobacco, cocaine, or other vasoconstrictive agents during pregnancy. Left-sided cases of gastroschisis have been reported, and the clinical demographics, prenatal findings, and postnatal course differ substantially from the classic right-sided gastroschisis. For this reason, left-sided cases with bowel herniation may be more accurately simply referred to as left-sided abdominal wall defects.[1]

The prenatal diagnosis of gastroschisis cannot be made until the second trimester after 12 to 14 weeks, when the physiologic bowel herniation is expected to have resolved.[2] The majority of mothers will have elevated AFP levels. Surgical repair is performed within the first day of life to avoid infection. The postnatal course is variable and depends upon the extent of bowel and peritoneal inflammation in utero. Any UGI study performed on an infant or child with a history of gastroschisis will show malposition of the DJJ, as all of these patients are malrotated and remain so following surgical repair.

Questions for Further Thought

1. What are the implications for the general health of a neonate with gastroschisis as opposed to a newborn with omphalocele?
2. List some congenital abnormalities associated with gastroschisis.

Reporting Responsibilities

- The second or third trimester fetal ultrasound reporting on gastroschisis should document the side of the abdominal wall defect relative to the umbilical cord insertion, patency of the mesenteric vessels, and appearance of the herniated bowel, including dilatation and wall thickening.
- Abdominal radiographs and contrast studies serve to identify the presence of bowel dysfunction or obstruction, and locate the presence and site of stenoses.

What the Treating Physician Needs to Know

- Any associated congenital anomalies evident by prenatal imaging should be conveyed to the treating pediatrician.
- The postsurgical course for these patients may be quite complex, and the treating physician will utilize radiography and fluoroscopy for the diagnosis of bowel obstruction and localization of bowel stenoses.

Answers

1. In contrast to gastroschisis, omphalocele is not thought to be caused by a weakening of the abdominal wall by a vascular insult, but is instead an early embryologic developmental defect that may be small or large and leads to herniation of abdominal viscera into the base of the cord. In approximately 60% of cases of omphalocele, there are other congenital defects affecting other systems, including cardiac, renal, musculoskeletal, gastrointestinal (GI) and respiratory, and the central nervous system (CNS).

2. Approximately 15% of gastroschisis cases may be associated with jejunal or ileal atresia, or cryptorchidism. As mentioned above, all affected neonates are malrotated.

REFERENCES

1. Maurel A, Harper L, Knezynski S, et al. Left-sided gastroschisis: Is it the same pathology as on the right side? *Eur J Pediatr Surg.* 2010;20:60–62.
2. Barisic I, Clementi M, Hausler M, et al. Evaluation of prenatal ultrasound diagnosis of fetal abdominal wall defects by 19 European registries. *Ultrasound Obstet Gynecol.* 2001;18:309–316.

Teresa Chapman

CASE 3.13

CLINICAL HISTORY *Newborn with prenatal diagnosis of chest mass born with respiratory distress*

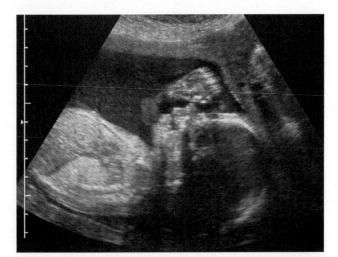

FIGURE **3.13A**

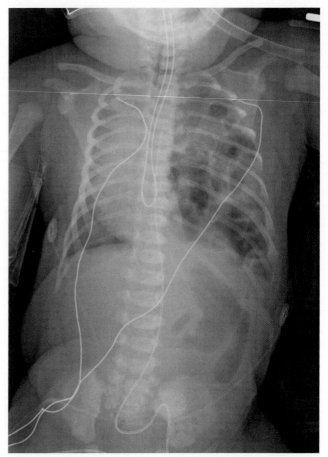

FIGURE **3.13B**

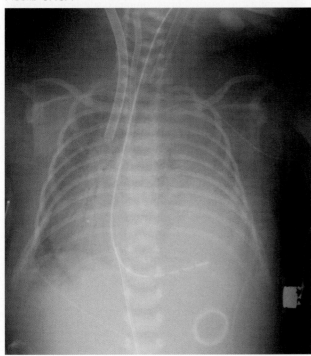

FIGURE **3.13C**

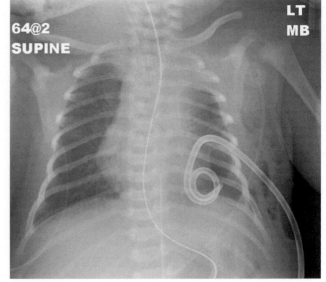

FIGURE **3.13D**

FINDINGS Second trimester fetal ultrasound (**A**) demonstrates an echogenic area in the fetal chest, which appears masslike and displaces the heart centrally. Postnatal chest radiograph (**B**) shows multiple large lucencies occupying the left hemithorax, with mediastinal shift toward the right, aberrant looping of an endogastric tube in the esophagus, and a paucity of bowel gas.

DIFFERENTIAL DIAGNOSIS CDH, congenital pulmonary airway malformation (macrocystic type), pulmonary sequestration, congenital hybrid chest lesion

DIAGNOSIS CDH

DISCUSSION CDH affects approximately 1 in every 2,000 to 5,000 live births.[1] Prenatal diagnosis may be made in the second or third trimester sonographically. Fetal ultrasound and MR findings that assist in predicting severity and prognosis include intrathoracic stomach or liver, polyhydramnios, small abdominal circumference, abnormally low lung-to-head ratio, and abnormally low percentage of the predicted lung volume. The congenital defect leads to pulmonary hypoplasia, pulmonary hypertension, and right heart failure, and therefore requires intensive care at a specialized tertiary care center. Survival has gradually improved over time, as attention moved from pulmonary ventilation to optimizing the right heart function by avoiding pulmonary hypertension.[2] Patients with documented severe pulmonary hypoplasia and a cardiac lesion may have improved survival with the combined use of ex utero intrapartum treatment (EXIT) and extracorporeal membrane oxygenation (ECMO).[3] Definitive surgical repair of the diaphragmatic defect is performed primarily if the defect is small and requires a synthetic graft if the defect is large.

Figure 3.13C and D show the radiographic findings of the same patient while on ECMO (**C**) and subsequently following surgical repair (**D**). Figure 3.13C is a chest radiograph of the same patient as in Figure 3.13B, following placement of extracardiac life support (ECLS) catheters in the right internal jugular and right common carotid vessels. There is opacification of the bilateral lungs, left more than right, as is expected with ECLS. The mediastinum remains shifted toward the right, due to the mass effect by the left-sided hernia. Figure 3.13D is a postsurgical chest radiograph following repair of the left CDH showing a small lucency in the lower left hemithorax consistent with a small pneumothorax. Extensive subcutaneous air is present in the right lateral chest wall. The hypoplasia is of the left lung is easily appreciable.

Questions for Further Thought

1. What percentage of affected infants with CDH will have other congenital malformations?
2. What is the most common type of CDH?

Reporting Responsibilities

- The prenatal imaging report should describe hernia contents, specifically stomach and liver. Quantitative information regarding pulmonary volume, such as lung-to-head ratio, is useful. Additional imperative information includes the amniotic fluid index and the presence or absence of hydrops. Because of the high incidence of associated anomalies, all fetal systems should be commented upon.
- Postnatal radiographic imaging will be for the monitoring of ventilation and ECLS complications. Evaluate carefully for signs of barotrauma including pulmonary interstitial emphysema and pneumothorax.

What the Treating Physician Needs to Know

- Prenatal assessment should attempt to differentiate a CDH from a lung mass. If the imaging findings are not straightforward for diagnosis of CDH, offer a differential including other congenital lung masses.
- Additional associated abnormalities, including cardiac, genitourinary (GU), GI, and CNS anomalies, should be conveyed clearly to the clinician.

Answers

1. More than one-third of affected patients will have other congenital abnormalities. The most commonly affected system is cardiac, with a significant cardiac defect lowering the survival rate. Other systems involved may include GU, GI, and CNS. CDH in the setting of chromosomal anomalies is also well documented and has a higher incidence of mortality.[4]
2. The Bochdalek hernia, a posterolateral diaphragmatic hernia, accounts for the vast majority of CDH. Approximately 80% are on the left side. Morgagni hernia refers to herniation of abdominal contents through the foramina of Morgagni, located just lateral to the lower sternum, usually on the right side. Diaphragm eventration, or focal thinning of the diaphragm due to abnormal development, may result in protrusion of the abdominal viscera upward. This latter form is usually asymptomatic.

REFERENCES

1. Weinstein S, Stolar CJ. Newborn surgical emergencies. Congenital diaphragmatic hernia and extracorporeal membrane oxygenation. *Pediatr Clin North Am.* 1993;40:1315–1333.
2. Downard CD, Wilson JM. Current therapy of infants with congenital diaphragmatic hernia. *Semin Neonatol.* 2003;8:215–221.
3. Kunisaki SM, Barnewolt CE, Estroff JA, et al. Ex utero intrapartum treatment with extracorporeal membrane oxygenation for severe congenital diaphragmatic hernia. *J Pediatr Surg.* 2007;42:98–104.
4. Fauza DO, Wilson JM. Congenital diaphragmatic hernia and associated anomalies: Their incidence, identification, and impact on prognosis. *J Pediatr Surg.* 1994;29:1113–1117.

CLINICAL HISTORY *A 14-year-old child with recurrent abdominal pain and bloody diarrhea*

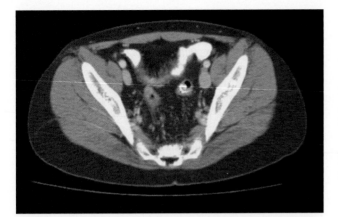

FIGURE **3.14A**

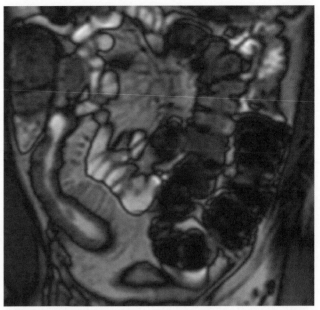

FIGURE **3.14B**

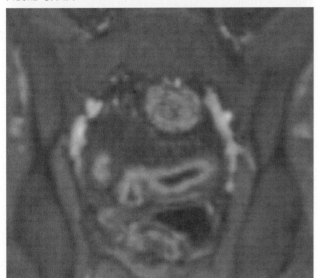

FIGURE **3.14C**

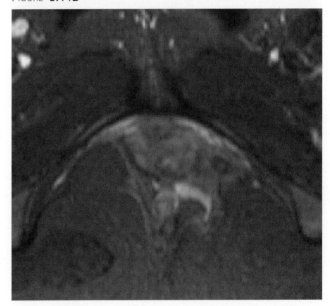

FIGURE **3.14D**

FINDINGS Contrast-enhanced CT and MRI images through the pelvis show ileal inflammation. By CT (**A**), fibrofatty proliferation and engorged vasa recta (referred to as the comb sign) surrounding distal ileum and the sigmoid colon are evident. By MRI, precontrast coronal steady-state free precession (FISP; **B**) and postcontrast T1-weighted (**C**) sequences show wall thickening and layering mucosal enhancement of the distal ileum.

DIFFERENTIAL DIAGNOSIS Crohn disease with acute on chronic inflammation, acutely inflammatory bowel disease, infectious enteritis, Langerhans cell histiocytosis

DIAGNOSIS Crohn disease with acute on chronic inflammation

DISCUSSION Crohn disease is a transmural inflammatory disease of the GI tract that may affect the system anywhere from the mouth to the anus and most commonly affects the terminal ileum. The incidence is 1 in 50,000. The disease tends to present in the teenage years and early adulthood, although the disease can occur at any age. Clinical signs and symptoms include abdominal pain, diarrhea, vomiting, and weight loss. The disease may also affect systems outside of the GI tract, leading to skin rashes, joint and eye inflammation, and fatigue.[1]

Cross-sectional imaging by CT and MR enterography (MRE) have assumed a greater role than fluoroscopic imaging in the evaluation of the small bowel for diagnosis and monitoring of Crohn disease. The sensitivity and specificity for the depiction of abnormal bowel segments is reported at 65% and 92% for CT and 85% and 91% for MRE.[2] Bowel wall thickening of the small bowel is defined as greater than 4 mm, and normal is 1 to 3 mm. The colon wall is normally 3- to 4-mm thick. The postcontrast findings on MRE are more useful than the T2-weighted findings, and can help in differentiating acute inflammation (homogenous wall enhancement) from acute-on-chronic disease (layered enhancing pattern) or fibrosis (dark signal with delayed enhancement).[3] Both CT and MRE may depict the complications of Crohn disease in the small bowel, which include stricture, obstruction, sinus formation, and abscess.

MRI is useful in the Crohn patient complaining of anorectal pain for the evaluation of perianal fissures and abscesses. Postcontrast fat-suppressed images allow for description of inflammation according to the following grading scheme: intersphincteric fistula without abscess (grade I) or with abscess (grade II); transsphincteric fistula without abscess (grade III; see **D**) or with abscess lateral to the external sphincter (grade IV); and transsphincteric fistula extending into the pelvis (grade V).[4]

Questions for Further Thought

1. What are the epidemiologic factors associated with development of Crohn disease?
2. What are aphthous ulcers?

Reporting Responsibilities

- Fluoroscopic imaging should document all sites of disease. In the UGI tract, detection of subtle mucosal abnormalities such as ulceration will be important. The small bowel follow-through may show skip lesions. Fibrofatty proliferation manifesting as displacement of bowel is a clue to additional sites of disease.
- Cross-sectional imaging should reveal the sites of affected bowel, degree of bowel-wall thickening, classic features such as fibrofatty proliferation, and complications of transmural inflammation including stricture/obstruction, sinus/fistula formation, or abscess.

What the Treating Physician Needs to Know

- Clearly convey any detectable complications of disease. Management of fistulizing Crohn disease includes antibiotic therapy and modification of anti-inflammatory medical agents. Indications for surgery include fibrotic strictures leading to bowel obstruction, internal fistulas leading to abdominal abscess, enterovesical fistulas, and enterocutaneous fistulas.
- The stage of inflammation of the affected small bowel will influence medical management. Therapy for induction of remission for active disease is different from maintenance therapy.

Answers

1. The disease is seen more commonly in western industrialized nations, and smokers are three times more likely to develop the disease than nonsmokers.
2. Aphthous ulcers, when they occur in the mouth, are also referred to as canker sores. In children, these are associated with poor nutrition or vitamin deficiencies, trauma, stress, malabsorption, Crohn disease, and food allergies. Aphthous ulcers may occur lower in the GI tract and on fluoroscopy, appear as a small superficial ulcer with a surrounding rim of edema. These are found in Crohn disease, gluten-sensitive enteropathy, Behcet disease, and cyclic neutropenia.

REFERENCES

1. Baumgart DC, Sandborn WJ. Inflammatory bowel disease: Clinical aspects and established and evolving therapies. *Lancet.* 2007;369:1641–1657.
2. Low RN, Francis IR, Politoske D, et al. Crohn disease evaluation: Comparison of contrast-enhanced MR imaging and single-phase helical CT scanning. *J Magn Reson Imaging.* 2000; 11:127–135.
3. Sempere GAJ, Sanjuan VM, Chulia EM, et al. MRI evaluation of inflammatory activity in Crohn disease. *AJR Am J Roentgenol.* 2005;184:1829–1835.
4. Morris J, Spencer JA, Ambrose NS. MR imaging classification of perianal fistulas and its implications for patient management. *Radiographics.* 2000;20:623–635.

CLINICAL HISTORY *A 13-year-old child with bloody stools following meals, crampy abdominal pain*

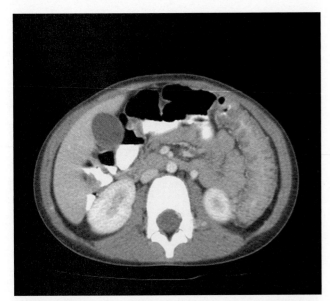

FIGURE 3.15A

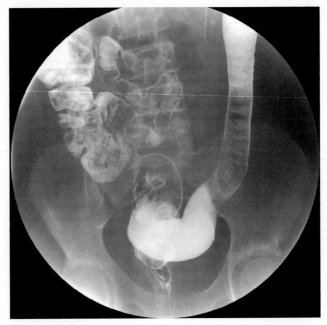

FIGURE 3.15B

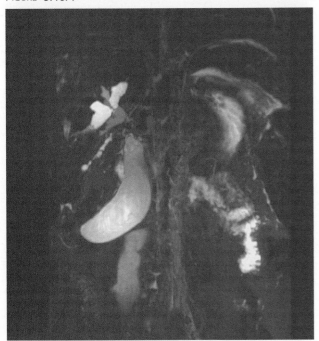

FIGURE 3.15C

FINDINGS Contrast-enhanced abdominal CT and contrast enema images show left colon inflammation. By CT (**A**), seen on this single axial image there is a long segment of colon with wall thickening and no periluminal abnormality. Contrast enema performed at a later date (**B**) shows a normal right colon and cecum in contrast to a tubular left colon and sigmoid colon with widespread subtle granular mucosal abnormality reflecting mucosal and submucosal hyperemia.

DIFFERENTIAL DIAGNOSIS Ulcerative colitis (UC), infectious colitis, Crohn disease, chronic constipation, laxative use

DIAGNOSIS UC

DISCUSSION Pediatric cases of UC usually begin in adolescence, and earlier cases typically are associated with a family history of the disease. UC, unlike Crohn disease, is a nontransmural inflammatory disorder that is restricted to the colon. Involvement may be limited to the more distal colon (proctitis or left-sided colitis) or the disease may affect the entire colon (pancolitis). A small percentage of cases involve the terminal ileum (called backwash ileitis), which can mimic Crohn disease. The disease relapses and remits. Histologically, the inflammation leads to crypt architectural distortion and crypt abscesses. Fissures or skip lesions are seen only rarely.[1]

The diagnosis is usually made clinically and based on endoscopy and biopsy of the colonic mucosa. Cross-sectional imaging by CT of a patient with UC will show a continuous segment of colon affected from the rectum more proximally. Concentric wall thickening is observed and may be smooth or nodular. Nodular wall thickening, or pseudopolyp formation, reflects active disease and is created by extensive ulceration of the mucosa and submucosa amidst isolated islands of normal tissue. It is useful to keep in mind that the most severe wall thickening of the colon tends to be seen in pseudomembranous colitis and Crohn disease, not UC.[2] Common extraintestinal manifestations of inflammatory bowel disease include inflammatory diseases of the eye, sensorineural hearing loss, myocarditis, primary sclerosing cholangitis (**C**), arthritis, and erythema nodosum. Figure 3.15C is a thick-slab coronal T2-weighted image from an MRCP study of a 15 year old with UC and primary sclerosing cholangitis shows central intrahepatic bile duct stenoses alternating with aneurismal dilatation of the ducts. In the right-sided branches, small, rounded, low-signal structures are outlined by fluid signal and represent small intraductal stones or sludge.

Questions for Further Thought

1. What is the fatty halo sign?
2. When is emergency colectomy indicated in patients with UC?

Reporting Responsibilities

• Document the extent of the involved colon, including pertinent absent findings, such as complications of transmural inflammation seen in Crohn disease.
• Identify any visualized extraintestinal manifestations of inflammatory bowel disease in the abdomen or pelvis, such as primary sclerosing cholangitis, nephrolithiasis, pancreatitis, ankylosing spondylitis, and sacroiliitis.

What the Treating Physician Needs to Know

• If the diagnosis has not already been established, the clinician needs to know that the findings may be due to UC versus other etiologies, such as infection (bacterial, parasitic, viral, or fungal), eosinophilic gastroenteritis, graft-versus-host disease, radiation changes, Behcet disease, or laxative abuse. Clinical history will narrow the differential diagnosis effectively.
• Abnormal bowel dilatation in addition to concentric wall thickening is a worrisome finding and requires close attention.

Answers

1. The fatty halo sign is a CT finding of submucosal fatty deposits that is visualized by low attenuation deep to the mucosa. The chronicity of UC may lead to these fatty deposits, resulting in a fatty "halo". This pattern on CT has also been described in graft-versus-host disease and asymptomatic obese patients.[2]
2. Toxic megacolon is a life-threatening inflammatory complication of UC manifesting as rapid dilation (within a few days) of the colon. Clinical symptoms include abdominal tenderness, fever, dehydration, and shock. Supportive medical therapy is given initially, and if not enough to reverse the megacolon, surgery is required to avoid a bowel perforation.

REFERENCES

1. Baumgart DC, Sandborn WJ. Inflammatory bowel disease: Clinical aspects and established and evolving therapies. *Lancet.* 2007;369:1641–1657.
2. D'Almeida M, Jose J, Oneto J, et al. Bowel wall thickening in children: CT findings. *Radiographics.* 2008;28:727–746.

CASE 3.16

CLINICAL HISTORY *An 8-year-old child with history of acute leukemia, status post–bone marrow transplant, presenting with abdominal pain and diarrhea*

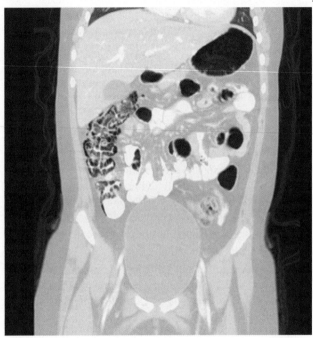

FIGURE **3.16A**

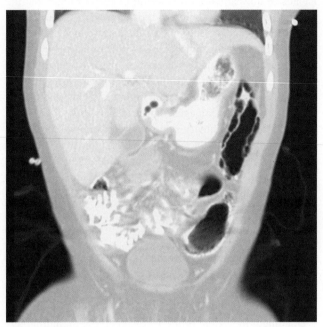

FIGURE **3.16B**

FINDINGS Coronal reconstructions of abdominal and pelvic CT studies in two different patients affected by the same process. Images shown in lung windows demonstrate an abnormal appearance of the ascending colon (**A**) and the descending colon (**B**). Intramural air is seen extensively. No portal venous gas is present.

Differential Diagnosis Pneumatosis intestinalis secondary to BMT, NEC, idiopathic pneumatosis cystoides intestinalis

DIAGNOSIS Pneumatosis of the colon, secondary to BMT

DISCUSSION Pneumatosis intestinalis refers to the abnormal presence of gas in the submucosal or subserosal space of the intestines. In the pediatric population, pneumatosis most commonly arises in the neonatal population with NEC, and the entity is otherwise rare. An exception to this observation is in allogeneic BMT patients, in which pneumatosis intestinalis occurs in a small percentage of patients. The passage of air

into the wall of the bowel following BMT is thought to be a result of mucosal injury or bowel ischemia related to the chemotherapy, irradiation, or infection associated with this procedure. High-dose corticosteroid use required for the treatment of graft-versus-host-disease may also result in pneumatosis intestinalis.[1] Pneumoperitoneum may develop as a result of rupture of a pneumatocele rather than bowel perforation. Pneumatosis and pneumoperitoneum generally resolve with conservative management. However, even though they recover through the acute disorder, the mortality rate of BMT patients who develop pneumatosis is considerably higher than the mortality rate of unaffected BMT patients.[2]

Questions for Further Thought

1. Name some clinical factors associated with development of pneumatosis intestinalis in BMT patients?

2. What segment of the GI tract does primary pneumatosis intestinalis typically affect?

Reporting Responsibilities

- If pneumatosis is suspected on a radiograph of a BMT patient, the finding should be reported to the referring physician urgently.
- Pneumatosis intestinalis visualized by CT should be described by its location and extent. Other pertinent findings would include free air, portal venous gas, and findings of other BMT complications such as intra-abdominal infection, typhlitis, and graft-versus-host disease.

What the Treating Physician Needs to Know

- Radiographically detected or suspected pneumatosis merits further evaluation with abdominal CT to fully evaluate extent of disease and to identify other intra-abdominal complications that could contribute to the presentation.
- Conservative management is used to treat pneumatosis intestinalis, even if free air is present.

Answers

1. Neutropenia, corticosteroid administration, and graft-versus-host disease are all conditions that tend to be present in BMT patients with pneumatosis intestinalis and may contribute to its development.
2. Primary pneumatosis intestinalis, the idiopathic benign form of intramural gas, is rare in adults and even rarer in the pediatric population. This form tends to affect the descending colon.

REFERENCES

1. Benya EC, Sivit CJ, Quinones RR. Abdominal complications after bone marrow transplantation in children: Sonographic and CT findings. *AJR Am J Roentgenol.* 1993;161:1023–1027.
2. Ade-Ajayi N, Vyes P, Stanton M, et al. Conservative management of pneumatosis intestinalis and pneumoperitoneum following bone marrow transplantation. *Pediatr Surg Int.* 2002; 18:692–695.

Teresa Chapman

CLINICAL HISTORY *A 10-month-old infant with abdominal distention*

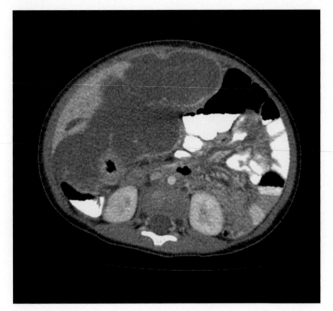

FIGURE **3.17A**

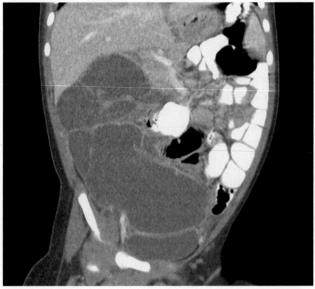

FIGURE **3.17B**

FINDINGS Axial (**A**) and coronal (**B**) contrast-enhanced CT images through the abdomen and pelvis show a large intraperitoneal multilobulated low-attenuation mass with enhancing walls and some internal thick septations. The mass creates some mass affect, although it also encompasses a few loops of bowel without compressing them. There is no associated bowel obstruction.

DIFFERENTIAL DIAGNOSIS Mesenteric lymphatic malformation, cystic germ cell tumor, ovarian cyst

DIAGNOSIS Lymphatic malformation

DISCUSSION The majority of lymphatic malformations occur in the axilla and neck. Uncommonly (1 in 140,000), they occur in the abdomen and they most likely arise from an aberrantly sequestered section of the embryonic retroperitoneal lymph sac.[1,2] Mesenteric and omental lymphatic malformations tend to present acutely as abdominal distention or pain in young children, whereas retroperitoneal lymphatic malformations tend to present with slowly progressive symptoms in adult patients.[3] The mesenteric lymphatic malformations have been reported to cause bowel obstruction, intestinal volvulus, intussusception, and may mimic ascites.[1,4]

Ultrasound is often the initial imaging modality to evaluate suspected abdominal masses in young children. Classic sonographic features of intra-abdominal lymphatic malformations include a multilocular cystic lesion with thin septations. Hemorrhage or infection may occur, in which case internal echoes may be observed. By CT, the lymphatic malformation insinuates among solid abdominal organs and may wrap around loops of bowel. If the involved bowel is narrowed, obstruction may develop.

Questions for Further Thought

1. What are the possible management options for intra-abdominal lymphatic malformations?
2. Name a reasonable differential for cystic mass in the pediatric abdomen.

Reporting Responsibilities

- An intra-abdominal cystic mass should be described by its size, borders, intracystic contents, presence of septations, and mass effect upon adjacent structures.
- Describe findings which pertain to the differentiation of a mesenteric or omental cyst from a solid abdominal organ cyst.

What the Treating Physician Needs to Know

- Urgent and emergent complications such as bowel obstruction or volvulus need to be conveyed immediately as critical findings.

- For treatment planning, sclerotherapy may be more optimal than a laparotomy. The treating physician will need to know the extent of the lesion and the amount of internal loculations. Ultrasound is ideal for this evaluation.

Answers

1. Surgical excision may be definitive if the malformation is small. Marsupialization refers to opening up the cyst and allowing direct communication with the peritoneal cavity. For large lesions, sclerotherapy by interventional radiology using an irritating agent such as alcohol or doxycycline may be therapeutic. However, this can only be attempted if there is confidence that the lesion is isolated, to avoid drug toxicity by direct contact with other intra-abdominal structures.

2. Purely cystic intraperitoneal masses are uncommon in children. Cystic neoplasms such as germ cell tumor, undifferentiated embryonal sarcoma of the liver, and cystic rhabdomyosarcoma should all be considered if there is substantial soft tissue associated with the mass. The size, location, and enhancement pattern will all be helpful information in the differentiation of the following intra-abdominal cystic masses in young children: ovarian cyst, enteric duplication cyst, Meckel diverticulum, urachal remnant, and mesenteric hamartoma.

REFERENCES

1. Traubici J, Daneman A, Wales P, et al. Mesenteric lymphatic malformation associated with small-bowel volvulus—Two cases and a review of the literature. *Pediatr Radiol.* 2002;32:362–365.

2. Egozi EI, Ricketts RR. Mesenteric and omental cysts in children. *Am Surg.* 1997;63:287–290.

3. De Perrot M, Rostan O, Morel P, et al. Abdominal lymphangioma in adults and children. *Br J Surg.* 2003;85:395–397.

4. Nett MH, Vo NJ, Chapman T. Large omental cyst. *Radiol Case Rep.* 2010;5(2).

CLINICAL HISTORY *Newborn with abdominal distention*

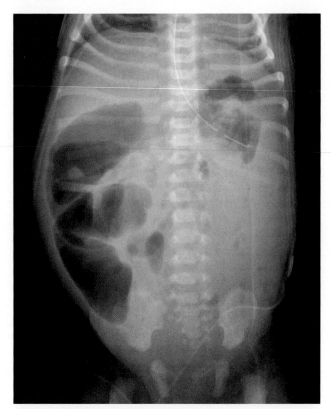

FIGURE **3.18A**

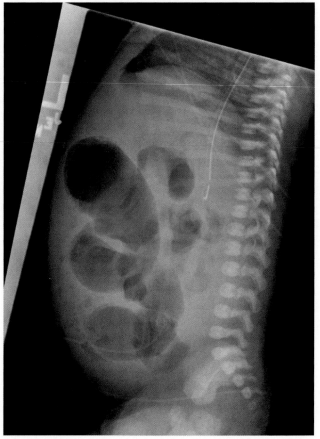

FIGURE **3.18B**

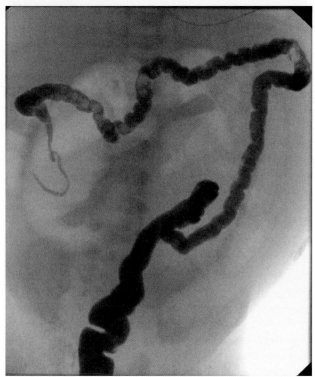

FIGURE **3.18C**

FINDINGS The left lateral decubitus and lateral abdominal radiographs (**A** and **B**) show multiple loops of bowel throughout the abdomen that are abnormally distended. Single fluoroscopic image from a water-soluble contrast enema (**C**) shows a very small-caliber colon (microcolon) and scattered filling defects in the right colon consistent with meconium.

DIFFERENTIAL DIAGNOSIS Meconium ileus, ileal atresia, ileal stenosis, Hirschsprung disease

DIAGNOSIS Meconium ileus

DISCUSSION Meconium ileus is obstruction of the small bowel due to abnormally thick meconium. The majority of patients with meconium ileus have CF, although non-CF cases do occur.[1] Prenatal ultrasound findings that may signify meconium ileus include bowel that is dilated (greater than 7 mm intraluminal diameter) and/or echogenic (brighter than bone).[2] The most concerning complication of meconium ileus is bowel perforation, which occurs either during fetal life or soon after birth. The release of meconium into the peritoneum triggers an inflammatory response that can lead to development of ascites, calcification, fibrosis, and cyst formation.[3]

Meconium peritonitis should be suspected in the newborn if there is ascites, abdominal distention, or failure to pass meconium in the first 24 hours. Initial imaging includes supine, lateral, and decubitus radiographs of the abdomen. Lower GI obstruction evidenced radiographically by numerous loops of dilated bowel throughout the abdomen could signify meconium ileus, small bowel atresia, Hirschsprung disease, or left colon syndrome. Loops of bowel that are larger in diameter than the vertebral bodies are tall should be considered dilated. The next appropriate imaging study is a contrast enema. In the setting of meconium ileus, the colon will be very small in caliber, and the microcolon observed with meconium ileus tends to be smaller than that seen with other neonatal distal bowel obstruction. The meconium plugs seen with ileus are predominantly in the proximal colon.

Questions for Further Thought

1. Do fetal intraperitoneal echogenic foci seen by ultrasound suggest perforated meconium ileus?
2. In addition to meconium ileus, what are other neonatal manifestations of CF?

Reporting Responsibilities

- The abdominal radiograph of a newborn should comment on degree of gaseous distention of the bowel. If the entirety of the bowel does not contain gas by 24 hours of life, then GI obstruction should be suspected and the clinician should be alerted. Bowel perforation may be evident by free air or by calcification that occurs following meconium peritonitis.
- The contrast enema report should contain information regarding the negative findings pertinent to the other diagnoses in the differential for a newborn with lower GI obstruction, including absence of a transition point (as

would be seen with Hirschsprung disease or left colon syndrome) and absence of stenoses or atresias in the colon.

What the Treating Physician Needs to Know

- The diagnosis of meconium ileus merits testing for CF.
- Repeat water-soluble contrast enema may be therapeutic for bowel obstruction.

Answers

1. Intra-abdominal echogenic foci may be seen in the fetus during routine fetal ultrasound screening and often spontaneously resolve. Fetal meconium peritonitis is a chemical reaction to antenatal bowel perforation and will be diagnosed not simply based on intraperitoneal echogenicities, but also ascites and abnormal bowel dilatation.
2. CF may not be immediately recognized, and therefore newborn screening programs are being developed in an increasing number of countries. There is evidence that newborn screening decreases the prevalence of severe malnutrition, and it remains unclear if there is any long-term benefit to respiratory health.[4]

REFERENCES

1. Buonomo C. Neonatal gastrointestinal emergencies. *Radiol Clin North Am.* 1997;35:845–864.
2. Jackson CR, Orford J, Minutillo C, et al. Dilated and echogenic fetal bowel and postnatal outcomes: A surgical perspective. Case series and literature review. *Eur J Pediatr Surg.* 2010;20:191–193.
3. Tsai MH, Chu SM, Lien R, et al. Clinical manifestations in infants with symptomatic meconium peritonitis. *Pediatr Neonatol.* 2009;50(2):59–64.
4. Southern KW, Merelle MM, Dankert-Roelse JE, et al. Newborn screening for cystic fibrosis. *Cochrane Database Syst Rev.* 2009;(1):CD001402.

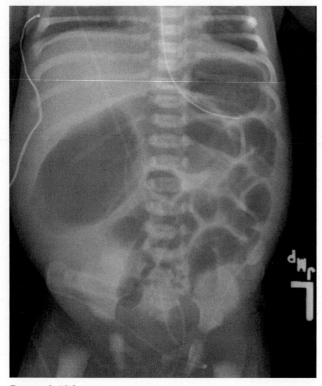

FIGURE **3.19A**

FIGURE **3.19B**

FINDINGS The supine abdominal radiograph (**A**) shows multiple loops of bowel throughout the abdomen that are abnormally distended. Single fluoroscopic image from a water-soluble contrast enema (**B**) shows a small-caliber colon (microcolon) and reflux of contrast through the ileocecal valve into the terminal ileum. The contrast column abruptly terminates and cannot be introduced further.

DIFFERENTIAL DIAGNOSIS Ileal atresia, ileal stenosis, meconium ileus, Hirschsprung disease, left colon syndrome

DIAGNOSIS Small bowel atresia

DISCUSSION Small bowel atresia is a congenital absence of a segment of duodenum, jejunum, or ileum. Duodenal atresia is the most common upper bowel obstruction in the neonate and typically affects the second or third portion of the duodenum. If the affected segment is stenotic rather than atretic, there may be some distal gas on the initial radiograph, as opposed to duodenal atresia. With atresia, the classic "double bubble" sign may be seen and is due to distention of both the stomach and the duodenal bulb. About one-third of patients with duodenal atresia have Down syndrome (trisomy 21). Additional associations include malrotation and annular pancreas. More distal small bowel atresias may present with failure to pass meconium in the first 24 to 48 hours of life, abdominal distention, or bilious emesis. Jejunoileal atresia is much more common than colonic atresia, which is very rare. The prognosis depends on the amount of residual functional bowel following surgical repair.[1]

Initial imaging includes supine, lateral, and decubitus radiographs of the abdomen. In the newborn, small and large bowels cannot be reliably distinguished from one another. A lower GI obstruction manifests radiographically by numerous loops of dilated bowel throughout the abdomen, as opposed to an UGI obstruction, which may show a paucity of bowel gas or may be normal. Loops of bowel that are larger in diameter than the vertebral bodies are tall should be considered dilated. If a distal bowel obstruction is suspected, the next appropriate imaging study is a contrast enema. In the setting of small bowel atresia, the colon will be small in caliber, a reflection of its lack of use during fetal life.[2]

Questions for Further Thought

1. When performing a contrast enema on a newborn, what aspects of the procedural technique differ from that of enemas performed on older infants or young children?

2. How does the enema findings of small bowel atresia differ from the findings seen with left colon syndrome?

Reporting Responsibilities

• The abdominal radiograph of a newborn should comment on degree of gaseous distention of the bowel. If the entirety of the bowel does not contain gas by 24 hours of life, then GI obstruction should be suspected and the clinician should be alerted. Bowel perforation may be evident by free air or by calcification that occurs following meconium peritonitis.

• The contrast enema should determine if there are additional atresias in the colon, and attempt should be made to identify the atretic end or a stenosis in the terminal or distal ileum.

What the Treating Physician Needs to Know

Presence of a small bowel obstruction in the neonate based on abdominal radiograph merits further evaluation with contrast enema. If malrotation with midgut volvulus is also a consideration, a UGI study should be performed first to avoid contrast from a lower GI study obscuring the visualization of an opacified ligament of Treitz.

Answers

1. A small-caliber tube, such as a 6-French or 8-French Foley catheter, should be selected, and it should be secured externally by tape alone. Inflating the retention balloon places the patient at risk for rupture. Water-soluble contrast should be used rather than barium, given the potential for surgical repair soon after the enema.

2. Left colon syndrome, also called meconium plug syndrome, is a transient dysfunction of bowel related to immaturity of the colon and is more commonly seen in hypotonic states as seen in infants born to mothers with diabetes or those treated with magnesium sulfate as a tocolytic agent. The enema of newborns with left colon syndrome shows a small-caliber colon up to the splenic flexure, and small filling defects consistent with meconium plugs are present in the left colon. This is in contrast to a complete microcolon seen in cases of small bowel atresia.

REFERENCES

1. Buonomo C. Neonatal gastrointestinal emergencies. *Radiol Clin North Am.* 1997;35:845–864.

2. Berdon WE, Baker DH, Santulli TV, et al. Microcolon in newborn infants with intestinal obstruction: its correlation with the level and time of onset of obstruction. *Radiology.* 1968;90: 878–885.

CLINICAL HISTORY *A 2-year-old male with abdominal pain*

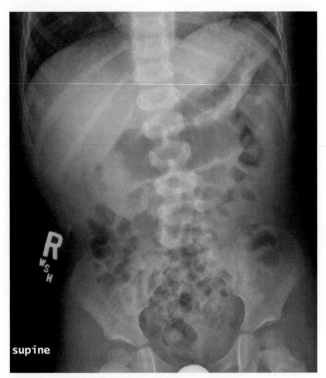

FIGURE **3.20A**

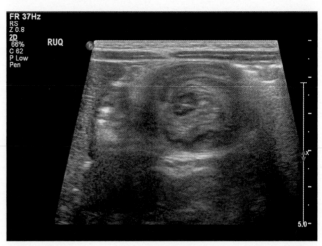

FIGURE **3.20B**

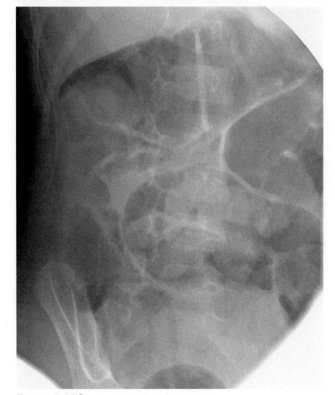

FIGURE **3.20C**

FINDINGS Frontal radiograph of the abdomen (**A**) demonstrates a soft-tissue density meniscus within the expected lumen of the transverse colon. Gray-scale image from limited abdominal ultrasound (**B**) demonstrates alternating concentric rings of hypoechoic and hyperechoic tissue. Spot image from air-contrast enema (**C**) demonstrates soft-tissue filling defect within the otherwise air-filled transverse colon.

DIFFERENTIAL DIAGNOSIS When examination is positive, findings are diagnostic. Etiology, however, may be considered idiopathic versus secondary

DIAGNOSIS Presumed idiopathic ileocolic intussusception

DISCUSSION Results from forward peristalsis of upstream bowel (intussuceptum) into downstream bowel (intussusceptiens). Most commonly the ileum telescopes into the colon (ileocolic). The majority are "idiopathic" with lead point of lymphoid hypertrophy (presumed related to viral illness).[1] Consequently, occurrence is seasonal: spring and winter. Clinical evaluation can be confusing, with classic findings of episodic pain and currant jelly stool absent in many.[2] Most commonly affects children 3 months to 1 year of age. If present in child older than 3, pathologic lead point (such as lymphoma, Meckel diverticulum, intramural hematoma) is suspected. Workup typically commences with radiographs, which variably demonstrate the intussusception and are important to demonstrate possible pneumoperitoneum. If radiographs are inconclusive, ultrasound is typically performed.

Questions for Further Thought

1. What are the absolute contraindications to image-guided reduction?
2. Which fluoroscopic technique has the lowest radiation?

Reporting Responsibilities

- Finding is urgent. Call to the clinician is highly recommended and will facilitate proper treatment.
- Findings which would contraindicate enema reduction (i.e., signs of perforation) should be relayed to the referring physician.

What the Treating Physician Needs to Know

- Intussusception is reliably diagnosed with imaging. No further workup indicated with confidently identified either radiographically or with ultrasound.
- Treatment of choice is air-contrast enema with surgery reserved for cases of failed reduction. Current efforts are investigating ultrasound-guided hydrostatic reduction, with main advantage being lack of ionizing radiation.

Answers

1. Shock which is unresponsive to corrective measures. Perforation (radiographically or clinical signs of peritonitis).
2. Air-contrast reduction. This is related to shortened time needed to reduce the intussusception and lower radiation technique (mA and kV) needed to image.

REFERENCES

1. Applegate KE. Intussusception in children: Evidence-based diagnosis and treatment. *Pediatr Radiol.* 2009;39(Suppl 2): S140–S143.
2. del-Pozo G, Albillos JC, Tejedor D, et al. Intussusception in children: Current concepts in diagnosis and enema reduction. *Radiographics.* 1999;19(2):299–319.

Marla Sammer

CLINICAL HISTORY *A 14-year-old female with abdominal pain and vomiting*

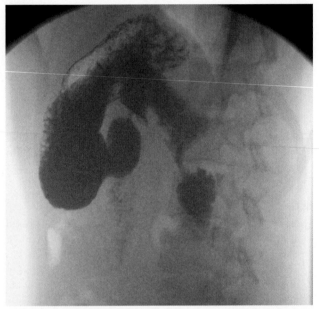

FIGURE **3.21A**

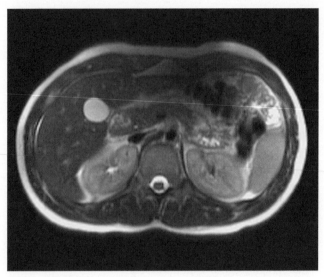

FIGURE **3.21B**

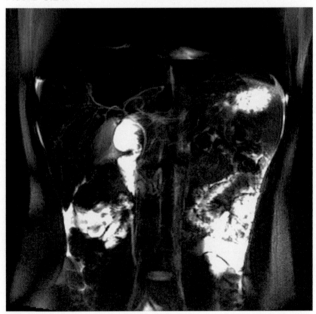

FIGURE **3.21C**

FINDINGS Right anterior oblique (RAO) fluoroscopic screen save image from single contrast barium UGI (**A**) demonstrates narrowing within the second portion of the duodenum. No mucosal irregularity is noted. On further dynamic imaging (not provided), lesion is seen to be fixed, though contrast readily traverses the narrowing. Axial T2 Haste (**B**) demonstrates pancreatic tissue encircling the second portion of the duodenum. Coronal MRCP maximum intensity projection (MIP) (**C**) corroborates duodenal narrowing, as demonstrated previously on UGI.

DIFFERENTIAL DIAGNOSIS Based on UGI: Annular pancreas, duodenal stenosis, duplication cyst, gastrointestinal stromal tumor (GIST), lymphoma, duodenal hematoma

DIAGNOSIS Annular pancreas

DISCUSSION On the basis of UGI, abnormality appears extrinsic, with differential listed above, though narrowing as seen here (second portion of duodenum) is fairly characteristic.[1] Further evaluation with MRI can help differentiate and was performed, confirming annular pancreas, an uncommon congenital anomaly in which incomplete embryonic rotation of the ventral anlage leads to pancreatic tissue surrounding the second portion of the duodenum.[2] Not all cases are symptomatic, but in at least 50% of symptomatic cases, findings manifest in neonate with GI obstruction, biliary duct obstruction, or pancreatitis. In adults, the condition often manifests with symptoms of GI distress (often confused with peptic ulcer disease), partial duodenal obstruction, or pancreatitis. The diagnosis can be suspected on fluoroscopic examinations, and confirmed with cross-sectional imaging.

Questions for Further Thought

1. Annular pancreas is in the differential diagnosis for the "double bubble" sign on neonatal abdominal radiographs. What are the other differential considerations for "double bubble"?
2. What additional findings on abdominal radiograph may help differentiate between the etiologies of the "double bubble"?

Reporting Responsibilities

- Signs of which may suggest obstruction should be reported.

- Associated pancreatic ductal anomalies (such as drainage of the annular pancreas directly into the duodenum versus into the major papilla) should be reported, as identifiable.

What the Treating Physician Needs to Know

- Finding can be incidental (i.e., patient is asymptomatic). Treatment should be based on clinical symptomatology.
- Surgical resection is recommended for symptomatic lesions.

Answers

1. Duodenal atresia (most commonly), malrotation, duodenal/pyloric stenosis.
2. With duodenal atresia, no gas should be identified within the distal bowel. If present, one of the other etiologies should be suggested. If there is relatively little gas within the duodenum compared with the stomach, malrotation (a more acute cause of obstruction) should be considered.

REFERENCES

1. Yu J, Turner MA, Fulcher AS, et al. Congenital anomalies and normal variants of the pancreaticobiliary tract and the pancreas in adults: part 2, Pancreatic duct and pancreas. *AJR Am J Roentgenol.* 2006;187(6):1544–1553.
2. Mortele KJ, Rocha TC, Streeter JL, et al. Multimodality imaging of pancreatic and biliary congenital anomalies. *Radiographics.* 2006;26(3):715–731.

CLINICAL HISTORY *A 4-year-old boy on chronic immunosuppression, presented to the emergency room with progressively worsening vomiting for 4 days*

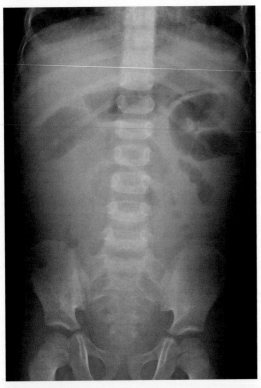

FIGURE **3.22A**

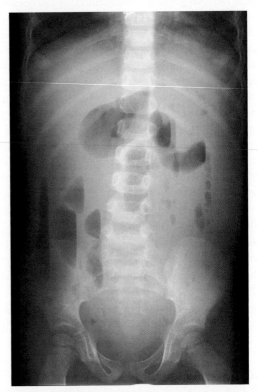

FIGURE **3.22B**

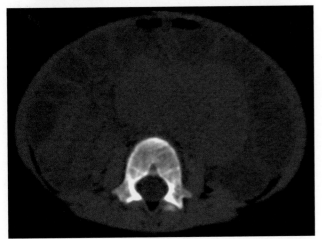

FIGURE **3.22C**

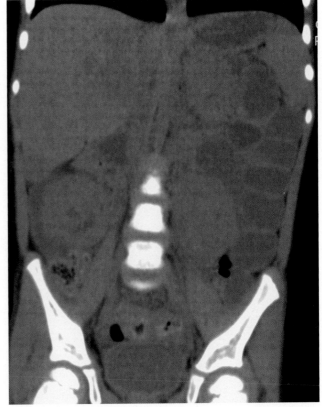

FIGURE **3.22D**

FINDINGS Figure 3.22A and B: Supine and upright views of the abdomen demonstrate dilated bowel loops in the upper abdomen with absence of air in the rectum. There is paucity of gas in the lower abdomen.

Figure 3.22C: Axial image from a non-contrast CT scan of the abdomen and pelvis demonstrates a large retroperitoneal soft-tissue mass with dilated small bowel loops and decompressed colon consistent with a bowel obstruction.

Figure 3.22D: Coronal reformation of the abdomen shows part of the retroperitoneal soft-tissue mass to the left of the spine. The right lower quadrant mass has the classic appearance of an intussusception with alternating layers of the bowel wall (soft-tissue density) and fat. Multiple dilated proximal small bowel loops are seen in the left upper quadrant.

DIFFERENTIAL DIAGNOSIS Lymphoma, neuroblastoma, retroperitoneal teratoma

DIAGNOSIS Non-Hodgkin lymphoma (NHL; Burkitt lymphoma)

DISCUSSION Primary GI malignancies are very rare in the pediatric age group comprising less than 1% of all pediatric malignancies. NHL, however, commonly involves the GI tract in children, comprising 74% of alimentary tract malignancies in one of the larger series. Tumors were found in the colon (50.9%), small bowel (21.8%), and stomach (1.8%). Other series have identified 50% to 93% of the primary intestinal lymphomas occurring in the ileocecal region.

Burkitt lymphoma is the most frequent subtype of NHL in children, accounting for about one-third of all cases. It is the fastest growing tumor in children with a doubling time of approximately 24 hours. The terminal ileum is the most common location.[1]

The WHO has categorized Burkitt lymphoma into endemic, sporadic, and immunodeficiency associated types. The sporadic or American form is the most common type seen in North America and is associated with Epstein–Barr virus infection in 15% of patients. The immunodeficiency type is seen in patients with HIV, allograft recipients, and patients with congenital immunodeficiency.

NHL occurs more commonly in males than in females with a ratio of 2:1.[2]

In children with NHL, extranodal sites are much more commonly involved than in adults. The clinical presentation depends on the site of involvement. The clinical history in patients with GI involvement is usually nonspecific such as chronic abdominal pain. The patient may present with an acute abdomen secondary to an intussusception, acute appendicitis, bowel obstruction, or perforation. A palpable abdominal mass may be evident on clinical examination. Systemic symptoms such as fever and weight loss are uncommon.

Definitive diagnosis of NHL is established by tissue diagnosis. Imaging is essential for the initial staging of the disease to determine prognosis and to direct therapy. Imaging is also important to monitor response to therapy and to exclude recurrence.

Ultrasound is usually the initial imaging modality used in a child presenting with an abdominal mass or an acute abdomen, to exclude intussusception or acute appendicitis. It is the best method to identify testicular involvement.[3] However, it is not accurate for staging purposes. CT is the primary modality used for initial staging of the disease. The role of MRI may increase in future secondary to concerns for radiation exposure in children.

Question for Further Thought

1. What is the role of positron emission tomography (PET) in NHL?

Reporting Responsibilities

Detailed description of the organs involved to accurately describe the full extent of the disease involvement and estimate the tumor burden. It is also important to report secondary findings such as associated bowel obstruction due to luminal narrowing (rare) or intussusception, bowel perforation, or abscess formation.

What the Treating Physician Needs to Know

The full extent or stage of disease at initial presentation since tumor burden is a reliable prognostic factor and directs future therapy.

The response to therapy on the follow-up studies since poor initial response indicates patients at higher risk of relapse or death due to the disease.

Answer

1. Fluorodeoxyglucose (FDG) PET is helpful in assessing the rate of response to therapy and confirming posttherapy remission. In children with residual soft-tissue mass on CT or MR, PET may help differentiate between active disease and nonactive residual soft-tissue mass.

REFERENCES

1. Biko DM, Anupindi SA, Hernandez A, et al. Childhood Burkitt lymphoma: Abdominal and pelvic imaging findings. *AJR Am J Roentgenol.* 2009;192:1304–1315.

2. Kjeldsberg CR, Wilson JF, Berard CW. Non-Hodgkin's lymphoma in children. *Hum Pathol.* 1983;14:612–627.

3. Toma P, Granata C, Rossi A, et al. Multimodality imaging of Hodgkin disease and non-Hodgkin lymphomas in children. *Radiographics.* 2007;27:1335–1354.

CASE 3.23

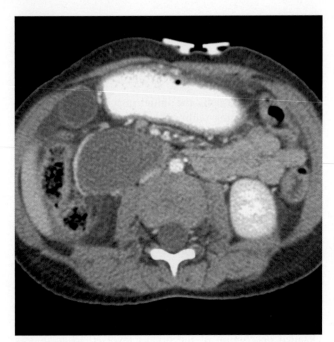

FIGURE **3.23A**

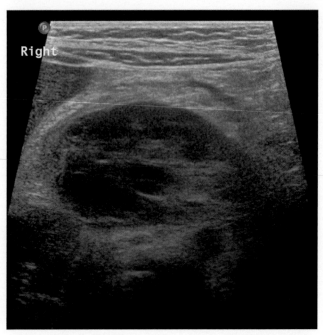

FIGURE **3.23B**

FINDINGS Axial postcontrast CT (**A**) demonstrates a heterogeneous retroperitoneal fluid collection within the second and third portions of the duodenum resulting in compression and obstruction of the duodenum. Findings are confirmed on ultrasonography (**B**), demonstrating a complex, primarily hypoechoic, fluid collection in the region of the duodenum. No internal vascular flow was demonstrated within this collection (not shown).

DIFFERENTIAL DIAGNOSIS Duodenal hematoma, retroperitoneal hematoma, duodenal rupture, pancreatic laceration

DIAGNOSIS Duodenal hematoma

DISCUSSION Intramural duodenal hematoma in children is most often seen following blunt abdominal trauma although duodenal hematoma can also occur with bleeding disorders, Henoch–Schonlein purpura (HSP), or after invasive endoscopic procedures.[1] Accidents involving motor vehicles and bicycles, as well as direct blows to the abdomen, account for most traumatic duodenal injuries in children. This is in contradistinction to adults where most duodenal injuries are due to penetrating trauma.[2] Children are at higher risk of duodenal injury because of weak abdominal musculature, which can cause compression of the duodenum against the spine and resultant mural hematoma. Symptoms and physical findings are often nonspecific, with abdominal pain and bilious vomiting often presenting in a delayed manner due to expanding hematoma.[3] Most cases of duodenal injury are evaluated with CT, which will show a heterogeneous, or high-attenuation mass in the wall of the duodenum. UGI examination will reveal intramural mass effect with a coiled spring appearance in the acute phase of the hematoma while fold thickening of the duodenum is seen during the resolving phase of hematoma. Ultrasound is useful in the follow-up of duodenal hematoma, showing a hypoechoic mass in the region of the pancreas. Most duodenal hematomas will resolve spontaneously with supportive care including bowel rest and parenteral nutrition. Stricture formation, life-threatening hemorrhage, and duodenal perforation are rare in children but require surgical correction when encountered.

Questions for Further Thought

1. Should children with duodenal hematoma be evaluated for possible abuse?
2. In what portions of the duodenum are injuries most likely to occur, and are duodenal injuries associated with other solid organ injury?

Reporting Responsibilities

- Describe the location and extent of hematoma as well as any evidence of obstruction.
- Report additional injuries associated with duodenal hematoma.

What the Treating Physician Needs to Know

- Duodenal hematoma is more common in children sustaining blunt abdominal trauma.
- Clinical symptoms can be delayed more than 48 hours after injury because of increasing hematoma and obstruction.[3]

Answers

1. Duodenal hematoma in children less than 4 years of age without convincing history of trauma should prompt evaluation of possible abuse. Visceral injuries are relatively uncommon in abused children; however, when present they are associated with high mortality, up to 50%.[4]

2. Hematoma and perforation are more frequent in the second and third segments of the duodenum, owing to the relative fixed position and the rich submucosal vascular supply at these points. Crushing injury of the duodenum between the spine and a blunt object can occur in isolation or with pancreatic injury.

REFERENCES

1. Sidhu MK, Weinberger E, Healey P. Intramural duodenal hematoma after blunt abdominal trauma. *AJR Am J Roentgenol.* 1998;170(1):38.
2. Shilyansky J, Pearl RH, Kreller M, et al. Diagnosis and management of duodenal injuries in children. *J Pediatr Surg.* 1997; 32(6):880–886.
3. You JS, Park S, Chung YE, et al. Images in emergency medicine. Duodenal hematoma. *Ann Emerg Med.* 2008;51(1):107, 116.
4. Kleinman PK, Brill PW, Winchester P. Resolving duodenal-jejunal hematoma in abused children. *Radiology.* 1986;160(3): 747–750.

CASE 3.24

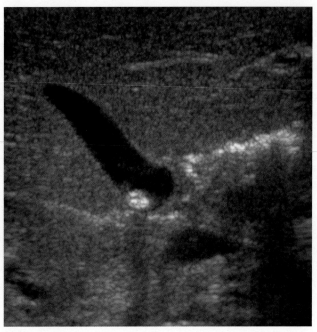

FIGURE **3.24**

FINDINGS Transverse gray-scale ultrasound image of the right upper quadrant in a 1-month-old male demonstrates an incidentally noted echogenic focus in the gallbladder with posterior acoustic shadowing. Gallbladder wall is of normal thickness.

DIFFERENTIAL DIAGNOSIS Cholelithiasis, gallbladder polyp, tumefactive sludge

DIAGNOSIS Cholelithiasis

DISCUSSION Cholelithiasis is a condition wherein the normally soluble elements of bile precipitate to form solid concretions known as gallstones. While traditionally considered a disease of adults, it is being diagnosed with increasing frequency in the pediatric population. The estimated prevalence in children is approximately 2%.[1] Unlike in adults, in whom the majority of the gallstones comprise cholesterol, black pigment stones are the most common stone type in children, accounting for greater than half of all pediatric stone disease.[2] The increased prevalence of black pigment stones reflects the etiologic contribution of hemolytic anemias and chronic parenteral nutrition, both of which are common in the pediatric population and predispose to black pigment stone formation. Other risk factors for stone formation include obesity, bowel resection, ileal disease, and CF. Although most stones in children are diagnosed in the second decade, approximately 15% of cholelithiasis is detected in the neonatal period, as in this case. In the neonatal population, specific risk factors include diuretic therapy, dehydration, phototherapy, prematurity, and NEC. Spontaneous resolution of gallstones has been demonstrated in up to three-quarters of infants, and up to a third of children less than a year of age.[3] Irrespective of patient age or stone type, the ultrasound appearance of gallstones is that of mobile, echogenic foci with posterior acoustic shadowing. This is in contrast to tumefactive sludge, which presents as mobile, nonshadowing echogenic foci. Gallbladder polyps are similar in ultrasound appearance to tumefactive sludge, but are characteristically adherent to the gallbladder wall and rarely occur in children. Radiographically, 20% to 40% of pediatric gallstones are radiopaque and appear as clustered lucent-centered calcifications in the right upper quadrant that layer dependently with upright positioning.[2]

Questions for Further Thought

1. What is pseudocholelithiasis?
2. Which forms of hemolytic anemia most commonly predisposed to stone disease in children?

Reporting Responsibilities

• Note the presence of echogenic foci, mobility, and posterior acoustic shadowing.

• Confirm the absence of ultrasound features of cholecystitis, including gallbladder wall thickening and pericholecystic fluid.

What the Treating Physician Needs to Know

• Approximately half of pediatric gallstones are asymptomatic, and conservative management is recommended. Cholecystectomy is advocated only in the setting of symptomatic cholelithiasis. In the neonatal period, low complication rates and high spontaneous resolution rates support nonoperative management of cholelithiasis, even in initially symptomatic patients.

• Complications of stone disease are similar to those seen in adults, and include acute and chronic cholecystitis, obstructive choledocholithiasis, and pancreatitis.

Answers

1. Pseudocholelithiasis refers to the transient formation of calcium ceftriaxone salt precipitates in the gallbladder that can simulate stones or biliary sludge. It occurs in up to 40% of children treated with ceftriaxone for greater than 10 days.[4]

2. Sickle cell disease, hereditary spherocytosis, and hereditary elliptocytosis. On average, half of those with sickle cell disease will develop gallstones by age 22.

REFERENCES

1. Wesdorp I, Bosman D, de Graaff A, et al. Clinical presentation and predisposing factors of cholelithiasis and sludge in children. *J Pediatr Gastroenterol Nutr.* 2000;31:411–417.

2. Stringer MD, Taylor DR, Soloway RD. Gallstone composition: Are children different? *J Pediatr.* 2003;142(4):435–440.

3. Bogue CO, Murphy AJ, Gerstle JT, et al. Risk factors, complications, and outcomes of gallstones in children: A single-center review. *J Pediatr Gastroenterol Nutr.* 2010;50(3):303–308.

4. Bor O, Dinleyici EC, Kebapci M, et al. Ceftriaxone-associated biliary sludge and pseudocholelithiasis during childhood: A prospective study. *Pediatr Int.* 2004;46:322–324.

Jason Nixon and Mahesh Thapa

CASE 3.25

CLINICAL HISTORY *A 6-week-old term infant with 4 weeks of worsening jaundice*

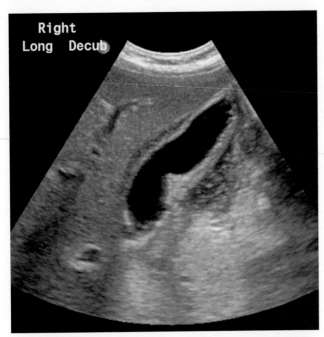

FIGURE **3.25A**

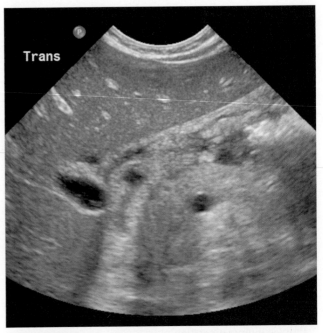

FIGURE **3.25B**

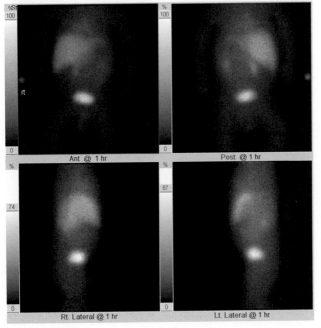

FIGURE **3.25C**

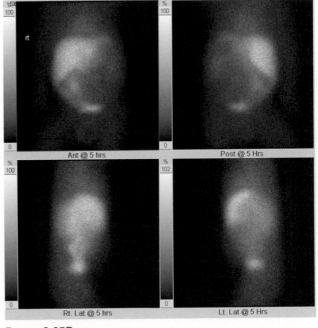

FIGURE **3.25D**

FINDINGS Sagittal (**A**) and transverse (**B**) gray-scale ultrasound images of the right upper quadrant demonstrate normal bile ducts, moderate gallbladder wall thickening, and mildly hypoechoic hepatic parenchyma. Planar abdominal images from a technetium (Tc)-99m hepatobiliary scan at 1 hour (**C**) and 5 hours (**D**) demonstrate poor hepatic radiotracer extraction with increased urinary clearance at 1 hour, with bowel activity in the right abdomen at 5 hours.

DIFFERENTIAL DIAGNOSIS Neonatal hepatitis (NH), extrahepatic biliary obstruction, extrahepatic biliary atresia (EHBA), cholestatic syndromes

DIAGNOSIS NH

DISCUSSION NH is a syndrome of cholestatic inflammation of the liver, and is among the commonest causes of conjugated hyperbilirubinemia in the first 2 months of life. Histologically, there is characteristic giant cell transformation with a mixed inflammatory infiltrate and periportal fibrosis. This pattern of neonatal giant cell hepatitis represents a nonspecific reaction of the neonatal liver to a variety of insults, including infectious, metabolic, and toxic.[1] In about a quarter of cases, it is idiopathic. The major goal of imaging in NH is to exclude alternate causes of conjugated hyperbilirubinemia that are surgically treated. Ultrasound is typically obtained first to exclude causes of extrahepatic obstruction such choledochal cysts or obstructing mass lesions. Gallbladder wall thickening and abnormal parenchymal echogenicity can be seen in NH but are nonspecific. Nonvisualization of the gallbladder or common duct can suggest EHBA, another surgically treated cause of conjugated hyperbilirubinemia, but neither finding alone is sensitive. If ultrasound is nondiagnostic, a hepatobiliary scintigram can be obtained to rule out EHBA. Visualization of radiotracer activity in the bowel at any point during the examination excludes the diagnosis, implicating either NH or a cholestatic syndrome. Poor hepatic extraction of the radiotracer with persistent blood pool activity beyond 10 minutes is a marker for hepatic dysfunction, and favors NH. Conversely, delayed hepatic clearance with parenchymal retention of radiotracer at 5- and 24-hour delayed imaging suggests primary cholestasis. Considerable overlap exists, however. Nonvisualization of the bowel by 24 hours is nonspecific, and can be seen in EHBA, cholestatic syndromes, and severely cholestatic NH.[2] The role of hepatobiliary scintigraphy and percutaneous liver biopsy are complementary, and the exact sequence of diagnostic evaluations will depend on the degree of local expertise, the age of the child at presentation, and the results of the individual investigations.[1]

Questions for Further Thought

1. What medication should be routinely used to increase the diagnostic accuracy of hepatobiliary scintigraphy in discriminating between EHBA and NH?
2. What are the commonest causes of NH?
3. What are the major cholestatic syndromes to cause neonatal jaundice?

Reporting Responsibilities

- Note the presence of obstructing lesions or duct dilation on ultrasound.
- Report presence of bowel activity on early or delayed hepatobiliary scintigraphy.

What the Treating Physician Needs to Know

- Ultrasound is generally considered relatively insensitive to the diagnosis of both EHBA and NH, but is useful in excluding extrahepatic obstruction.
- Presence of bowel activity on the hepatobiliary scan virtually excludes EHBA.

Answers

1. Phenobarbital at 5 mg/kg/day in two divided doses for 3 to 5 days before scan.
2. Congenital hepatic infection, hypopituitarism, hypothyroidism, alpha-1 antitrypsin deficiency, galactosemia, and tyrosinemia.
3. Alagille syndrome/paucity of interlobular bile ducts (PIBD), progressive familial intrahepatic cholestasis (PFIC), sepsis-related cholestasis, TPN-related cholestasis, inspissated bile syndrome in CF.

REFERENCES

1. Moyer V, Freese DK, Whitington PF, et al. Guideline for the evaluation of cholestatic jaundice in infants: Recommendations of the North American Society for Pediatric Gastroenterology, Hepatology and Nutrition. *J Pediatr Gastroenterol Nutr.* 2004; 39(2):115–128.
2. Gilmour SM, Hershkop M, Reifen R, et al. Outcome of hepatobiliary scanning in neonatal hepatitis syndrome. *J Nucl Med.* 1997;38(8):1279–1282.

Jason Nixon and Mahesh Thapa

CLINICAL HISTORY *A 3-year-old boy with hematemesis*

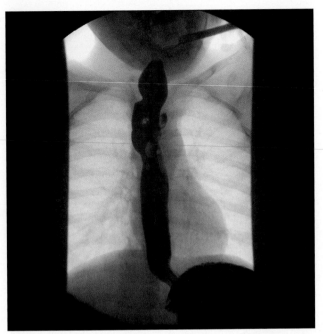

FIGURE **3.26A**

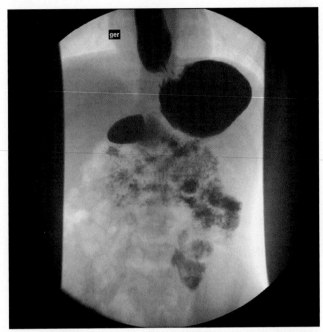

FIGURE **3.26B**

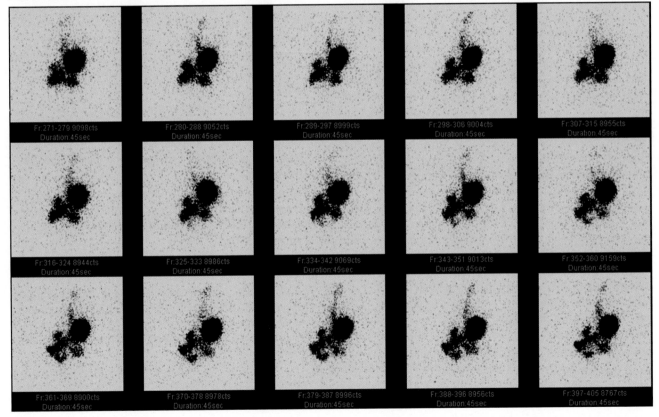

FIGURE **3.26C**

FINDINGS Coned frontal fluoroscopic spot view of the chest (**A**) during a single contrast barium study demonstrates two intraluminal polyps in the mid-esophagus adjacent to a small ulceration, and a patulous gastroesophageal junction. Fluoroscopic spot view of the abdomen (**B**) demonstrates spontaneous GER. Sequential anterior planar images from a Tc-99m sulfur colloid study (**C**) demonstrate multiple episodes of GER.

DIFFERENTIAL DIAGNOSIS GER disease (GERD), physiologic GER

DIAGNOSIS GERD

DISCUSSION GER refers to the retrograde passage of gastric contents into the esophagus, with or without regurgitation into the pharynx or oral cavity. GER is extremely common in healthy individuals of all ages, with asymptomatic episodes occurring up to 30 times daily.[1] When associated with no symptoms or evidence of secondary tissue injury, this reflux is considered physiologic. At most ages, physiologic GER is subclinical. Clinically evident GER manifests as "spitting" or regurgitation, and is common only during infancy. It is especially common among premature infants due to functional immaturity of the distal esophageal sphincter. Clinically evident GER occurs with peak prevalence at 4 months of life, when it is reported in between half and two-thirds of infants.[2] It subsequently decreases or resolves during the first year of life, and its presence is unusual in children beyond 18 months of age. No treatment is currently recommended for clinical or subclinical GER in children.[3]

The association of GER with symptoms or evidence of resultant tissue damage defines GERD. Symptoms depend on age at presentation, and are often nonspecific. Poor weight gain, feeding refusal, and irritability are often the only signs of GERD in infants. Heartburn, respiratory symptoms, and decreased food intake can be seen in the older children. Dysphagia secondary to stricture or hematemesis related to underlying esophagitis, as in this case, can be present at any age.

The role of imaging in the diagnosis of GER is limited. Although active reflux can be seen on both contrast UGI studies as well as nuclear scintigraphy, sensitivity is limited and absence of observed GER does not exclude the diagnosis. Further, the presence of GER on imaging does not imply GERD, with the exception of rare instances in which both GER and resulting pathology are concomitantly observed. Diagnosis is on the basis of pH monitoring, intraluminal impedance monitoring, manometry studies, and endoscopy with biopsy. UGI contrast studies are often used to identify anatomic abnormalities that might predispose to known GERD, and to evaluate for complications such as esophagitis, ulceration, or inflammatory polyps. Scintigraphy can be used to evaluate the contribution of delayed gastric emptying in cases of known or suspected GERD,[3] as well as to demonstrate aspiration as a result of GER in infants (the so-called "milk scan"). Treatment of GERD is with acid suppression and prokinetic agents, with surgical intervention in refractory cases.

Questions for Further Thought

1. What condition should be specifically excluded in infants with GER and poor weight gain or failure to thrive?
2. Which medical conditions predispose to severe, chronic GERD?

Reporting Responsibilities

- Describe the presence of GER noted on any imaging study.
- On contrast fluoroscopic studies of the UGI tract, assess for the presence of any structural abnormalities that may predispose to GER, such as hiatal hernia, and any complications, such as ulceration, stricture, or esophagitis.

What the Treating Physician Needs to Know

Presence of GER on UGI contrast study or nuclear scintigraphy does not imply GERD, nor does its absence exclude it.

Answers

1. Dietary protein induced gastroenteropathy, otherwise known as cow's milk protein intolerance. This condition can result in regurgitation and failure to thrive in infants. A trial of hypoallergenic formula in formula-fed infants, or maternal elimination of cow's milk and dairy in exclusively breast-fed infants, can be diagnostic.
2. Neurologic impairment, obesity, repaired esophageal atresia (EA), CF, repaired achalasia, hiatal hernia, and lung transplantation all predispose to GERD.

REFERENCES

1. Shay S, Tutuian R, Sifrim D, et al. Twenty-four hour ambulatory simultaneous impedance and pH monitoring: A multicenter report of normal values from 60 healthy volunteers. *Am J Gastroenterol.* 2004;99:1037–1043.
2. Campanozzi A, Boccia G, Pensabene L, et al. Prevalence and natural history of gastroesophageal reflux: Pediatric prospective study. *Pediatrics.* 2009;123(3):779–783.
3. Vandenplas Y, Rudolph CD, Di Lorenzo C, et al. Pediatric gastroesophageal reflux clinical practice guidelines: Joint recommendations of the North American Society for Pediatric Gastroenterology, Hepatology, and Nutrition (NASPGHAN) and the European Society for Pediatric Gastroenterology, Hepatology, and Nutrition (ESPGHAN). *J Pediatr Gastroenterol Nutr.* 2009;49:498.

Jennifer Williams

CLINICAL HISTORY *A 3-year-old male with right lower quadrant abdominal pain*

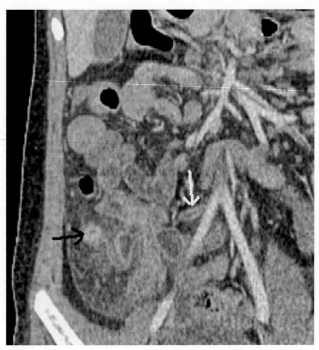

FIGURE **3.27A**

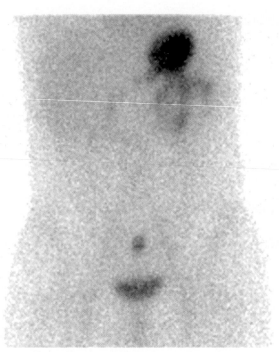

FIGURE **3.27B**

FINDINGS (**A**) Coronal CT of the abdomen and pelvis with IV and oral contrast reveals a broad-based blind-ending tubular structure arising from the antimesenteric portion of the ascending colon (*black arrow*). Note the separate tubular structure arising from the mesenteric aspect of the colon (*white arrow*). (**B**) Tc-99m pertechnetate scintigraphy in a separate patient shows a focus of radiotracer accumulation in the pelvis, which appeared at the same time as the gastric mucosa and increased in intensity over time.

DIFFERENTIAL DIAGNOSIS Meckel diverticulum, appendicitis with abscess, inflammatory bowel disease with abscess

DIAGNOSIS Meckel diverticulum

DISCUSSION Meckel diverticulum is a relatively rare developmental abnormality, which occurs when there is incomplete

regression of the omphalomesenteric duct.[1] It can present with variable symptoms including acute abdominal pain, diverticulitis, intussusception, perforation, bowel obstruction, and bleeding.[2] As these lesions typically occur within 40 to 60 cm of the cecum,[1] they can be difficult to distinguish from appendicitis both clinically and on imaging studies. Often, a Meckel diverticulum will contain ectopic tissue, with gastric and pancreatic tissue occurring most frequently. Lesions containing gastric mucosa can be imaged using Tc-99m pertechnetate studies; pertechnetate is taken up by gastric mucosa. Typically, a focal region of radiotracer accumulation is seen in the right lower quadrant, appearing simultaneously to stomach mucosa and increasing in intensity over time.[3]

Questions for Further Thought

1. What is the rule of two's?
2. How sensitive and specific is scintigraphy in diagnosing Meckel diverticulum?

Reporting Responsibilities

- Signs of acute abdomen (free air, free fluid, abscess, bowel obstruction, and so on).
- Incidental Meckel diverticulum should be reported to the referring physician.

What the Treating Physician Needs to Know

- Complicating features as described above.
- Relative location of lesion.

Answers

1. The rule of two's is a memory aid for Meckel diverticulum, and is as follows: 2% of the population, 2 years of age, 2 cm in size, 2 feet from the ileocecal valve, and 2 common forms of ectopic tissue (gastric and pancreatic).

2. Specificity of 95%[2]; sensitivity of 85% to 90% in children.[3] It should be noted that there are variable reports of the efficacy of scintigraphy which relate primarily to the presenting symptoms of the patient.

REFERENCES

1. Elsayes KM, Menias CO, Harvin HJ, et al. Imaging manifestations of Meckel's diverticulum. *AJR Am J Roentgenol.* 2007;189:81–88.
2. Thurley PD, Halliday KE, Somers JM, et al. Radiological features of Meckel's diverticulum and its complications. *Clin Radiol.* 2009;64:109–118.
3. Sfakianakis GN, Conway JJ. Detection of ectopic gastric mucosa in Meckel's diverticulum and in other aberrations by scintigraphy. I. Pathophysiology and 10-year clinical experience. *J Nucl Med.* 1981;22:647–654.

CLINICAL HISTORY *A 5-year-old male with severe abdominal pain*

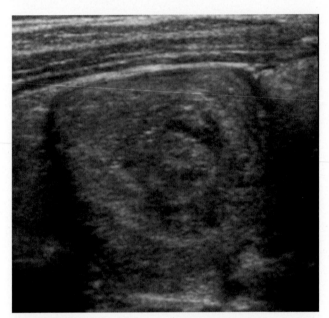

FIGURE **3.28A**

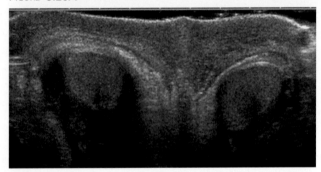

FIGURE **3.28C**

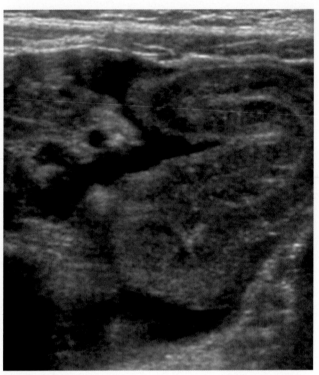

FIGURE **3.28B**

FINDINGS Sonographic evaluation of the abdomen demonstrates an ileoileal intussusception as well as significant bowel wall thickening and mild ascites (**A** and **B**). Scrotal ultrasound demonstrates severe scrotal wall edema (**C**).

DIFFERENTIAL DIAGNOSIS Henoch-Schonlein Purpura (HSP), trauma

DIAGNOSIS HSP

DISCUSSION HSP is a small vessel vasculitis presenting frequently in young children.[1] Its etiology is not known, and

it has been linked to multiple preceding events, including upper respiratory infection, drugs, and environmental exposures to name a few. As HSP is a vasculitis, any organ can be affected; however, the GI system is most frequently involved from the radiographic perspective. The most common finding is bowel wall thickening and edema secondary to hemorrhage. Other findings include ascites, lymphadenopathy, and intussusception (typically ileoileal).[2] Patients display a classic rash involving the lower extremities, and commonly present with symptoms relating to renal, joint, and/or GI involvement. Less frequently other organs are involved in HSP; for instance, occasionally children will present with severe scrotal edema secondary to hemorrhage or with pulmonary hemorrhage.[3,4]

Questions for Further Thought

1. Should reduction be attempted for ileoileal intussusception?
2. What is the classic sonographic imaging appearance for intussusception?

Reporting Responsibilities

- Describe the location of intussusception.
- In cases of scrotal edema, confirm normal flow within the testicles/epididymis.

What the Treating Physician Needs to Know

The radiographic findings of HSP are nonspecific. If the patient has a purpuric rash involving primarily the lower extremities and/or renal symptoms, however, the radiographic findings become nearly pathognomonic.

Answers

1. Air or contrast enema for intussusception reduction should only be performed in patients with ileocolic intussusception. Thus patients with HSP and ileoileal intussusception are not candidates for reduction.

2. The "target sign" or the "doughnut sign"; both are composed of alternating hyper- and hypoechoic bands corresponding to bowel, edema, and mesenteric fat.[5]

REFERENCES

1. Jeong YK, Ha HK, Yoon CH, et al. Gastrointestinal involvement in Henoch-Schonlein syndrome: CT findings. *AJR Am J Roentgenol.* 1997;168:965–968.

2. Sohagia AB, Gunturur SG, Tong TR, et al. Henoch-Schonlein purpura—A case report and review of the literature. *Gastroenterol Res Pract.* 2010;2010: 597–648.

3. Lee JS, Choi SK. Acute scrotum in 7 cases of Schonlein-Henoch syndrome. *Yonsei Med J.* 1998;39:73–78.

4. Nadrous HF, Yu AC, Specks U, et al. Pulmonary involvement in Henoch-Schonlein purpura. *Mayo Clin Proc.* 2004;79(9): 1151–1157.

5. Sorantin E, Lindbichler F. Management of intussusception. *Eur Radiol.* 2004;14: L146–L154.

Deborah Conway

CASE 3.29

CLINICAL HISTORY *A 1-day-old infant with grunting and abdominal distention*

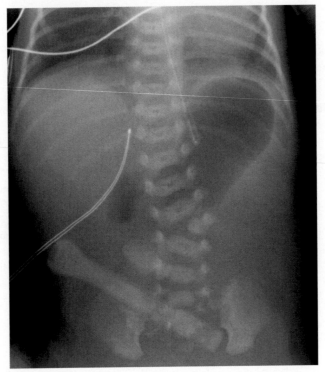

FIGURE 3.29

FINDINGS Portable kidney, ureter, and bladder (KUB) demonstrating gaseous distention of the stomach with a "double bubble" sign. There is a paucity of gas in the distal bowel. Additionally, there is a hemivertebral body in the lumbar spine.

DIFFERENTIAL DIAGNOSIS Duodenal atresia, annular pancreas, duodenal stenosis, severe duodenal web

DIAGNOSIS Duodenal atresia

DISCUSSION Duodenal atresia occurs in approximately 1 in 4,000 live births. It is considered a failure of recanalization, which normally occurs at 10 weeks of gestational age. Partial recanalization failure results in duodenal stenosis while complete failure results in duodenal atresia. Frequently, these patients have other congenital abnormalities, which include malpositioning of bowel, Down syndrome, tracheoesophageal fistula (TEF), imperforate anus, or congenital heart disease.[1] Clinical findings classically include bilious vomiting within the first day of life. Imaging findings include the classic "double bubble" sign as well as polyhydramnios seen in perinatal ultrasound. The proximal left-sided bubble is the air- and fluid-filled stomach. The proximal duodenum represents the second bubble to the right of the midline.[2] There are multiple surgical techniques for treatment and the prognosis is largely determined by associated abnormalities.

Questions for Further Thought

1. What is the etiology of bowel atresia distal to the duodenum?

2. What is the name of the classic radiographic finding seen on a UGI series in the setting of an intraluminal diverticulum?

Reporting Responsibilities

- Offer the most likely diagnosis, as well as a full evaluation of any other congenital abnormalities imaged.
- Identify any distal bowel gas to determine if there is complete atresia, stenosis, or bifid termination of the CBD with gas passing the atretic segment.

What the Treating Physician Needs to Know

- The differential diagnoses so that appropriate consultations may be obtained.
- Any other observed congenital abnormality that would alter immediate treatment.

Answers

1. A vascular accident or ischemic insult is the most common cause of bowel atresia distal to the duodenum.

2. The "windsock" deformity of the duodenum.

REFERENCES

1. Blickman H. *Pediatric Radiology: The Requisites.* 2nd ed. Boston: Mosby; 1997:106–125.

2. Traubici J. The double bubble sign. *Radiology.* 2001;220(2): 463–464.

CASE 3.30

CLINICAL HISTORY *A 6-week-old infant with abdominal distention*

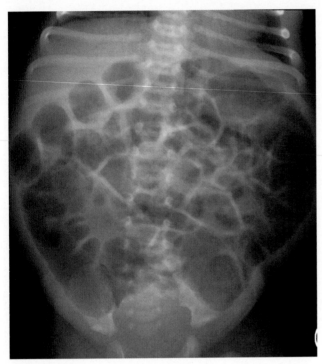

FIGURE **3.30A**

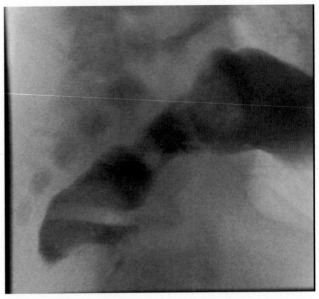

FIGURE **3.30B**

FINDINGS (**A**) Frontal radiograph of the abdomen demonstrates multiple loops of distended bowel with paucity of gas within the rectum. (**B**) Contrast enema in lateral position demonstrates the rectum to be of smaller caliber compared to the sigmoid colon.

DIFFERENTIAL DIAGNOSIS Hirschsprung disease, Meconium plug syndrome

DIAGNOSIS Hirschsprung disease

DISCUSSION During development, the neural crest cells in the GI tract migrate in a craniocaudal direction during the 5th to 12th weeks of gestation. With Hirschsprung disease, the parasympathetic ganglion cells are absent, which has been attributed to failure of this neural crest cell migration. The longer the segment of abnormally constricted colon, the earlier is the arrest of cell migration. The parasympathetic ganglion cells allow the colon to relax and distend. When they are absent, the colon will appear constricted due to the unopposed sympathetic tone, causing a functional obstruction. The more proximal colon becomes dilated secondary to this functional obstruction.[1] The neonate may present with abdominal distention and failure to pass little or no meconium. Older children may present with constipation and often have shorter segments of involvement. Hirschsprung disease is associated with trisomy 21 in 5% of cases. Boys are affected more often than girls when the disease only involves the rectosigmoid colon, which occurs in 75% of cases. Girls are affected more when longer segments of colon are involved.[2] A contrasted enema is the radiologic imaging of choice. If the entire colon is involved, it may mimic a microcolon. A rectal biopsy must be performed for a definitive diagnosis.[3] Treatment consists of removing the aganglionic segment. For short segment disease, a transanal mucosectomy may be an option.[2]

Questions for Further Thought

1. What is the principal cause of neonatal mortality associated with untreated Hirschsprung disease?
2. What is the most important view to evaluate for possible Hirschsprung disease?

Reporting Responsibilities

- Describe the lateral early filling findings on contrasted enema examination.
- Describe the length of the transition zone.

What the Treating Physician Needs to Know

- Definitive diagnosis is obtained by rectal biopsy.
- If a lateral early filling image is not performed on contrasted enema examination, suggest repeating the examination.

Answers

1. When Hirschsprung disease is untreated it may lead to enterocolitis. The neonate will appear ill with fever, abdominal distention, and foul-smelling watery bowel movements. A contrasted enema should be avoided in patients presenting with enterocolitis.

2. The first images obtained during the contrasted enema should be the early filling views, lateral position. This is the most important view to evaluate the transition zone from an abnormally small caliber rectum to a more dilated obstructed proximal colon.

REFERENCES

1. Holschneider A, Puri P, eds. *Hirschsprung's Disease and Allied Disorders.* 3rd ed. New York, NY: Springer Science + Business Media; 2008.
2. Norton JA, Barie PS, Bollinger R, et al. *Surgery: Basic Science and Clinical Evidence.* 2nd ed. New York, NY: Springer Science + Business Media, LLC; 2008.
3. Donnelly L. *Fundamentals of Pediatric Radiology.* Philadelphia, PA: W.B. Saunders Company; 2001.

Deborah Conway

CLINICAL HISTORY *A 5-year-old male with cough*

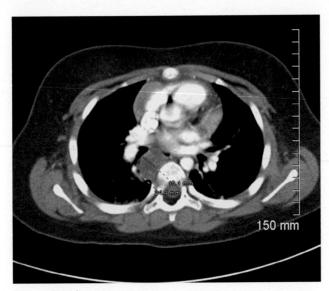

FIGURE 3.31A

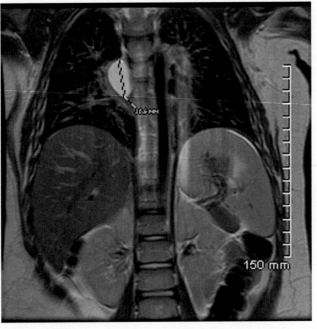

FIGURE 3.31B

FINDINGS CT scan of the chest with contrast (**A**) demonstrates a nonenhancing cystic lesion posterior to the right main stem bronchus in close approximation to the esophagus. MRI of the chest (**B**) shows a well-circumscribed posterior mediastinal lesion with homogeneous bright T2 signal.

DIFFERENTIAL DIAGNOSIS Esophageal duplication cyst, bronchogenic cyst, neurenteric cyst, pericardial cyst, cystic teratoma

DIAGNOSIS Esophageal duplication cyst

DISCUSSION GI duplication cysts are uncommon congenital anomalies that can be found anywhere along the alimentary tract. Ileal duplications are most common (33%), followed by duplications of the esophagus (20%), large bowel (13%), jejunum (10%), stomach (7%), and duodenum (5%). They have smooth muscle walls and are lined by alimentary tract mucosa, which may not be that of the adjacent segment of GI tract. In most cases, no connection exists between the duplication and the GI tract lumen. Duplication cysts are commonly asymptomatic, and are not discovered until adulthood in approximately 30% of patients. Presenting symptoms of mediastinal duplication cysts can include nonspecific respiratory symptoms (cough, wheezing, stridor, and respiratory distress) or dysphagia due to compression of

airways or the esophagus, respectively. Complications of GI duplication cysts include infection (most common), peptic ulceration, and GI bleeding if the cyst contains ectopic gastric mucosa, and pancreatitis if ectopic pancreatic tissue is present within the cyst.

Questions for Further Thought

1. What are the two most common congenital anomalies associated with esophageal duplication?
2. What nuclear medicine study can be useful in confirming GI tract duplication when the results of other imaging studies are equivocal?

Reporting Responsibilities

- Criteria used to differentiate benign congenital cysts from other cyst-like lesions include shape of the lesion; cyst wall thickness; presence of intracystic septations; presence of a solid component, fat, or calcifications; and infiltration of surrounding structures.

- Cysts containing non-serous fluid can have high attenuation on CT and may be mistaken for solid lesions. MRI can be useful in showing the cystic nature of a lesion, which is typically high signal intensity on T2-weighted sequences regardless of the cyst contents.

What the Treating Physician Needs to Know

Surgical excision of GI tract duplications is recommended to prevent associated complications and possibility of malignant transformation.

Answers

1. Thoracic vertebral anomalies and EA.
2. Tc-99m pertechnetate scintigraphy can confirm presence of a GI tract duplication when it contains ectopic gastric mucosa.

REFERENCES

1. Eisenberg R. *Gastrointestinal Radiology: A Pattern Approach.* 4th ed. Philadelphia, PA: Lippincott Williams & Wilkins; 2003: 108–109.
2. Fitch S, Tonkin I, Tonkin A. Imaging of foregut duplication cysts. *Radiographics.* 1986;6:189–201.
3. Jeung M, Gasser B, Gangi A, et al. Imaging of cystic masses of the mediastinum. *Radiographics.* 2002;22:S79–S93.
4. Macpherson R. Gastrointestinal tract duplications: Clinical, pathologic, etiologic, and radiologic considerations. *Radiographics.* 1993;13:1063–1080.

CASE 3.32

CLINICAL HISTORY *A 5-year-old female with history of heart transplant, now with intermittent abdominal pain*

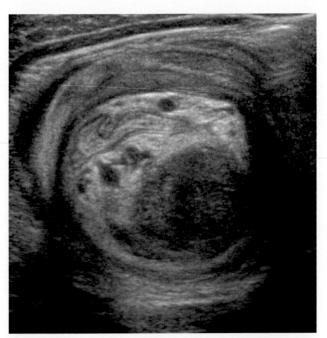

FIGURE **3.32A**

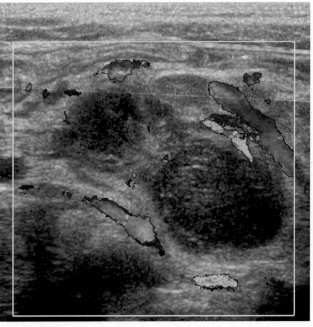

FIGURE **3.32B**

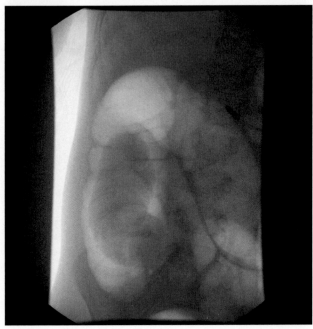

FIGURE **3.32C**

FINDINGS Transverse (**A**) and longitudinal (**B**) ultrasound images of the right lower quadrant demonstrate the bowel-in-bowel appearance of intussusception, centered around a hypoechoic, lobulated mass. Spot fluoroscopic view of the right lower quadrant during pneumatic reduction (**C**) demonstrates air outlining an ileocolic intussusception.

DIFFERENTIAL DIAGNOSIS Pathologic intussusception, idiopathic intussusception

DIAGNOSIS Pathologic intussusception secondary to post-transplant lymphoproliferative disorder

DISCUSSION Intussusception refers to the invagination of a portion of more proximal bowel, termed the intussusceptum, into the lumen of more distal bowel, termed the intussuscipiens. Intussusceptions are generally classified according to the bowel segments involved, and enteroenteric, ileocolic, ileoileocolic, and colocolic variants are described. Greater than 90% of those occurring in the pediatric population are ileocolic, with prolapse of the distal ileum through the ileocecal valve.[1] The majority of ileocolic intussusceptions are believed to result from the normal peristaltic action of bowel upon a masslike lead point within or adjacent to terminal ileum. When this lead point is related to normal lymphoid hypertrophy, the intussusception is considered idiopathic. When a mass or congenital abnormality serves as the lead point, a pathologic intussusception results. The majority of idiopathic intussusceptions occur in children between the ages of 2 months and 2 years. The incidence of pathologic intussusceptions increases sharply in older children, from less than 4% in children less than 2 years to greater than a third of patients beyond that age.[1] Common pathologic lead points include Meckel diverticula, intestinal polyps, and Burkitt lymphoma. Radiographs are frequently obtained to exclude pneumoperitoneum, and infrequently will identify a colonic mass silhouetted by gas. Sonography is the imaging of choice for presumed intussusception, however. The sonographic appearance of pathologic intussusception is the classic bowel-in-bowel appearance of the idiopathic variety associated with a cystic or solid mass at the leading edge of the intussusceptum.[2] Risks associated with all forms of intussusception include bowel obstruction and mesenteric vascular compromise with associated bowel necrosis. Pneumatic or contrast enema serves as both diagnostic confirmation as well as a means of reduction, with surgical reduction reserved for refractory or recurrent cases.

Questions for Further Thought

1. Which systemic conditions increase the risk of pathologic intussusception?
2. What is the importance of enteroenteric intussusception?

Reporting Responsibilities

• Describe the presence and type of the intussusception, and any associated pathologic lead point.

• Note the presence or absence of color flow within the intussuscepting bowel.

What the Treating Physician Needs to Know

• Intussusception is a true pediatric emergency, and is second only to appendicitis as the most common cause of acute abdominal emergency in children. Risk is for bowel necrosis and perforation with peritoneal contamination, sepsis, and shock.

• The risk for pathologic intussusception increases sharply beyond 2 years of age.

Answers

1. HSP, CF, Peutz–Jeghers syndrome, familial polyposis, nephritic syndrome, and mesenteric adenopathy all predispose to intussusception.

2. Enteroenteric intussusceptions are often incidentally noted on sonography, CT, and MR of the abdomen. In isolation and without associated obstruction, these are typically transient phenomena without clinical importance. When multiple, diffuse small bowel diseases such as polyposis syndromes, HSP or malabsorption syndromes such as celiac disease should be considered.[3]

REFERENCES

1. Waseem M, Rosenberg HK. Intussusception. *Pediatr Emerg Care.* 2008;24(11):793–800.
2. Williams H. Imaging and intussusception. *Arch Dis Child Educ Pract Ed.* 2008;93(1):30–36.
3. Horton KM, Fishman EK. MDCT and 3D imaging in transient enteroenteric intussusceptions: Clinical observations and review of the literature. *AJR Am J Roentgenol.* 2008;191(3):736–742.

Marguerite T. Parisi

CLINICAL HISTORY *(Fig. 3.33A and B): Two newborns, each presenting with respiratory distress from birth. (Fig. 3.33C and D): A 5-month-old child who has choking and cyanosis with feeds*

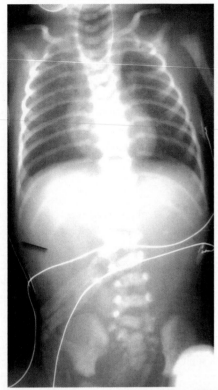

FIGURE **3.33A**

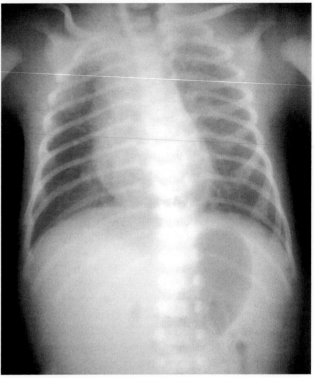

FIGURE **3.33B**

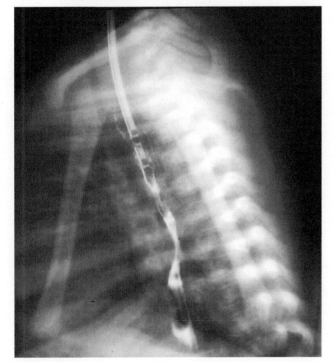

FIGURE **3.33C**

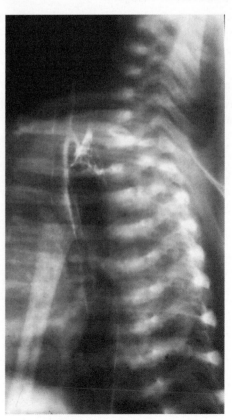

FIGURE **3.33D**

FINDINGS In the first infant (**A**), plain film radiograph of the chest and abdomen reveals a large paratracheal air collection overlying the cervical spine containing a tube coiled within. This air collection represents a dilated proximal esophageal pouch due to EA. There is an absence of bowel gas in the abdomen, indicating either isolated EA or EA with only a proximal TEF. Sacral vertebral anomalies are present.

In the second newborn (**B**), a similar air collection is present overlying the cervical spine and displacing the trachea to the right, again consistent with EA. There is a subtle right upper lobe opacity, likely aspiration. Bowel gas is present within the upper abdomen; consequently, there is an associated distal TEF present. No vertebral anomalies identified in field of view.

In the third child (**C** and **D**), true lateral views from a contrast esophagram are presented. In the initial image (**C**), contrast is being injected into the esophagus via an enteric tube. A thin string of contrast is noted anterior to the upper esophagus, coursing toward the trachea. After removal of the enteric tube (**D**), contrast is noted in both the trachea and the esophagus, clearly demonstrating a classic H- or N-type TEF.

DIFFERENTIAL DIAGNOSIS In the newborn presenting with respiratory distress from birth, the presence of air in a distended pharyngeal pouch, particularly when the tip of an enteric tube is present within, is pathognomonic of EA.

In the older child who presents with cough, choking, or cyanosis with feeds, the clinical considerations include dysphasia with recurrent aspiration, vascular ring, laryngotracheal cleft, and an isolated TEF. Attention to detail during the performance of a contrast esophagram will distinguish between these entities.

DIAGNOSES (**A**) EA with distal TEF; (**B**) EA without distal TEF; (**C** and **D**) isolated TEF

DISCUSSION EA, a complete interruption in the continuity of the esophageal lumen, and TEF, a congenital fistulous connection between the proximal or distal esophagus and the airway, are common congenital anomalies, occurring in 1 in 2,400 to 4,500 live births.[1] These anomalies are due to the disordered formation and separation of the primitive foregut, which occurs during the fourth and fifth weeks of gestation.

Clinically, patients with EA present with increased pharyngeal secretions and respiratory distress due to recurrent aspiration. The single best radiologic clue to the diagnosis on chest film is the presence of a paratracheal (frontal view) or retropharyngeal (lateral view) air collection, which represents the dilated proximal esophageal pouch. The presence of air within the abdomen on plain film imaging will help to distinguish those patients who have an associated distal TEF, the most common form of this malformation (82% to 88% of cases), from those who have isolated EA (8% to 9%) or EA with proximal TEF (1%) in which there is absence of gas within the abdomen.

Approximately 5% of patients have an isolated H- or N-type TEF (**C** and **D**). Cough, choking, or cyanosis with feeds and recurrent pneumonias are the classic clinical presentations in these patients. Although most patients with isolated TEF are symptomatic at birth, diagnosis is often delayed, sometimes even until adulthood. In their series, Kanak et al.[2] reported a mean age of diagnosis of 8 months in their patents with isolated TEF.

Associated anomalies in those with EA and TEF are common, with an incidence ranging from 25% to 75%. The occurrence of any of a combination of vertebral, anal, cardiac, tracheoesophageal, renal, or limb anomalies is termed VACTERL syndrome.

Unless there is a wide separation of the esophageal ends, most infants with EA/TEF undergo repair early in infancy with division of the TEF and primary esophageal anastomosis.[1,3] Surgical correction of those with isolated H- or N-type TEF tends to occur later, related to delay in diagnosis.[3]

Despite best practices and a significant decrease in mortality over the past 40 years,[3] there are numerous sequelae following surgical repair of EA/TEF with long-term clinical implications.[1] Complications of repair include leak, obstruction or stricture at the anastomotic site, disturbances in esophageal motility, GER, recurrent TEF, and respiratory complications. Anastomotic leak, an uncommon early complication of surgical repair, occurs in approximately 17%; postoperative strictures in 6% to 40%. Esophageal dysmotility is a nearly uniform occurrence; while dysphagia occurs in up to 92% of these patients, both of which conditions may contribute to recurrent aspiration or esophageal obstruction by food. Esophageal strictures near the anastomotic site occur in between 6% and 40% of patients and are more likely when GERD is present. Between 35% and 66% of children after repair of EA/TEF will develop GERD, which can lead to the additional complications of esophageal strictures, recurrent aspiration, tracheal inflammation, bronchial hyperreactivity, and permanent airway or lung parenchymal damage. Recurrent TEF occurs in about 9% of cases, is more common after a previous anastomotic leak, and requires reoperation. Recurrent TEF is usually located near the site of the original fistula and typically manifests 2 to 18 months after initial repair.[1]

Other respiratory complications or comorbidities which occur in those with of EA/TEF include tracheomalacia, which is found in up to 75% in path specimens but is clinically significant in about 20% of patients.[4] Recurrent infections are common, becoming less frequent over time. Likewise, wheezing, asthma, and persistent pulmonary function abnormalities are common.[5]

Questions for Further Thought

1. What imaging is recommended for the newborn with suspected EA and TEF?
2. What is the protocol for performing a contrast study (either esophagram or, preferably, a UGI) for those suspected of isolated TEF?

Reporting Responsibilities

In the newborn with EA, plain film evaluation should include an assessment of heart size as an indicator of associated cardiac anomalies. Include a statement identifying the side of the aortic arch as surgical approach for repair is typically on the side opposite the aortic arch. Pulmonary opacities may reflect aspiration rather than infectious pneumonias. Search for the presence of vertebral or limb anomalies that may be part of a VACTERL association. Once EA is diagnosed, suggest the performance of renal ultrasound. Avoid the performance of barium or water-soluble contrast studies for diagnosis as these rarely identify proximal fistulas and typically result in recurrent aspiration.

What the Treating Physician Needs to Know

EA and TEF are a spectrum of abnormalities which can be classified as follows: EA with distal TEF: 82% to 88% of cases; isolated EA: 8% to 9% of cases; isolated H- or N-type TEF: 5% of cases; EA with proximal and distal TEF: 2% of cases; EA with proximal TEF: 1% of cases.

Associated anomalies are common in these patients (VACTERL and CHARGE syndromes) and appropriate evaluation includes a thorough physical examination for musculoskeletal, cardiac, and craniofacial anomalies. Screening radiographs should be obtained to search for vertebral anomalies. Renal ultrasound is mandated for detection of GU malformations.

While newborns present with respiratory distress from birth and classic plain film findings, the diagnosis of those with isolated TEF is often delayed. UGI should be considered in those patients with cough, chocking, or cyanosis with feeds or who present with recurrent pneumonias.

Finally, awareness of the commonly encountered respiratory and GI sequelae in those with EA/TEF will allow early intervention, appropriate management, and lead to improved quality of life in these patients.

Answers

1. The best imaging test for diagnosis in the newborn suspected of EA is plain film radiography of the chest and abdomen. The presence of air in the distended pharyngeal pouch is diagnostic of this entity, particularly if the distal tip of an enteric tube is present within the pouch. The presence or absence of air in bowel determines if there is an associated distal TEF.

If further diagnostic confirmation is desired, one can inject a small amount of air (10 cc or so) in the pouch and obtain anteroposterior (AP) and lateral radiographs of the neck/chest or perform fluoroscopy during the air injection. Neither water-soluble nor barium contrast agents are warranted in the initial evaluation of these patients.

However, a contrast study using nonionic water-soluble agents should be performed approximately 5 to 10 days following primary surgical repair to evaluate for leak or other early complications.

2. Protocol suggestions for performing aUGI in the child suspected of isolated TEF include the following. Place patient in the true lateral projection using meticulous technique. Although many patients can swallow sufficient amounts of barium for diagnosis, do not hesitate to place a 5 or 8 French feeding tube in the esophagus when necessary to obtain adequate distention. During contrast bolus, fluoroscope continuously in expected region of fistula with field of view to include the pharynx to just below the carina before acquiring images to exclude aspiration. Obtain confirmatory images or demonstrate normalcy.

Ensure that you do not confuse aspirated contrast from dysphasia or from a laryngotracheal cleft with an isolated TEF. Image the stomach and ligament of Treitz (DJJ) to exclude malrotation.

REFERENCES

1. Kovesi T, Rubin S. Long-term complications of congenital esophageal atresia and/or tracheoesophageal fistula. *Chest.* 2004; 126:915–925.

2. Kanak I, Senocak ME, Hicsonmez A, et al. The diagnosis and treatment of H-type tracheoesophageal fistula. *J Pediatr Surg.* 1997;32:1670–1674.

3. Orford J, Cass DT, Glasson MJ. Advances in the treatment of oesophageal atresia over three decades: The 1970s and the 1990s. *Pediatr Surg Int.* 2004;20:402–407.

4. Spitz L. Esophageal atresia and tracheoesophageal atresia in children. *Curr Opin Pediatr.* 1993;5:347–352.

5. Couriel JM, Hibbert M, Olinsky A, et al. Long term pulmonary consequences of oesophageal atresia with tracheoesophageal fistula. *Acta Pediatr Scand.* 1982;71:973–978.

CASE 3.34

Jason Nixon and Mahesh Thapa

CLINICAL HISTORY *A 6-year-old child with abdominal pain and lethargy following a fall*

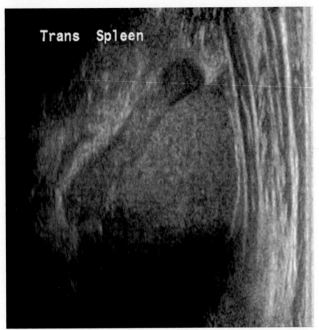

FIGURE **3.34A**

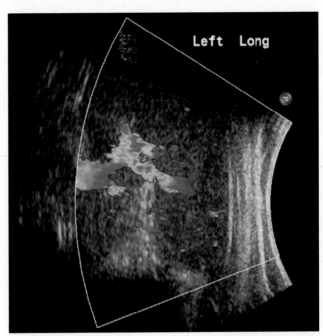

FIGURE **3.34B**

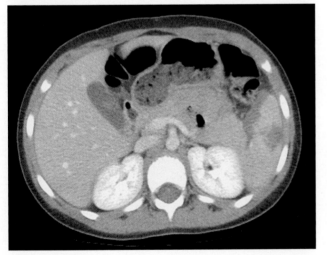

FIGURE **3.34C**

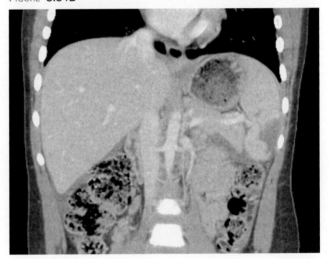

FIGURE **3.34D**

FINDINGS Transverse gray-scale (**A**) and coronal color Doppler (**B**) sonographic images of the left upper quadrant demonstrate a subtle, avascular peripheral hypodensity in the spleen with an associated subcapsular collection. Axial (**C**) and coronal (**D**) images from a contrast-enhanced CT demonstrate a peripheral wedge shaped area of hypoenhance-ment in the spleen with associated subcapsular hematoma. Sonographic images have been reoriented to match the accompanying CT images. Note that the hypoenhancing abnormality on the axial CT image (**C**) appears essentially isoechoic to surrounding spleen on the corresponding sonographic image (**A**).

DIFFERENTIAL DIAGNOSIS Splenic laceration, splenic infarction

DIAGNOSIS Splenic laceration

DISCUSSION The spleen is the most commonly injured abdominal organ following blunt abdominal trauma, accounting for up to 45% of resultant visceral injury.[1] The spectrum of clinical presentation in children with splenic injury is broad, varying from abdominal pain and hemodynamic instability to an essentially asymptomatic state. Imaging thus assumes an important role in diagnosis and characterization of splenic injury. Though historically treated with splenectomy, there has recently been a dramatic evolution in the clinical approach to blunt splenic trauma with a trend toward nonoperative management. This approach is favored due to its high success rate in the pediatric population, allowing for minimization of operative risk, surgical costs, blood transfusions, length of hospital stay, and risk of overwhelming postoperative sepsis. Nonoperative treatment of splenic injury is now the preferred management strategy in children, and is generally pursued if the patient is hemodynamically stable regardless of injury grade.[2] This is in contrast to adult patients, in whom management is guided primarily by grade of injury.

Contrast-enhanced CT is the imaging modality of choice to evaluate possible splenic injury in the pediatric population, with significantly higher sensitivity than ultrasound,[1] as is illustrated in this case. The spectrum of splenic injury seen with blunt abdominal trauma includes laceration, rupture, devascularization, subcapsular hematoma, and hemoperitoneum. Splenic lacerations are evident as irregular, hypodense defects in the periphery of the spleen on contrast-enhanced CT of the abdomen, with similarly configured subtle hypoechoic defects seen on abdominal ultrasound. Splenic rupture is similar in appearance but more extensive in degree, with multiple fragments of splenic tissue separated by hypoenhancing or hypoechoic lacerations. Splenic devascularization is evident as complete transection of the splenic vessels at the hilum, with associated nonenhancement of the splenic parenchyma following contrast administration and absent color Doppler signal at ultrasound. Subcapsular hematoma and hemoperitoneum are evident as collections of blood in the subcapsular space or within the peritoneum. Active contrast extravasation indicates a more severe injury and is characterized by a contrast blush within the hemorrhagic

collection. Though in adults this finding is often a specific indication for embolization or surgical management, hemodynamically stable children are still successfully managed nonoperatively with good long-term outcomes.[3]

Questions for Further Thought

1. What are the delayed complications that can occur following blunt splenic injury?
2. How does the management of penetrating splenic injury differ from that of blunt trauma?

Reporting Responsibilities

- Describe the type and extent of splenic injury.
- Assess for any additional intra-abdominal injuries, most commonly of the liver, kidneys, bowel, or mesentery.

What the Treating Physician Needs to Know

- Contrast-enhanced CT of the abdomen is the preferred imaging modality of choice for the detection of splenic injury following blunt abdominal trauma.
- Unlike in adults, management of blunt splenic injury in children is driven mainly by assessment of hemodynamic stability, with injury grade considered less important.

Answers

1. Pseudocyst, abscess, and pseudoaneurysm formation, as well as delayed splenic rupture. Unlike in adults in whom it is reported in close to 5% of nonoperatively managed patients, delayed splenic rupture in children is extremely rare.[1]
2. Penetrating splenic injury is routinely treated with splenectomy due to unacceptably high failure rates with nonoperative management.

REFERENCES

1. Lynn KN, Werder GM, Callaghan RM, et al. Pediatric blunt splenic trauma: A comprehensive review. *Pediatr Radiol.* 2009; 39:904–916.
2. Moore HB, Vane DW. Long-term follow-up of children with nonoperative management of blunt splenic trauma. *J Trauma.* 2010;68:522–525.
3. Davies DA, Ein SH, Pearl R, et al. What is the significance of contrast "blush" in pediatric blunt splenic trauma? *J Pediatr Surg.* 2010;45:916–920.

CLINICAL HISTORY *An 8-year-old boy with recurrent severe abdominal pain*

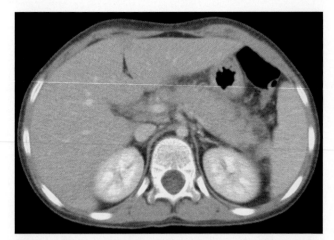

Figure **3.35A**

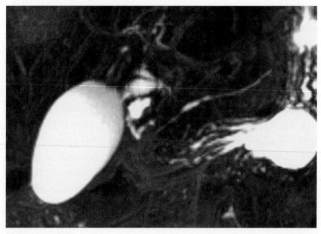

Figure **3.35B**

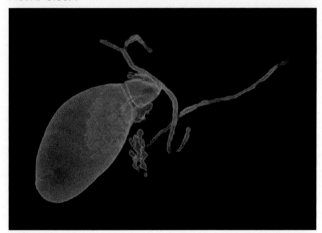

Figure **3.35C**

FINDINGS Axial contrast-enhanced CT (**A**) demonstrates an enlarged, edematous pancreas with peripancreatic fluid consistent with acute interstitial pancreatitis. Coronal oblique MIP (**B**) and volume rendered (**C**) reconstructions from a subsequent MRCP demonstrate a short duct of Wirsung medially, draining into the major papilla along with the CBD. The duct of Santorini is visualized separately, draining into the minor papilla more superiorly. Note mild irregularity of the Santorini duct contour related to chronic pancreatitis.

DIFFERENTIAL DIAGNOSIS PD, annular pancreas

DIAGNOSIS PD

DISCUSSION The pancreatic gland forms from the fusion of two separate anlagen or primordial buds during early embryogenesis. The smaller ventral anlage is initially positioned anterior to the distal foregut, but migrates to the right and posteriorly, rotating 180° around the bowel to fuse with the undersurface of the larger dorsal anlage and form the hook-shaped pancreatic gland proper. The gland as a whole then continues to rotate until it comes to lie in its expected position to the left of the duodenum in the retroperitoneal space. The ventral primordium gives rise to the uncinate process and portions of the pancreatic head, while the neck, body, tail, and remainder of the head are formed by the dorsal primordium. Each anlage is initially drained by a distinct ductal system. The duct of Santorini drains the dorsal bud into the foregut proximally, while the duct of Wirsung drains the ventral bud into the gut lumen slightly more distally, joining with the CBD at its enteric insertion. As the two anlagen merge, an anastomosis is formed between the two ducts and the upstream segment of the Santorini duct becomes continuous with the Wirsung duct distally. This forms the main pancreatic duct, composed of elements of both original duct systems. The short segment of the Santorini duct downstream from the point of anastomosis variably regresses, and if persistent is termed the accessory pancreatic duct.

Failure of fusion of the Santorini and Wirsung ducts results in the pathologic condition known as PD. This represents the most common pancreatic duct anomaly, and is present in an estimated 5% to 10% of individuals based on large postmortem series.[1] Classically, the importance of PD has been that it was considered a risk factor for chronic recurrent pancreatitis. However, there has been considerable debate in the literature as to whether this association is true. Multiple past studies reached conflicting conclusions regarding this association, though the majority was based on endoscopic evaluation with resulting selection bias. More recent studies based on MRCP have demonstrated that between 13% and 44% of patients with recurrent idiopathic pancreatitis had underlying PD, versus only 3% to 7% of community controls.[1,2] Historically, PD was considered to predispose to pancreatitis based upon presumed stenosis at the minor papilla. Emerging evidence suggests that the role of PD in chronic intermittent pancreatitis is not causal, however, but that occurrence of PD associates with underlying genetic mutations that result in pancreatitis. In fact, after excluding these genetic causes for pancreatitis, there remains no statistically significant difference in the rate of PD in those with recurrent idiopathic pancreatitis and controls.[1]

The imaging appearance of PD is that of unfused dorsal and ventral ducts within the pancreas as visualized on thin-section CT, MR, or MRCP. MRCP performed after secretin administration results in improved visualization of the duct system due to increased pancreatic fluid secretion and duct distension, and is reported to have the greatest sensitivity in detecting this and other pancreatic duct anomalies.[3] In contrast to PD, annular pancreas refers to an uncommon ring-like remnant of the ventral anlage left encircling the foregut after it has completed its rotation. This condition results in an obstructive constriction of the duodenum, and is unassociated with pancreatitis.

Questions for Further Thought

1. PD is associated with which types of pancreatitis?
2. What are the types of PD?

Reporting Responsibilities

- Describe the presence and type of PD.
- Note the presence of any imaging signs of acute or chronic pancreatitis, including gland edema, peripancreatic fluid collections, gland necrosis, duct dilation, or gland calcification.

What the Treating Physician Needs to Know

PD is believed to associate with genetic mutations responsible for chronic recurrent pancreatitis, including *CFTR, SPINK1,* and *PRSS1,* and genetic evaluation should be considered if this anatomic anomaly is found.

Answers

1. PD is implicated as a risk factor for both recurrent acute pancreatitis as well as chronic pancreatitis.
2. Three forms of PD have been described: (1) classical PD, in which the ventral duct is visualized but there is failure of fusion; (2) PD with absent ventral duct, in which the ventral duct is nonvisualized; and (3) incomplete PD, in which a rudimentary communication is observed between the dorsal and ventral ducts.

REFERENCES

1. Bertin C, Pelletier AL, Vullierme MP, et al. Pancreas divisum is not a cause of pancreatitis by itself, but acts as a partner of genetic mutations. *Am J Gastroenterol.* 2012;107:311–317.
2. Gonoi W, Akai H, Hagiwara K, et al. Pancreas divisum as a predisposing factor for chronic and recurrent idiopathic pancreatitis: Initial in vivo survey. *Gut.* 2011;60:1103–1108.
3. Mosler P, Akisik F, Sandrasegaran K, et al. Accuracy of magnetic resonance cholangiopancreatography in the diagnosis of pancreas divisum. *Dig Dis Sci.* 2012;57:170–174.

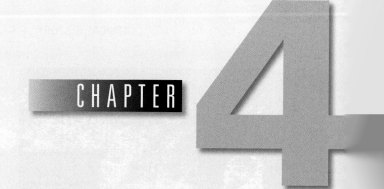

CHAPTER 4

Genitourinary Imaging

CASE 4.1

CLINICAL HISTORY *A 3-year-old child with palpable abdominal mass*

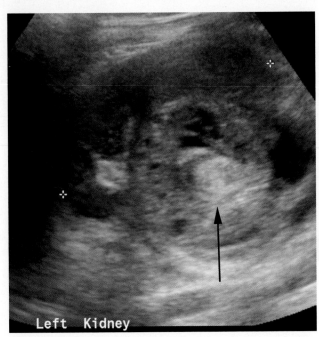

FIGURE **4.1A**

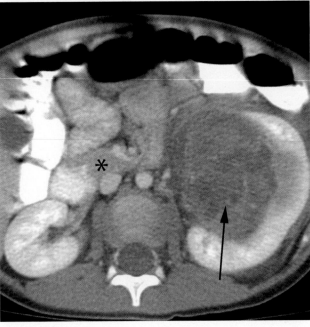

FIGURE **4.1B**

FINDINGS Sagittal ultrasound (US) image of the left kidney (**A**) demonstrates a complex, solid, echogenic mass (*arrow*) arising from the left kidney. Axial computed tomography (CT) image of the abdomen with contrast (**B**) demonstrates an exophytic left renal mass (*arrow*) with perinephric stranding. Enlarged lymph nodes (*) are also shown between the inferior vena cava (IVC) and superior mesenteric vein (SMV).

DIFFERENTIAL DIAGNOSIS Wilms' tumor, mesoblastic nephroma, renal cell carcinoma (RCC), clear cell sarcoma, malignant rhabdoid tumor

DIAGNOSIS Wilms' tumor

DISCUSSION Wilms' tumor is the most common pediatric renal malignancy and occurs most frequently in children 5 years and younger. It is rare in the neonate. It is bilateral in approximately 10%. Most common clinical presentation is a palpable mass. The tumor can arise in any portion of the kidney. The tumor spreads by direct extension and may invade the renal vein and IVC and occasionally extends into the right atrium. Unlike neuroblastoma, Wilms' tumor does not typically elevate or encase the aorta. Most common sites of metastases are the lung, liver, and regional lymph nodes and rarely bone and brain.[1]

Questions for Further Thought

1. What genetic syndromes are associated with Wilms' tumor?

2. What extrarenal abnormalities occur in up to 8% of patients with Wilms' tumor?

3. What is the staging of Wilms' tumor?

Reporting Responsibilities

- Size and location of tumor
- Presence of vascular invasion; surgical management changes if the tumor extends into the right atrium
- Presence of enlarged lymph nodes and/or distant metastasis

What the Treating Physician Needs to Know

- Screening for Wilms' tumor in patients with associated syndromes should begin at 6 months of age with a contrast CT of the abdomen, followed by renal USs every 3 months until 7 years of age. Screening is no longer needed after 7 years because the incidence of Wilms' tumor after the age of 7 decreases significantly.[1]
- Staging is a surgical diagnosis.
- Prognosis is based on surgical staging and histology of the tumor. Cure rate is now over 90%.

Answers

1. Beckwith–Wiedemann syndrome, Denys–Drash syndrome, Trisomy 18, and Bloom syndrome

2. Hemihypertrophy, sporadic aniridia, hypospadias, and cryptorchidism

3. Stage I: Limited to the kidney and completely resectable

    Stage II: Tumor extends beyond the kidney and completely resectable

    Stage III: Residual tumor in the abdomen including lymph nodes, peritoneal implants, or non-resected tumor

    Stage IV: Hematogenous metastasis

    Stage V: Bilateral disease initially or during treatment. Each side is staged independently.[2]

REFERENCES

1. Lowe L, Isuani B, Heller R, et al. Pediatric renal masses: Wilm's tumor and beyond. *Radiographics.* 2000;20:1585–1603.

2. Barnewolt C, Paltiel H, Lebowitz R, et al. Genitourinary tract. In: Kirks D, ed. *Practical Pediatric Imaging.* 3rd ed. Philadelphia, PA: Lippincott-Raven; 1998:1111–1126.

CASE 4.2

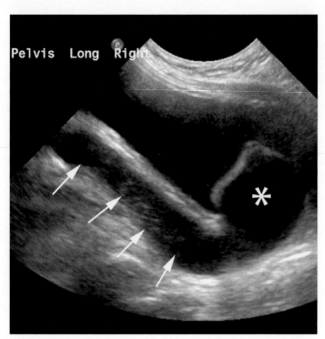

FIGURE 4.2A

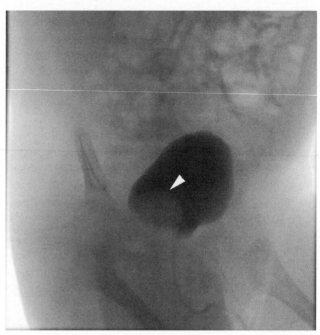

FIGURE 4.2B

FINDINGS Longitudinal US image of the bladder (**A**) shows a thin-walled cystic mass (*) near the trigone and dilation of the distal right ureter (*arrows*). Lateral voiding cystourethrogram (VCUG) image of the bladder (**B**) shows a round, negative filling defect (*arrowhead*) in the contrast-filled bladder near the right trigone.

DIFFERENTIAL DIAGNOSIS Ureterocele, urachal cyst, paraureteral diverticula

DIAGNOSIS Ureterocele

DISCUSSION A ureterocele results from cystic dilatation of the intravesical portion of the distal ureter related to a distal congenital stricture. They can be simple or ectopic and associated with a single or duplex ureter. Duplication of the ureters is demonstrated in approximately 75% of children with ureteroceles. An ectopic ureterocele is most often associated with a duplicated collecting system and represents the distal portion of the ureter of the upper renal moiety. By definition, it inserts more inferiorly and medially compared with a normal insertion. Girls are more commonly affected than boys.[1] If large, the ureterocele can prolapse into the bladder neck resulting in obstruction. Alternatively, a ureterocele can evert during the voiding phase of a VCUG and can be mistaken for a paraureteral diverticulum.[2]

Questions for Further Thought
1. What is the cobra sign?
2. What is a cecoureterocele?

Reporting Responsibilities

- Report if simple or ectopic and if associated with a single or duplex ureter.
- Describe degree of collecting system obstruction.

What the Treating Physician Needs to Know

- If a ureterocele is demonstrated on a screening US for recurrent UTIs, a VCUG should be ordered to evaluate for vesicoureteral reflux (VUR) and possible bladder neck obstruction.

Answers

1. A classic sign on intravenous urogram (IVU), the cobra head sign, consists of a radiolucent halo of the wall of the ureterocele surrounding the rounded area of contrast in the ureterocele.[3]

2. A cecoureterocele is an uncommon presentation of an ectopic ureterocele that extends submucosally below the trigone and produces a mass-like protrusion upon the bladder and urethra.[1]

REFERENCES

1. Berrocal T, Lopez-Pereira P, Arjonilla A, et al. Anomalies of the distal ureter, bladder and urethra in children: Embryologic, radiologic, and pathologic features. *Radiographics.* 2002;22: 1139–1164.

2. Bellah R, Long F, Canning D. Ureterocele eversion with vesicoureteral reflux in duplex kidneys: Findings at voiding cystourethrography. *AJR Am J Roentgenol.* 1995;165:409–413.

3. Chavhan G. The cobra head sign. *Radiology.* 2002;225: 781–782.

CASE 4.3

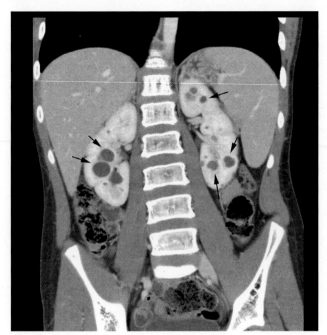

FIGURE **4.3A**

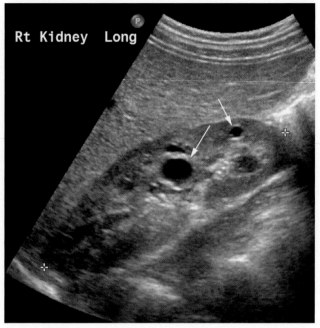

FIGURE **4.3B**

FINDINGS Coronal CT of the abdomen with contrast (**A**) and sagittal US (**B**) of the right kidney show multiple simple renal cysts of varying sizes (*arrow*) in the cortex and medulla.

DIFFERENTIAL DIAGNOSIS Autosomal dominant polycystic kidney disease (ADPKD), tuberous sclerosis, von Hippel–Lindau disease, autosomal recessive polycystic kidney disease (ARPKD)

DIAGNOSIS ADPKD

DISCUSSION ADPKD is a systemic disease that is dominantly inherited. Characteristically, it presents with renal and extrarenal cyst development in an age-dependent manner. The development of multiple renal cysts results in gradual, slow enlargement of the kidneys. These cysts communicate directly with the collecting ducts and the nephrons. Progressive cystic replacement of the renal parenchyma results in hematuria, hypertension, and renal insufficiency. ADPKD has a highly variable disease progression, with onset of end-stage renal disease ranging from childhood to old age.[1]

Questions for Further Thought
1. What are common associated findings?
2. What is the cause for hypertension?
3. Is there an increased incidence of RCC?

Reporting Responsibilities
- Number, size, and location of renal cysts
- Presence or absence of cysts in liver, pancreas, and spleen
- Presence or absence of cyst complications, including hemorrhage, infection, or calcification

What the Treating Physician Needs to Know
- Generally, this disease presents in the fourth or fifth decade of life with hematuria or hypertension.
- If clinically symptomatic in the neonate, the kidneys can be echogenic and enlarged with small cysts making it indistinguishable from ARPKD.[2]
- Establishing if at least one affected family member is a first-degree relative is key to the diagnosis. However, up to 50% of patients have no family history of the disease.
- Renal failure develops in 50% of patients.[3]

Answers

1. (a) Liver (especially in women), pancreatic, and splenic cysts (b) Cysts in thyroid, ovary, endometrium, seminal vesicles, lung, brain, pituitary, breast, and epididymis (c) Cerebral berry aneurysms in approximately 10% (d) Abdominal aortic aneurysm (e) Colonic diverticula

2. The attenuation and stretching of intrarenal vessels around cysts cause activation of the renin–angiotensin–aldosterone system.[4]

3. No. However, if they go on to dialysis, then they have increased risk associated with cystic disease of dialysis.[3]

REFERENCES

1. Siegal MJ. *Pediatric Sonography.* 2nd ed. Philadelphia, PA: Lippincott-Raven; 1996:377–378.

2. Pei Y. Diagnostic approach in autosomal dominant polycystic kidney disease. *Clin J Am Soc Nephrol.* 2006;1:1108–1114.

3. Currie R, Freeman S, McCormick F, et al. Polycystic kidneys: a cautionary story. *Br J Radiol.* 2007;80:305–309.

4. Chapman ABN, Johnson A, Gabow PA, et al. The renin-angiotensin-aldosterone system and autosomal dominant polycystic kidney disease. *N Engl J Med.* 1990;323:1091–1096.

Angelisa Paladin

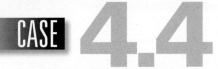

CASE 4.4

CLINICAL HISTORY *Prenatal diagnosis of cystic kidneys*

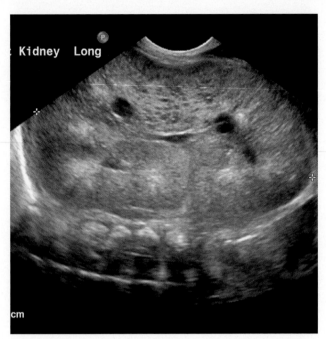

FIGURE **4.4A**

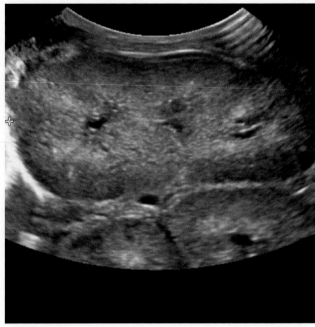

FIGURE **4.4B**

FINDINGS Sagittal US images of the right and left kidneys (**A**) and (**B**) demonstrate that they are grossly enlarged, diffusely echogenic, and have loss of the corticomedullary differentiation. Both kidneys show several subcentimeter diameter cysts as well as many other scattered smaller cysts.

DIFFERENTIAL DIAGNOSIS ARPKD, ADPKD, cystic renal dysplasia

DIAGNOSIS ARPKD

DISCUSSION ARPKD is a disease of non-obstructive renal tubular ectasia and malformation. Usually, the ducts dilate and elongate in a bilateral and symmetric pattern. Interstitial fibrosis also occurs and, in combination with the tubular ectasia, renal function may be impaired. This results in decreased urinary concentration, hypertension, and renal insufficiency. If the degree of renal collecting duct involvement is severe, renal failure may occur resulting in the need for dialysis and transplantation.

Congenital hepatic fibrosis is also a hallmark of this disease. Findings include abnormal formation of the bile ducts, which are often dilated and increased in number. The portal tracts may be fibrotic and enlarged as well. Clinically, this may lead to portal hypertension.[1]

The presentation of ARPKD is variable depending on the degree of kidney and liver involvement. The severity of the hepatic disease is often inversely proportional to the severity of the kidney disease.[2]

Questions for Further Thought

1. Why are the kidneys large?
2. Why are the kidneys echogenic?
3. Why do cysts develop?

Reporting Responsibilities

- Size and degree of echogenicity of the kidneys
- Presence or absence of biliary duct dilatation
- Evidence of liver fibrosis, including increase of liver echogenicity and findings of portal hypertension

What the Treating Physician Needs to Know

• Renal size and echogenicity do not correlate with renal function.[1]

• Early in life, the liver may appear normal or may have some dilated intrahepatic biliary ducts.[2]

Answers

1. The dilated ducts enlarge the kidney and the degree of enlargement is directly proportional to the number of dilated ducts.[1]

2. Hyperechogenicity is related to the large number of fluid–tubular wall interfaces

3. Renal cysts develop from focal epithelial proliferation primarily in the collecting duct, resulting in tubular dilatation and lengthening of the collecting duct. The abnormal epithelial proliferation changes its function from resorptive to secretory and creates discrete macrocysts.[1]

REFERENCES

1. Lonergan G, Rice R, Suarez E. Autosomal recessive polycystic kidney disease: Radiologic-pathologic correlation. *Radiographics.* 2000;20:837–855.

2. Siegal MJ. *Pediatric Sonography.* 2nd ed. Philadelphia, PA: Lippincott-Raven; 1996:377–378.

Angelisa Paladin

CASE 4.5

CLINICAL HISTORY *A 1-day-old infant with bilateral hydroureteronephrosis on prenatal US*

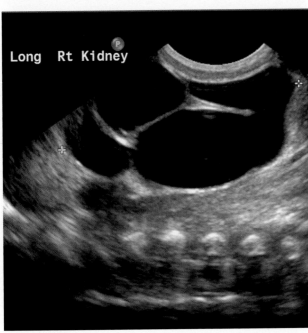

FIGURE 4.5A

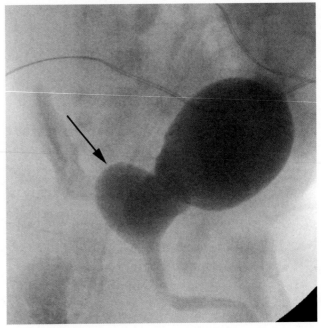

FIGURE 4.5B

FINDINGS Sagittal US image of the right kidney (**A**) shows severe hydronephrosis. Left lateral image of the pelvis during a VCUG (**B**)[1] shows dilatation and elongation of the posterior urethra (*arrow*) and narrowing of the bladder neck.

DIFFERENTIAL DIAGNOSIS Posterior urethral valves (PUVs), anterior urethral valves, congenital urethral polyp, congenital urethral stricture, prune belly syndrome

DIAGNOSIS PUVs

DISCUSSION PUVs are the most common cause of congenital bladder outlet obstruction, occurring exclusively in boys. Unlike its name, the obstruction is secondary to a membranous rather than a valvular lesion.[2] It originates from wolffian duct tissue that forms a thick membrane that courses obliquely from the distal portion of the prostatic urethra to the verumontanum. Increased mechanical pressure with voiding results in progressive dilatation of the posterior urethra and

bladder trabeculation and thickening. VUR is demonstrated in 50% of patients. Renal function is often impaired and is likely a result of several insults. Associated renal dysplasia is common and the increased pressure may contribute to a decrease of renal tubular function.[3]

Questions for Further Thought

1. Does the presence of a urethral catheter obscure the diagnosis of PUV on a VCUG?
2. What other abnormalities maybe present with PUV?

Reporting Responsibilities

- Renal US: Describe size of kidneys, evidence of renal dysplasia, presence or absence of collecting system dilatation, and bladder wall changes
- VCUG: Presence or absence of VUR, degree of bladder trabeculation, approximate bladder capacity, and degree of posterior urethral dilatation

What the Treating Physician Needs to Know

- An indicator of a good prognosis for long-term renal function is a serum creatinine level less than 0.8 mg/dl at age 1 year.[4]
- Lack of definitive documentation of PUV on radiologic studies does not exclude their presence. If there is a high index of suspicion, a catheter should be placed until a cystourethroscopy can be performed.

Answers

1. No. Studies have shown that the urethral catheter does not obscure PUV in boys and does not need to be removed during the voiding phase of voiding cystourethrography.
2. Pulmonary hypoplasia, urinary ascites, and perinephric urinomas.

REFERENCES

1. Lebowitz R. Voiding cystourethrography in boys: does the presence of the catheter obscure the diagnosis of posterior urethral valves? *AJR Am J Roentgenol.* 1996;166:724–725.
2. Imaji R, Dewan P. The clinical and radiological findings in boys with endoscopically severe congenital posterior urethral obstruction. *BJU Int.* 2001;88:263–267.
3. Berrocal T, Lopez-Pereira P, Arjonilla A, et al. Anomalies of the distal ureter, bladder and urethra in children: Embryologic, radiologic, and pathologic features. *Radiographics.* 2002;22:1139–1164.
4. Sarhan O, El-Dahshan K, Sarhan M. Prognostic value of serum creatinine levels in children with posterior urethral valves treated by primary valve ablation. *J Pediatr Urol.* 2010;6(1):11–14.

Angelisa Paladin

CLINICAL HISTORY *A 10-year-old male with swelling and pain in left testicle*

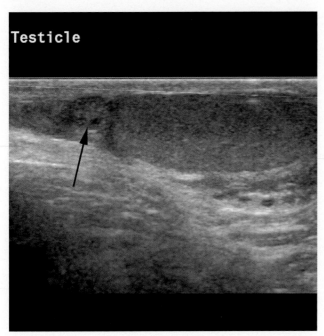

FIGURE 4.6A

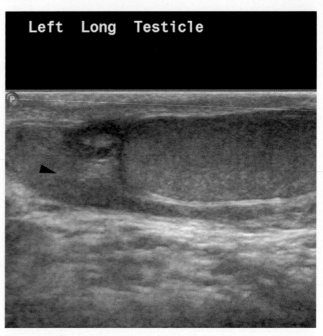

FIGURE 4.6B

FINDINGS Longitudinal US image of the left testicle (**A**) shows a hypoechoic, avascular mass (*arrow*) between the epididymal head and testicle. Longitudinal image of the left testicle (**B**) shows swelling of the epididymal head (*arrowhead*).

DIFFERENTIAL DIAGNOSIS Torsion of the appendix testis, epididymitis, orchitis, testicular torsion

DIAGNOSIS Torsion of the appendix testis

DISCUSSION Torsion of the testicular appendages is a common cause of acute scrotum in prepubertal boys. The appendages are pedunculated embryonic remnants of the mesonephric and paramesonephric ducts, which predispose them to torsion. There is a higher incidence in the left testicle.

There are four appendages, with the appendix testis most commonly involved.[1] US is the most sensitive test for diagnosis and shows an avascular paratesticular mass. Echogenicity varies dependent on time of imaging after presenting symptoms. Common associations include a reactive hydrocele, thickened overlying skin, and a swollen and hyperemic epididymis. Treatment is nonsteroidal anti-inflammatory medications and bed rest.[2]

Questions for Further Thought

1. If this patient has a follow-up US examination in a few months after the symptoms have resolved, what finding could be seen?
2. What finding on clinical examination is pathognomonic for torsion of a testicular appendage?

Reporting Responsibilities

- Document blood flow in the testicle with Doppler color flow imaging and spectral waveform to exclude testicular torsion
- Describe abnormality and any associated findings

What the Treating Physician Needs to Know

- Exclude epididymitis if the torsed appendage is not clearly identified
- Symptoms resolve with conservative management

Answers

1. Sometimes the torsed appendage will detach and calcify, leaving a scrotal calcification, called a scrotolith.[2]

2. The "blue dot" sign, which is a palpable nodule in the upper scrotum with bluish skin discoloration, is found in up to one-third of patients.[2]

REFERENCES

1. Rakha E, Puls F, Saidul I, et al. Torsion of the testicular appendix: importance of associated acute inflammation. *J Clin Pathol.* 2006;59:831–834.
2. Aso C, Enriquez G, Fité M, et al. Gray-Scale and color Doppler sonography of scrotal disorders in children: an update. *Radiographics.* 2005;25(5):1197–1214.

CASE 4.7

Molly E. Raske

CLINICAL HISTORY *A 3-year-old female with UTI*

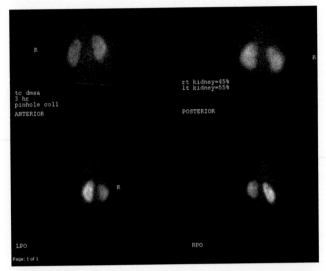

FIGURE **4.7A**

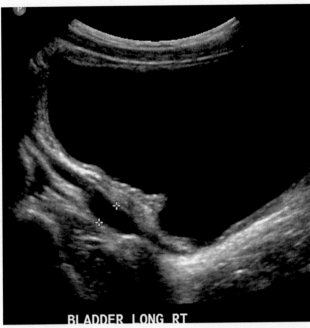

FIGURE **4.7B**

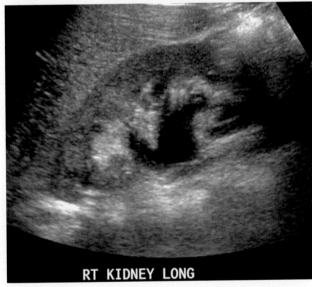

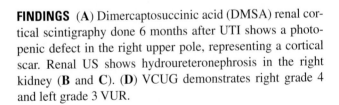

FIGURE **4.7C**

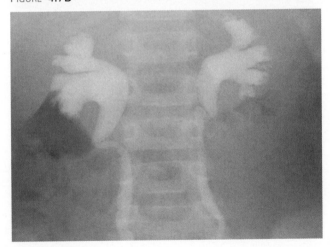

FIGURE **4.7D**

FINDINGS (**A**) Dimercaptosuccinic acid (DMSA) renal cortical scintigraphy done 6 months after UTI shows a photopenic defect in the right upper pole, representing a cortical scar. Renal US shows hydroureteronephrosis in the right kidney (**B** and **C**). (**D**) VCUG demonstrates right grade 4 and left grade 3 VUR.

DIFFERENTIAL DIAGNOSIS DMSA: Acute pyelonephritis, renal cortical scar; US: Ureteropelvic junction (UPJ) and concurrent ureterovesicular junction (UVJ) obstruction, VUR

DIAGNOSIS Bilateral VUR, high grade on the right side, with cortical scarring

DISCUSSION VUR is a common pediatric diagnosis, the primary form due to an abnormally decreased ureteral diameter to intramural length ratio and the secondary form due to elevated storage and/or emptying bladder pressures from anatomic or functional bladder outlet obstruction.[1] Imaging goals are to diagnose secondary causes of reflux and to detect renal damage, presumably caused by recurrent ascending infections. Guidelines from the American Academy of Pediatrics support obtaining a renal US with either a VCUG or a radionuclide cystography in children <2 years of age after UTI.[2] As most patients with low-grade primary reflux will spontaneously resolve with time, they are treated with observation and prophylactic antibiotics. Surgery is performed for patients with high-grade reflux, breakthrough pyelonephritis during prophylactic antibiotic treatment, and/or signs of renal damage.

Below is the grading classification for VUR:

Grade I: Reflux into nondilated ureter only

Grade II: Reflux into the renal pelvis and calyces without dilatation

Grade III: Mild/moderate dilatation of the ureter, renal pelvis, and calyces with minimal blunting of the fornices

Grade IV: Dilation of the renal pelvis and calyces with moderate ureteral tortuosity

Grade V: Gross dilatation of the ureter, pelvis, and calyces; ureteral tortuosity; loss of papillary impressions

Questions for Further Thought

1. How does the method of performing VCUG differ in a child less than 1 year of age compared to an older child?
2. Is DMSA the best test to evaluate for cortical scarring?

Reporting Responsibilities

- US: Describe renal size and growth, appearance of cortex, presence or absence of hydroureteronephrosis or anatomic anomalies

- VCUG: Describe the bladder capacity, contour, presence and grade of reflux, appearance of urethra, and presence of post-contrast residual volume
- DMSA: Presence and location of photopenic defects, any new defects

What Treating Physician Needs to Know

- Does the patient have reflux nephropathy (asymmetrically small kidney, no growth, cortical scarring)?
- Reflux grade. Are there abnormalities to suggest a secondary cause for reflux?

Answers

1. Perform cyclic bladder fillings in patients less than 1 year old to increase the exam's sensitivity.
2. DMSA is more sensitive than US. However, resolution of magnetic resonance urography (MRU) is far superior to DMSA, providing the ability to differentiate dysplasia from scar.[3]

REFERENCES

1. Wein AJ, Kavoussi LR, Novick AC, et al., eds. *Campbell-Walsh Urology.* 9th ed. Philadelphia, PA: Saunders Elsevier; 2007.
2. Lim R. Vesicoureteral reflux and urinary tract infection: Evolving practices and current controversies in pediatric imaging. *AJR Am J Roentgenol.* 2009;192:1197–1208.
3. Grattan-Smith JD, Little SB, Jones RA. Evaluation of reflux nephropathy, pyelonephritis and renal dysplasia. *Pediatr Radiol.* 2008;38(suppl):S83–S105.

Molly E. Raske

CLINICAL HISTORY *A 7-year-old female with 2 days of abdominal pain*

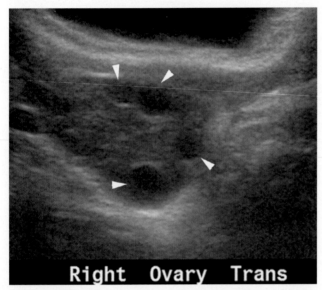

FIGURE **4.8A**

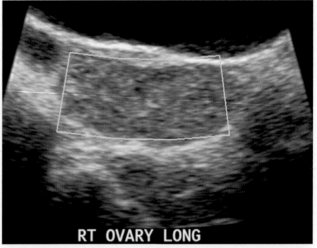

FIGURE **4.8B**

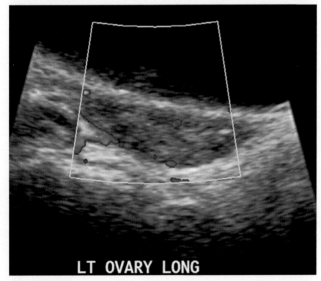

FIGURE **4.8C**

— R Ovary —	
R Ov Volume	8.47 ml
R Ov Length	4.35 cm
R Ov Height	1.78 cm
R Ov Width	2.09 cm
— L Ovary —	
L Ov Volume	4.11 ml

FIGURE **4.8D**

FINDINGS (**A**) Transabdominal pelvic US demonstrates an enlarged right ovary with peripheral cystic structures (*arrowheads*). Color Doppler image demonstrates no detectable vascular flow within the right ovary (**B**), but flow is seen in the left ovary at a similar depth (**C**). (**D**) The right ovary is enlarged, twice the volume of the left ovary.

DIFFERENTIAL DIAGNOSIS Ovarian torsion, adnexal mass

DIAGNOSIS Ovarian torsion (right side)

DISCUSSION Ovarian torsion is defined by rotation of the ovary and/or the fallopian tube about its vascular pedicle. It affects females of all ages, even occurring prenatally. The symptoms include pain, fever, leukocytosis, anorexia, and vomiting, and can mimic other gastrointestinal and genitourinary abnormalities such as acute appendicitis, urolithiasis, pyelonephritis, tubo-ovarian abscess, endometriosis, ectopic pregnancy, and ruptured ovarian cyst to name a few. The onset of pain is often sudden, which can distinguish it clinically from several of the other common differential diagnoses. Torsion can be primary or secondary to an adnexal mass that predisposes the ovary to rotate. In children, the relatively long vascular pedicle and mobile adnexa make it prone to torse. Pregnancy is another predisposing condition for torsion. Pelvic US is the most appropriate radiologic study, with the most reliable imaging feature being an enlarged ovary compared to the contralateral, normal side. The torsed ovary can have a variety of appearances, including solid, heterogeneous, or cystic. Peripheral cysts can be seen, representing congestion and transudative filling of follicles.[1] Often pelvic free fluid will be present. The Doppler examination is unreliable since arterial flow does not exclude torsion. Indeed, on several series, arterial and/or venous flow was detected in pathologically proven torsed ovaries.[1,2] In suspected ovarian torsion, the patient is emergently taken for surgical exploration, either open or laparoscopic. If detected early, some ovaries remain viable and, therefore, are able to be saved by untwisting. Often, an oophoropexy will be performed.

Questions for Further Thought

1. Which ovary is more likely to undergo torsion?
2. Do malignant ovarian neoplasms cause torsion as often as benign neoplasms or cysts?

Reporting Responsibilities

- The abnormal side and degree of suspicion for torsion. Is the contralateral ovary normal?
- Reporting of an associated mass is helpful but not essential, as it does not change the management of a suspected torsion.

What the Treating Physician Needs to Know

- Whether the sonographic findings suggest torsion.
- If torsion is unlikely by imaging appearance, are there other diagnoses suggested by imaging?

Answers

1. Ovarian torsion is more common on the right side. It is hypothesized that the presence of the sigmoid colon helps to prevent left ovarian torsion.
2. No. Malignant neoplasms rarely cause ovarian torsion, possibly due to ovarian fixation from associated fibrosis or extraovarian tumor invasion.

REFERENCES

1. Servaes S, Zurakowski D, Laufer M, et al. Sonographic findings of ovarian torsion in children. *Pediatr Radiol.* 2007;37:446–451.
2. Albayram F, Hamper U. Ovarian and adnexal torsion: Spectrum of sonographic findings with pathologic correlation. *J Ultrasound Med.* 2001;20:1083–1089.

CLINICAL HISTORY *A 3-week-old male with prenatal hydroureteronephrosis*

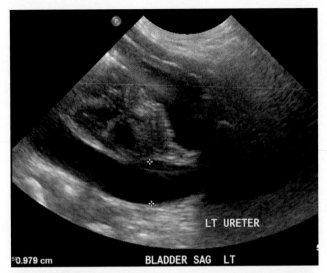

FIGURE **4.9A**

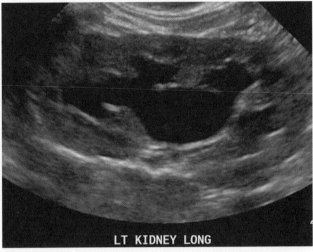

FIGURE **4.9B**

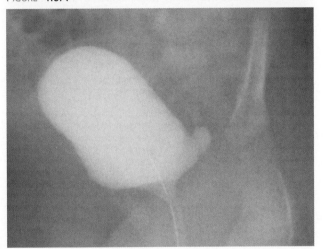

FIGURE **4.9C**

FINDINGS Images from a renal US demonstrate a dilated distal left ureter (**A**) and hydronephrosis (**B**). VCUG done that day shows a left periureteral diverticulum with only mild reflux (**C**).

DIFFERENTIAL DIAGNOSIS Primary megaureter, secondary megaureter

DIAGNOSIS Primary megaureter

DISCUSSION Megaureter is a general descriptive term for an enlarged ureter that in and of itself does not ascribe a cause. Normal ureteral width is usually less than 5 mm.[1] The term primary megaureter is used when ureteral dilation is due to an intrinsic abnormality of the ureter. Secondary megaureter is when dilation is caused by obstruction to bladder outflow (e.g., PUVs, urethral stricture, neurogenic bladder).[1] Primary megaureter can be classified as obstructed, refluxing, unobstructed, nonrefluxing, and various combinations of these terms. An obstructed primary megaureter is caused by a normal caliber, aperistaltic segment of distal ureter just above the UVJ, which causes functional obstruction and upstream dilation. The cause of the adynamic segment is unknown. A refluxing primary megaureter is due to an absent or extremely shortened distal ureter at the UVJ or a periureteral diverticulum. It is hypothesized that the chronic increase in pressure can progressively enlarge the ureter.[2] The nonrefluxing, unobstructed megaureter is idiopathic and often detected by prenatal US. It is thought to reflect a normal developmental variant, and common practice is to follow this condition as it usually spontaneously resolves.[3]

Questions for Further Thought

1. How can you differentiate between an obstructed and nonrefluxing, unobstructed megaureter?
2. What syndrome is associated with a primary refluxing megaureter? What condition is associated with a secondary non-obstructive, nonrefluxing megaureter?

Reporting Responsibilities

- Size of ureter and intrarenal collecting system
- Suggest the appropriate additional tests to help discern the etiology

What the Treating Physician Needs to Know

- Whether the megaureter is primary or secondary.
- If primary, is there reflux, obstruction, both, or neither?

Answers

1. A US and VCUG can define the megaureter and determine if it has reflux. If needed, a nuclear medicine renogram may help determine an obstructed versus unobstructed megaureter. MRU may help answer this question as well.
2. Prune belly syndrome can be associated with refluxing, unobstructed primary megaureter. A secondary cause of unobstructed, nonrefluxing megaureter is infection, with certain endotoxins inhibiting peristalsis.[2]

REFERENCES

1. Berrocal T, Lopez-Pereira P, Arjonilla A, et al. Anomalies of the distal ureter, bladder and urethra in children: Embryologic, radiologic and pathologic features. *Radiographics.* 2002;22:1139–1164.
2. Wein AJ, Kavoussi LR, Novick AC, et al., eds. *Campbell-Walsh Urology.* 9th ed. Philadelphia, PA: Saunders Elsevier; 2007.
3. Shukla A, Cooper J, Patel R, et al. Prenatally detected primary megaureter: A role for extended follow-up. *J Urol.* 2005;173:1353–1356.

CLINICAL HISTORY *A 6-year-old female with hypercalciuria*

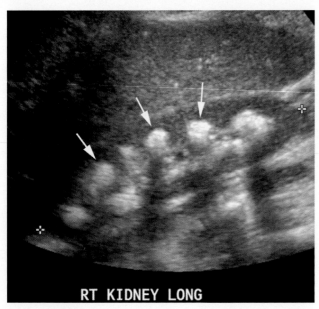

FIGURE 4.10A

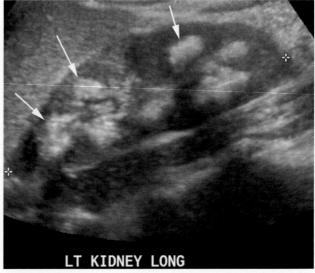

FIGURE 4.10B

FINDINGS (**A** and **B**) Renal US images demonstrate abnormal echogenicity of all of the medullary pyramids with associated acoustic shadowing (*arrows*).

DIFFERENTIAL DIAGNOSIS Medullary nephrocalcinosis, fungus infection

DIAGNOSIS Medullary nephrocalcinosis

DISCUSSION Medullary nephrocalcinosis is a radiographic finding of echogenic medullary pyramids with or without posterior acoustic shadowing. The finding is typically bilateral and represents deposits of calcium of varying sizes within the renal tubules or the interstitium. US is usually the most sensitive radiographic examination to detect this finding as the calcifications may be unapparent on plain radiographs and poorly visible on CT scan. The three most common causes of medullary nephrocalcinosis are medullary sponge kidney, hyperparathyroidism, and distal renal tubular acidosis. Other etiologies include sarcoidosis, furosemide, steroid or amphotericin treatment, Cushing's disease, hypomagnesuria, and hyperoxaluria. It is not possible to determine the etiology by imaging. In some cases, stones will precipitate and migrate into the collecting system. Renal failure can also be seen depending on the underlying etiology of the hypercalciuria. Medullary nephrocalcinosis can also be an incidental finding in asymptomatic patients.

Questions for Further Thought

1. How are nephrolithiasis and urolithiasis different?
2. Is nephrolithiasis reversible?

Reporting Responsibilities

- Correctly identify that the location of the increased echogenicity is in the medullary pyramids rather than the cortex or collecting system.
- Are there any concomitant collecting system stones?

What the Treating Physician Needs to Know

- Is the process bilateral?
- Are there any collecting system stones present?

Answers

1. Nephrolithiasis refers to calcium deposits in the medullary pyramids whereas in urolithiasis, the calcium deposits are within the collecting system.
2. Nephrolithiasis is potentially reversible, depending on the cause for the condition.

REFERENCES

1. Stechman MJ, Loh NY, Thakker RV. Genetic causes of hypercalciuric nephrolithiasis. *Pediatr Nephrol.* 2009;24(12):2321–2332.
2. Wein AJ, Kavoussi LR, Novick AC, et al., eds. *Campbell-Walsh Urology.* 9th ed. Philadelphia, PA: Saunders Elsevier; 2007.

Molly E. Raske

CLINICAL HISTORY *A 16-year-old male with acute onset of left testicular pain and swelling*

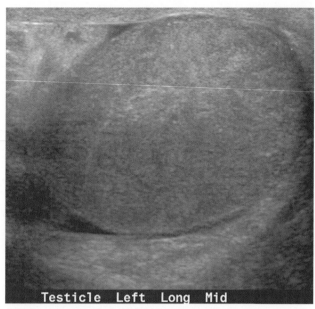

Testicle Left Long Mid

FIGURE **4.11A**

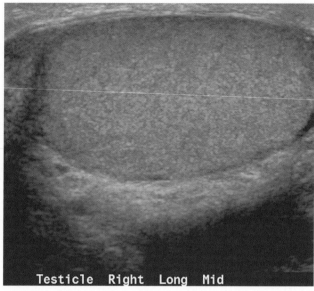

Testicle Right Long Mid

FIGURE **4.11B**

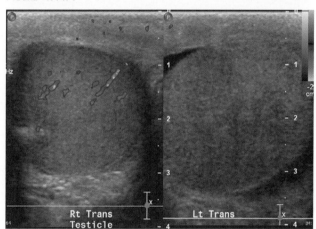

Rt Trans
Testicle   Lt Trans

FIGURE **4.11C**

FINDINGS Images from a scrotal US demonstrate an enlarged, heterogeneous left testis (**A**). The asymptomatic, right testis demonstrates a normal, homogeneous echotexture (**B**). Color Doppler evaluation shows the absence of internal arterial and venous blood flow in the left testis (**C**).

DIFFERENTIAL DIAGNOSIS Testicular torsion, testicular neoplasm, testicular trauma

DIAGNOSIS Acute left testicular torsion

DISCUSSION Testicular torsion, or more specifically torsion of the spermatic cord, is a surgical emergency that can

affect males of all ages, even occurring in the prenatal time period. Torsion more frequently occurs post-puberty, possibly because the heavier testis predisposes it to twist on its vascular stalk. Torsion can be secondary to trauma but is more often spontaneous.[1] The patient with torsion usually presents with an acute onset of pain, tenderness, and swelling.[1] Prompt diagnosis is essential. Within 2 hours after torsion, hemorrhagic infarction begins, followed by irreversible damage to the testis at 6 hours and complete infarction by 24 hours.[2] Adolescent males with torsion tend to come to medical attention later than males of other age groups and thus are more likely to lose the affected testis. Differential diagnosis of the acute scrotum includes torsion as well as incarcerated hernia, epididymo-orchitis, and torsion of the appendix testis or of the appendix epididymis. Color Doppler US can be helpful to discriminate torsion from these other causes. However, if the history and physical examination are highly suspicious for torsion, the surgeon may forgo imaging so as not to delay scrotal exploration. In the acute time period, the gray scale appearance of the affected testis may not have distinguishing features. However, at approximately 8 hours after onset, the testis and epididymis appear enlarged and heterogeneous or abnormally hyperechoic. The color Doppler examination in all stages will show no flow to the affected side. If the history is congruent with torsion but vascular flow is seen, the diagnosis of intermittent torsion should be considered. Surgical management includes untwisting the spermatic cord and suture fixation of the testis if it appears viable. Orchiopexy of the contralateral testis is also performed.

Questions for Further Thought

1. What developmental variant is associated with spontaneous testicular torsion?
2. What are the physical examination findings in torsion?

Reporting Responsibilities

- Side affected, gray scale appearance, and size of the testes
- Presence or absence of vascular flow in the testes

What the Treating Physician Needs to Know

- Whether the Doppler findings support a diagnosis of testicular torsion.
- Whether the findings correlate with the expected chronicity of the torsion.

Answers

1. The bell clapper deformity—improper fixation of the tunica vaginalis that allows mobility of the testis. This anomaly can be bilateral, necessitating orchiopexy of the contralateral testis.
2. Classically, the affected testis is high riding and transversely oriented with an absence of the cremasteric reflex. The examination is confounded in later stages by a reactive hydrocele and scrotal edema.

REFERENCES

1. Wein AJ, Kavoussi LR, Novick AC, et al., eds. *Campbell-Walsh Urology.* 9th ed. Philadelphia, PA: Saunders Elsevier; 2007.
2. Waldert M, Klatte T, Schmidbauer J, et al. Color Doppler sonography reliably identifies testicular torsion in boys. *Urology.* 2010; 75:1170–1174.

CLINICAL HISTORY *A 16-year-old male with palpable mass in the right testis*

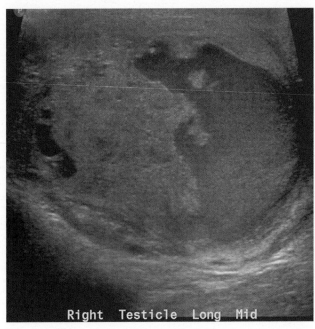

Right Testicle Long Mid

FIGURE **4.12A**

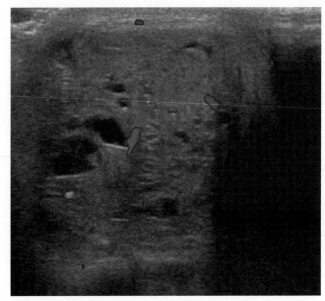

FIGURE **4.12B**

FINDINGS (**A** and **B**) Two sonographic images through the right hemiscrotum show an enlarged right testis with a heterogeneous, partially cystic echotexture. There are no well-defined borders defining the abnormal regions, and little normal parenchyma is seen. Internal vascular flow is present. The left testis (not shown) appeared normal.

DIFFERENTIAL DIAGNOSIS Malignant neoplasm, nonmalignant neoplasm, metastasis

DIAGNOSIS Testicular mass

DISCUSSION An adolescent male presenting with a painless, palpable testicular mass needs an emergent physical examination and US. An intratesticular mass, with rare exception, will be treated with orchiectomy, usually performed promptly after detection, as these malignancies rapidly grow. In 95% of cases, the testicular neoplasm will be a germ cell tumor. Other considerations include stromal tumors such as Sertoli and Leydig cell tumors, lymphoma, metastases, and an epidermoid cyst.[1,2] Testicular lymphoma is uncommon in the pediatric patient and if seen, is often bilateral, involving the epididymis and spermatic cord. If unilateral, the appearance can be similar to a seminoma and history will help guide the correct diagnosis. An epidermoid cyst has a characteristic appearance with well-defined borders of concentric rings. With these specific features, a benign process can be suggested and a biopsy instead of orchiectomy might be performed. Other non-neoplastic processes are unlikely to be confused with a neoplasm as there is little overlap in their imaging appearances. These include tubular ectasia, cysts, sarcoidosis (also uncommon in the pediatric population), and adrenal rests. Other processes such as infection, infarction, and trauma share some imaging features with a malignant neoplasm but will be differentiated by their history.

Questions for Further Thought

1. What is the most common malignant testis neoplasm in a young adult male?
2. What laboratory tests are usually ordered as part of the workup? What are other imaging tests?

Reporting Responsibilities

- Describe whether the abnormality is intra- or extratesticular, its size, and echotexture
- Determine if the abnormality is unilateral or bilateral

What the Treating Physician Needs to Know

- Whether the abnormality appears to represent a malignant or benign process.
- Whether the process is unilateral or bilateral.

Answers

1. Nonseminoma is the most common testis neoplasm in this age group, with histology most often being "mixed," meaning multiple cell types. Yolk sac tumor is the most common in childhood. Seminoma does not occur before 5 years of age.[2]
2. Alpha-fetoprotein (AFP), human chorionic gonadotropin (HCG), and lactate dehydrogenase serve as tumor markers with their values correlating with prognosis. Further imaging involves an abdominal/pelvic CT scan to assess for retroperitoneal metastases. If none are seen, thoracic metastases are unlikely and a chest radiograph can complete the workup. If abdominal metastases are present, a thoracic CT scan is needed.

REFERENCES

1. Wein AJ, Kavoussi LR, Novick AC, et al., eds. *Campbell-Walsh Urology.* 9th ed. Philadelphia, PA: Saunders Elsevier; 2007.
2. Bahrami A, Ro JY, Ayala AG. An overview of testicular germ cell tumors. *Arch Pathol Lab Med.* 2007;131(8):1267–1280.

CASE 4.13

CLINICAL HISTORY *A 3-day-old infant with ambiguous genitalia*

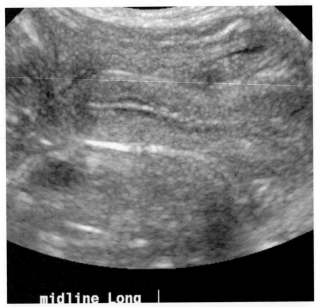

FIGURE 4.13A

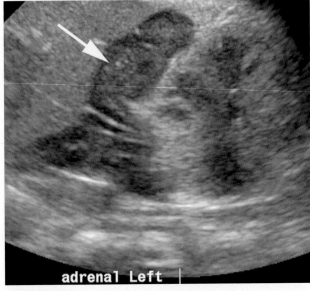

FIGURE 4.13B

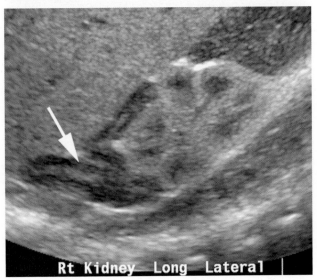

FIGURE 4.13C

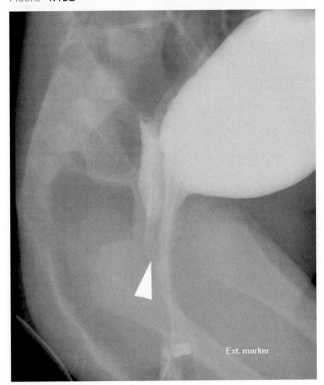

FIGURE 4.13D

FINDINGS Pelvic (**A**) and abdominal US (**B** and **C**) show a uterus with no visible gonads and enlarged adrenal glands (*arrow*), respectively. Fluoroscopic genitogram (**D**) shows a common urogenital sinus.

DIFFERENTIAL DIAGNOSIS Female pseudohermaphroditism, true hermaphroditism, gonadal dysgenesis

DIAGNOSIS Female pseudohermaphroditism secondary to congenital adrenal hyperplasia (CAH).

DISCUSSION Ambiguous genitalia, defined by the lack of typical male or female anatomy, are one feature seen in a group of anomalies called disorders of sexual differentiation (DSD). DSD are due to "congenital conditions in which development of chromosomal, gonadal, or anatomic sex is atypical."[1] By using gonadal morphology, disorders are classified into four types: Gonadal dysgenesis, female pseudohermaphrodite (46, XX with two ovaries), male pseudohermaphrodite (46, XY with two testes), and unclassified forms. This case illustrates female pseudohermaphroditism due to CAH, a disorder most commonly responsible for ambiguous genitalia in a newborn. In CAH, one of the five enzymes used to produce cortisol is deficient. To compensate, adrenocorticotropic hormone rises and adrenal steroid precursors upstream from the enzyme defect are overproduced and diverted to a pathway producing testosterone.[2] Clitoromegaly, labial fusion, and a common urogenital sinus occur to varying degrees. Adrenal hyperplasia can be seen, with a limb length more than 20 mm and width more than 4 mm. A lobular contour, termed a "cerebriform" appearance is thought to be specific. Absence of hyperplasia does not exclude CAH. Males are also afflicted with CAH and can present with salt wasting (also seen in females) or isosexual precocity.

Questions for Further Thought

1. Do all patients with DSD have ambiguous genitalia?
2. What is another cause for female pseudohermaphroditism?

Reporting Responsibilities

• Are müllerian structures present?
• Presence and morphology of gonads.

What the Referring Clinician Needs to Know

• Gonadal appearance and location.
• A magnetic resonance imaging (MRI) might demonstrate the location of gonads if they are not seen by US.

Answers

1. No. Ambiguous genitalia is not seen in patients with Klinefelter and Turner syndromes or with complete androgen insensitivity.
2. Transplacental maternal androgen exposure secondary to certain maternal tumors.

REFERENCES

1. Chavhan GB, Parra DA, Oudjhane K, et al. Imaging of ambiguous genitalia: Classification and diagnostic approach. *Radiographics*. 2008;28:1891–1904.
2. Wein AJ, Kavoussi LR, Novick AC, et al., eds. *Campbell-Walsh Urology*. 9th ed. Philadelphia, PA: Saunders Elsevier; 2007.

CLINICAL HISTORY *A 15-year-old male with mental retardation and skin rash*

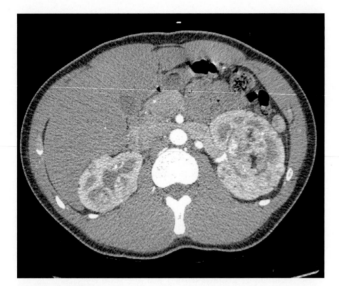

FIGURE **4.14A**

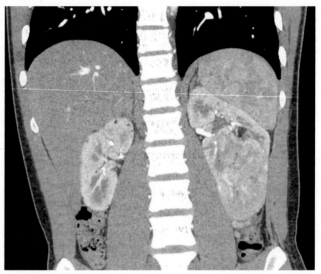

FIGURE **4.14B**

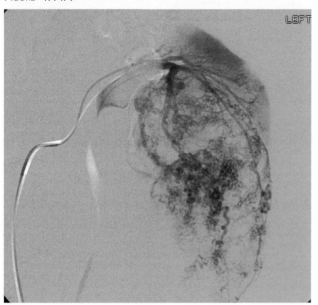

FIGURE **4.14C**

FINDINGS Axial and contrast-enhanced CT images of the abdomen (**A** and **B**) demonstrate several circumscribed, intraparenchymal, and exophytic renal masses. These enhance avidly and demonstrate multiple foci of macroscopic fat. Subsequent digitally subtracted angiographic image (**C**) of the left kidney shows a highly vascular mass with multiple pseudoaneurysms.

DIFFERENTIAL DIAGNOSIS Angiomyolipoma, Wilms' tumor, lymphoma, RCC

DIAGNOSIS Angiomyolipoma

DISCUSSION Angiomyolipoma (AML) is a benign renal neoplasm that derives its name from its combination of elements: Abnormal blood vessels, smooth muscle, and macroscopic fat. The presence of gross, focal intralesional fat on a CT scan (Hounsfield units <0) is considered diagnostic of an AML and will differentiate this tumor from the more aggressive Wilms' tumor, RCC, or renal lymphoma.

These can occur sporadically, most often in middle-aged women. Most of these are found incidentally on abdominal imaging for some other reason. In children, sporadic tumors are rare, and most AMLs are found in patients with tuberous sclerosis (TS). TS is an autosomal dominant multiorgan systemic disease characterized by hamartoma formation. The classically associated lesions are cortical tubers and subependymal giant cell astrocytomas, facial angiofibromas known as "adenoma sebaceum," and renal AMLs, which tend to be multifocal, bilateral, and large. About 80% of patients with TS will develop a renal AML.

As histologically benign lesions, AMLs do not undergo malignant degeneration. Small lesions are most often simply watched for stability, and these lesions are slow growing. Large lesions, those >4 cm in size, have a high likelihood of spontaneous retroperitoneal hemorrhage that can be life threatening (Wunderlich syndrome). In these cases, arterial coil embolization is frequently used either prophylactically or to treat the spontaneous bleed. Partial nephrectomy is another treatment option.

Questions for Further Thought

1. What percentage of patients found to have an AML will have TS? What further imaging should be done?
2. Can these lesions be confused with RCC or Wilms' tumor?

Reporting Responsibilities

- Documenting the presence of macroscopic fat to be certain this is AML not RCC or Wilms' tumor.
- Size of the lesion must be documented to stratify risk for spontaneous hemorrhage.

What the Treating Physician Needs to Know

- In a child, AML is a strong predictor of the TS spectrum. Imaging of the brain with MR should be recommended to screen for cortical tubers and subependymal giant cell astrocytomas.
- For AMLs larger than 4 cm, consideration for prophylactic embolization should be recommended.

Answers

1. Of all patients with AML, 20% will have TS. Pediatric patients and those with multiple lesions have a much higher likelihood.

2. The presence of macroscopic fat is diagnostic for AML, and excludes RCC or Wilms' tumor. Case reports of RCC engulfing medullary fat have been reported, but integral fat = AML. Wilms' tumor will be a predominantly solid mass, often with central necrosis and low attenuation, but will not have negative Hounsfield units. AMLs can have minimal fatty components, in which case biopsy and/or partial nephrectomy will be required for diagnosis.

REFERENCES

1. Lowe LH, Isuani BH, Heller RM, et al. Pediatric renal masses: Wilms tumor and beyond. *Radiographics.* 2000;20:1585–1603.
2. Logue LG, Acker RE, Sienko AE. Best cases from the AFIP: Angiomyolipomas in tuberous sclerosis. *Radiographics.* 2003; 23:241–246.
3. Yamakado K, Tanaka N, Nakagawa T, et al. Renal angiomyolipoma: Relationship between tumor size, aneurysm formation and rupture. *Radiology.* 2002;225:78–82.

Ho Nguyen and Sandra L. Wootton-Gorges

CASE 4.15

CLINICAL HISTORY *An 18-month-old asymptomatic female with palpable abdominal mass*

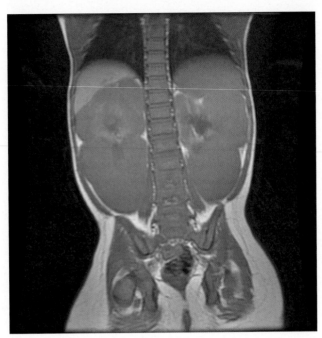

FIGURE 4.15A

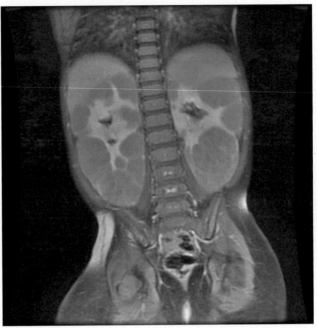

FIGURE 4.15B

FINDINGS Large bilateral kidneys with lobular peripheral soft tissue masses distorting the normal renal contours. These masses are T1 hypointense (**A**) and enhance less than normal renal parenchyma after gadolinium (**B**). The lesions are homogeneous but exhibit a striated enhancement pattern.

DIFFERENTIAL DIAGNOSIS Nephroblastomatosis, renal lymphoma

DIAGNOSIS Nephroblastomatosis

DISCUSSION Nephroblastomatosis are foci of metanephric blastema that persist beyond 36 weeks' gestation. They have the potential for malignant transformation into Wilms' tumor. Histologic classifications reflect biologic behavior and include dormant, sclerosing (regressing), hyperplastic, and neoplastic. Dormant and sclerosing rests are microscopic in size, while hyperplastic and neoplastic rests are visible by imaging. Nephrogenic rests can also be classified by location. Perilobar rests lie in the peripheral cortex and are associated with Beckwith–Wiedemann syndrome and hemihypertrophy, Perlman syndrome, and Trisomy 18. Intralobar rests are much less common, but have higher association with Wilms' tumor development. They are seen in Denys–Drash syndrome, sporadic aniridia, and WAGR (Wilms' tumor, aniridia, genitourinary tract abnormalities, and mental retardation) syndrome.

By US, nephroblastomatosis appears as iso- to hypoechoic homogeneous ovoid or subcapsular renal masses. At CT, the masses are hypodense and enhance less than the normal kidney. By MR, they are homogeneous and hypointense to normal renal cortex on T1-weighted images, and have variable intensity on T2-weighted images. Like CT, at MR they enhance less than the normal kidney. With diffuse nephroblastomatosis, there is diffuse renal enlargement with a thick peripheral rind of tissue that often shows striated enhancement. Lymphoma can mimic nephroblastomatosis but is unusual in infants and young children.

Patients with nephroblastomatosis or the syndromes described above typically undergo screening every 3 to 6 months (until about age 7) for development of Wilms' tumor. Lack of homogeneity of the mass, a mass with spherical shape and mass effect, and increase in heterogeneous enhancement all suggest development of Wilms' tumor. When lesions regress, they become smaller, lentiform, and dark on T1- and T2-weighted images.

Management is controversial. It is unclear if chemotherapy will reduce the risk of malignant transformation. This patient belongs to the category of diffuse hyperplastic perilobar nephroblastomatosis (DHPLN). Such patients have a high risk of developing Wilms' tumor, 46% in one retrospective analysis.

Questions for Further Thought

1. What syndromes are associated with increased risk of Wilms' tumor and/or nephrogenic rests?
2. How common are nephrogenic rests?

Reporting Responsibilities

- Describe locations and extent of involvement
- Evaluate for features which suggest development of Wilms' tumor, such as lesions with spherical shape with mass effect, and heterogeneous enhancement
- Describe other abnormalities that may suggest association with a syndrome

What the Treating Physician Needs to Know

- Offer an alternative diagnosis if not nephroblastomatosis (e.g., lymphoma).
- Wilms' tumor may develop in children with nephroblastomatosis.

Answers

1. Beckwith–Wiedemann syndrome (macroglossia, macrosoma, midline abdominal wall defects, neonatal hypoglycemia, ear creases or pits), WAGR, Denys–Drash syndrome (gonadal dysgenesis, renal failure), Perlman syndrome (nephromegaly, macrosomia, polyhydramnios, abnormal facies), and Trisomy 18 (cardiac abnormalities, clenched hands, rocker bottom feet, choroid plexus cysts).

2. Nephrogenic rests are found incidentally in 1% of infant kidneys at autopsies. Transformation to Wilms' tumor occurs in less than 1% of infants with nephrogenic rests. However, they are believed to give rise to 30% to 40% of Wilms' tumors and are found in up to 99% of bilateral Wilms' tumors.

REFERENCES

1. Lonergan GJ, Martínez-León MI, Agrons GA, et al. Nephrogenic rests, nephroblastomatosis, and associated lesions of the kidney. *Radiographics.* 1998;18:947–968.

2. Lowe LH, Isuani BH, Heller RM, et al. Pediatric renal masses: Wilms tumor and beyond. *Radiographics.* 2000;20:1585–1603. Erratum in: *Radiographics* 2001;21:766.

3. Perlman EJ, Faria P, Soares A, et al. Hyperplastic perilobar nephroblastomatosis: Long-term survival of 52 patients. *Pediatr Blood Cancer.* 2006;46:203–221.

CLINICAL HISTORY *A 10-year-old male with left flank pain*

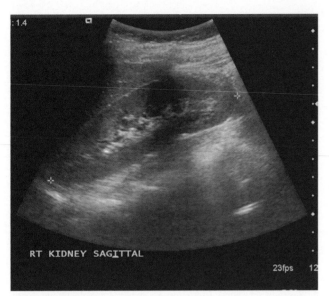

FIGURE **4.16A**

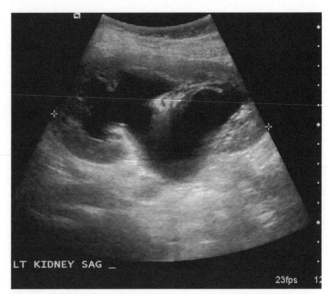

FIGURE **4.16B**

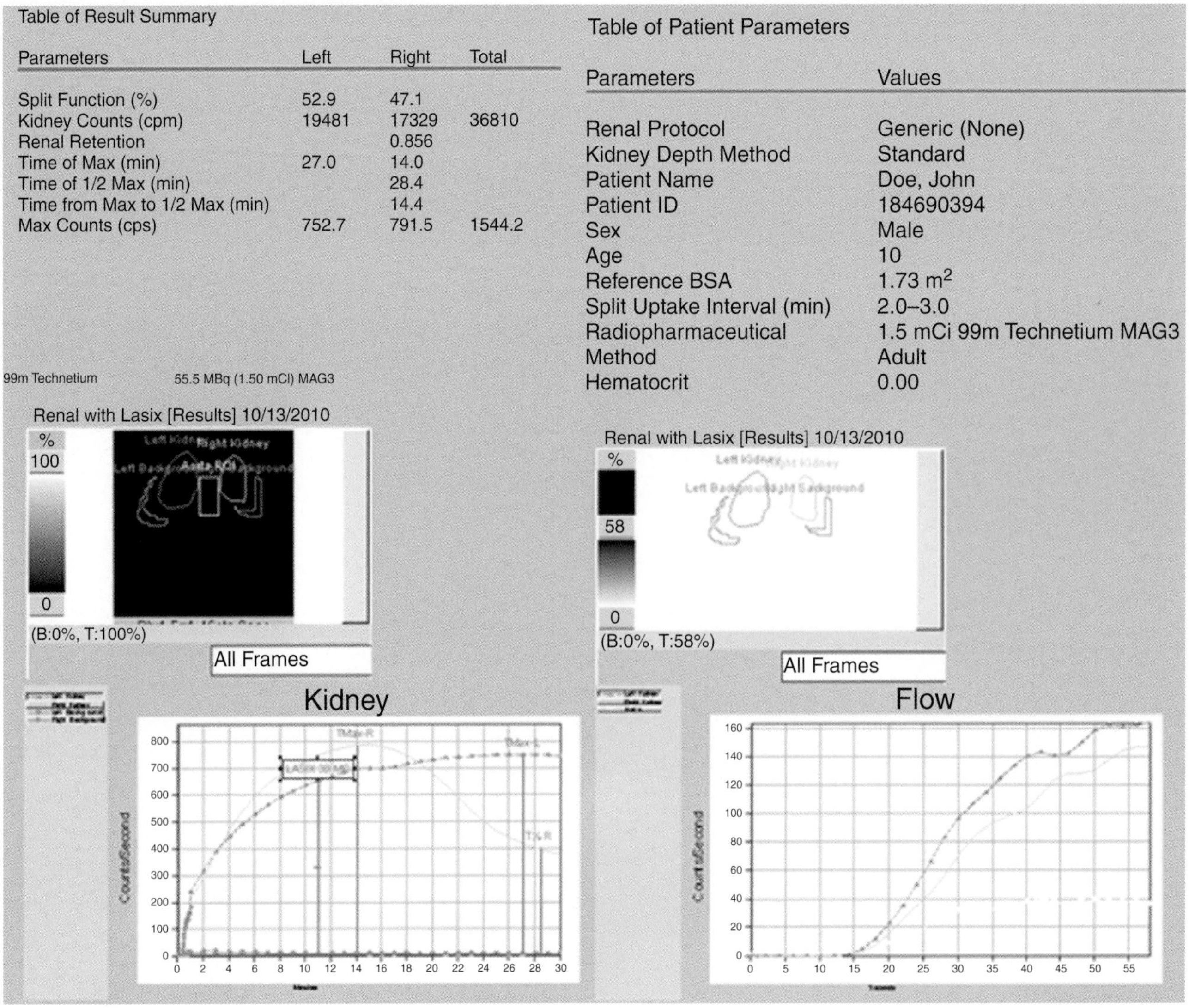

Table of Result Summary

Parameters	Left	Right	Total
Split Function (%)	52.9	47.1	
Kidney Counts (cpm)	19481	17329	36810
Renal Retention		0.856	
Time of Max (min)	27.0	14.0	
Time of 1/2 Max (min)		28.4	
Time from Max to 1/2 Max (min)		14.4	
Max Counts (cps)	752.7	791.5	1544.2

99m Technetium   55.5 MBq (1.50 mCi) MAG3

Table of Patient Parameters

Parameters	Values
Renal Protocol	Generic (None)
Kidney Depth Method	Standard
Patient Name	Doe, John
Patient ID	184690394
Sex	Male
Age	10
Reference BSA	1.73 m^2
Split Uptake Interval (min)	2.0–3.0
Radiopharmaceutical	1.5 mCi 99m Technetium MAG3
Method	Adult
Hematocrit	0.00

Renal with Lasix [Results] 10/13/2010

%
100

0
(B:0%, T:100%)

All Frames

Renal with Lasix [Results] 10/13/2010

%
58

0
(B:0%, T:58%)

All Frames

Kidney

Flow

FIGURE **4.16C**

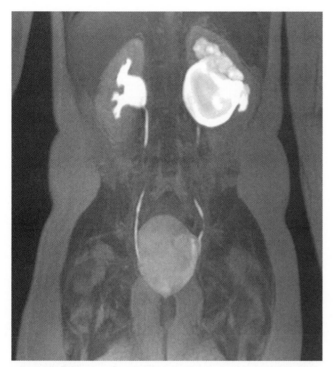

Figure **4.16D**

FINDINGS Renal sonography reveals moderate left hydrone-phrosis without ureteral dilation. Diuretic renal scintigraphy demonstrates prolonged intrarenal transit and poor response to diuresis concerning for UPJ obstruction. The findings are confirmed on MRU.

(**A** and **B**) Longitudinal sonographic images of the right and left kidneys. (**C**) Diuretic MAG-3 renal scintigraphy. (**D**) MRU maximum intensity projection (MIP) 20 minutes following contrast administration.

DIFFERENTIAL DIAGNOSIS Left UPJ obstruction, dilating VUR and reflux nephropathy, congenital megaureter, PUVs, multicystic dysplastic kidney (MCDK)

DIAGNOSIS Left UPJ obstruction

DISCUSSION Congenital UPJ obstruction is the most com-mon etiology of hydronephrosis in children. Explanations include extrinsic causes (15% to 20%), such as crossing ves-sels or retrocaval ureters, and intrinsic causes (80%), such as abnormal ureteric innervation, smooth muscle disorders, or scarring. Fetal folds at the UPJ may account for some milder forms of non-obstructive pelvicalyceal dilation.

The diagnosis is often made incidentally and at prenatal sonographic screening, while older patients may present with

infection or pain. The markedly dilated renal collecting system is also more susceptible to trauma. Males are more commonly affected (3 to 4:1) and one-third of the cases are bilateral.

Following US identification, the degree of UPJ obstruc-tion is traditionally defined with diuretic renal scintigra-phy, with post-diuretic T1/2 less than 10 minutes generally suggesting incomplete obstruction that can be conservatively managed, with T1/2 greater than 20 minutes suggesting a sig-nificant degree of obstruction requiring surgical intervention.

MRU offers superior anatomic and functional assessment without the use of ionizing radiation (although sedation is often required). Crossing vessels, fetal folds, other extrinsic etiolo-gies, and the precise level of obstruction are usually clearly delineated, and functional assessment, while less mature than scintigraphic analysis, will likely offer an expanded depiction of renal function as the methods improve.

Questions for Further Thought

1. What percentage of prenatal hydronephrosis is due to UPJ obstruction?
2. What ancillary MRU findings suggest the presence of UPJ obstruction?

Reporting Responsibilities

- Identification of any extrinsic etiology
- Quantitation of the degree of hydronephrosis and func-tional assessment of the degree of obstruction

What the Treating Physician Needs to Know

- Presence of extrinsic etiology
- Temporal course of hydronephrosis and degree of obstruc-tion in those cases managed conservatively

Answers

1. Approximately 50% of prenatal hydronephrosis is due to UPJ obstruction.
2. Atrophy of the medullary pyramids and extensive dilation of the renal pelvis. Fluid levels and swirling of excreted contrast material are also seen in UPJ obstruction.

REFERENCES

1. McDaniel BB, Jones RA, Scherz H, et al. Dynamic contrast-enhanced MR urography in the evaluation of pediatric hydrone-phrosis: Part 2, anatomic and functional assessment of uteropel-vic junction obstruction. *AJR Am J Roentgenol.* 2005;185(6): 1608–1614.
2. Shulkin BL, Mandell GA, Cooper JA, et al. Procedure guide-line for diuretic renography in children 3.0. *J Nucl Med Technol.* 2008;36(3):162–168.

CLINICAL HISTORY *A 16-day-old male with fever, fussiness, and decreased P.O. (by mouth) intake*

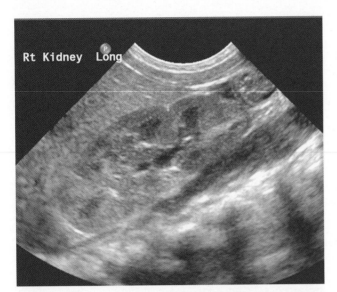

FIGURE **4.17A**

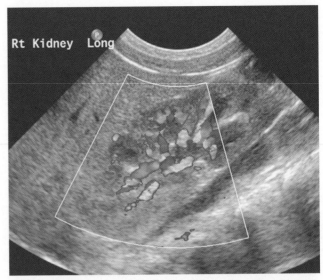

FIGURE **4.17B**

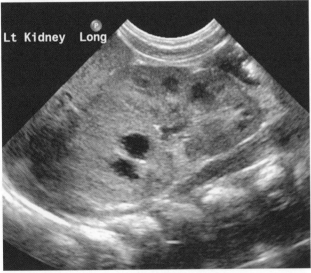

FIGURE **4.17C**

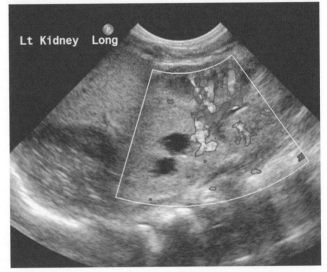

FIGURE **4.17D**

FINDINGS On the initial renal US examination, bilateral upper pole hyperechoic regions with diminished blood flow are identified, with two small rounded sonolucent abnormalities within the left upper pole. After 10 days, the hyperechoic zones have nearly resolved and vascularity is improved.

(**A–D**) Longitudinal images of both kidneys without and with color Doppler imaging. (**E** and **F**) Longitudinal images of both kidneys 10 days later following therapy.

DIFFERENTIAL DIAGNOSIS Pyelonephritis, renal dysplasia

DIAGNOSIS Acute pyelonephritis with calyceal diverticula or renal cysts

DISCUSSION Evaluation of pediatric UTI remains one of the most common and yet controversial indication for imaging in the pediatric population, despite decades of investigation.

Traditionally, a "bottom-up" approach has been used, with detection of associated VUR central to therapy. There is clearly an association between higher grades of VUR and risk for pyelonephritis and renal scarring. Renal US is the most common test used due to the noninvasive and non-ionizing characteristics of the examination.

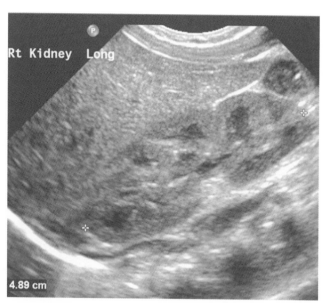

FIGURE 4.17E

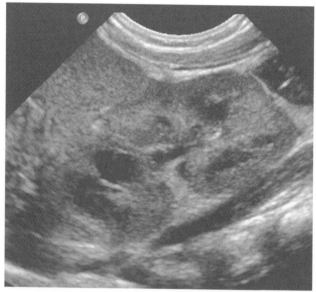

FIGURE 4.17F

More recent research has diversified the relationship of VUR and particularly its significance in the management of a pediatric UTI, while detection of renal parenchymal involvement (pyelonephritis) has become a more definitive parameter for prognosis.

Questions for Further Thought

1. What is the relative sensitivity of current imaging modalities for the detection of pyelonephritis?
2. What are the best predictors of future renal scarring?

Reporting Responsibilities

- Detection of acute pyelonephritis by renal US has reasonable sensitivity and provides the referring physician with useful information for managing pediatric UTI.
- Pertinent associated findings include an associated collecting system, ureteral, or urethral obstruction, renal or perinephric abscess, and calculi.

What the Treating Physician Needs to Know

- A negative renal US with Doppler does not reliably exclude pyelonephritis. Renal DMSA scintigraphy remains the gold standard for assessment of parenchymal involvement in the setting of UTI, although contrast-enhanced CT and MRI likely provide similar sensitivity.
- Detection of associated VUR has traditionally been addressed with VCU, but the association with UTI is still not well understood, and many practitioners currently advocate a "top-down" approach to imaging pediatric UTIs.
- The presence of a renal abscess or obstructed collecting system may require more acute urologic intervention.

Answers

1. Conventional renal US typically can detect approximately 40% to 50% of lesions seen on DMSA. The addition of power Doppler identifies approximately 80% of pyelonephritis in more recent studies (compared to DSMA). CT and MRI can identify roughly 85% to 90% of pyelonephritis, while renal DMSA remains the current gold standard, with sensitivity approximately 90% to 95%. These data continue to improve as technology improves and operator experience increases.

2. The presence of renal parenchymal DMSA defects and high-grade VUR are the best predictors of future scarring.

REFERENCES

1. Majd M, Nussbaum Blask AR, Markle BM, et al. Acute pyelonephritis: comparison of diagnosis with 99mTc-DMSA, SPECT, spiral CT, MR imaging, and power Doppler US in an experimental pig model. *Radiology.* 2001;218(1):101.
2. Stogianni A, Nikolopoulos P, Oikonomou I, et al. Childhood acute pyelonephritis: Comparison of power Doppler sonography and Tc-DMSA scintigraphy. *Pediatr Radiol.* 2007;37(7):685–690.
3. Smith EA. Pyelonephritis, renal scarring, and reflux nephropathy: A pediatric urologist's perspective. *Pediatr Radiol.* 2008; 38(Suppl 1):S76–S82.
4. Craig WD, Wagner BJ, Travis MD, et al. Pyelonephritis: Radiologic-pathologic review. *Radiographics.* 2008;28(1):255–277; quiz 327–328.
5. Lim R. Vesicoureteral reflux and urinary tract infection: Evolving practices and current controversies in pediatric imaging. *AJR Am J Roentgenol.* 2009;192(5):1197–1208.

CLINICAL HISTORY *A 2-day-old term infant with perinatal hypoxia, seizures, and renal insufficiency*

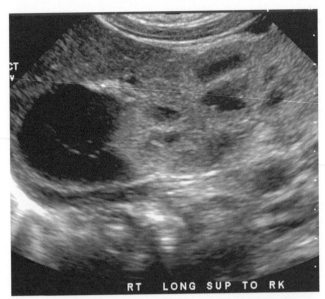

FIGURE **4.18A**

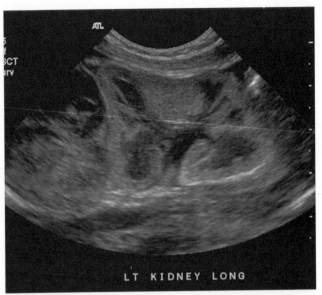

FIGURE **4.18B**

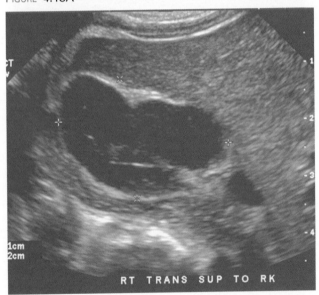

FIGURE **4.18C**

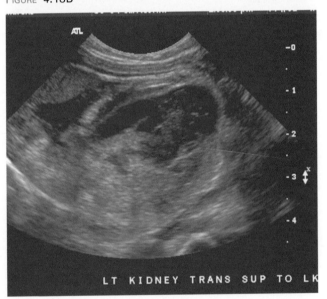

FIGURE **4.18D**

FINDINGS Bilateral moderately sized suprarenal well-circumscribed complex cystic masses

(**A**) Longitudinal right, (**B**) longitudinal left, (**C**) transverse right, and (**D**) transverse left sonographic images of the kidneys.

DIFFERENTIAL DIAGNOSIS Adrenal hemorrhage, congenital adrenocortical carcinoma, cystic neuroblastoma, subdiaphragmatic sequestration, dilated upper pole moiety of a duplex renal collecting system less likely

DIAGNOSIS Bilateral adrenal hemorrhage

DISCUSSION Neonatal adrenal hemorrhage is generally associated with intrauterine or perinatal stress, including hypoxia, birth trauma, renal vein thrombosis, and septicemia. The diagnosis is often made incidentally during examinations performed for other reasons. 70% occur on the right.

Initially, the hemorrhage may have a solid appearance, with ensuring liquefaction and diminishing size upon follow-up examinations. The intrinsic shape of the gland will be somewhat preserved, and rim calcifications may eventually develop.

Questions for Further Thought

1. What are the typical historical and clinical signs of adrenal hemorrhage?

2. What imaging examinations are most helpful in the diagnosis of adrenal hemorrhage?

3. What is the eventual clinical adrenal status of these affected patients?

Reporting Responsibilities

• Detection and characterization of the suprarenal mass.

• Recommendations for further imaging, typically sequential US examinations to demonstrate diminishing size of the hemorrhage.

What the Treating Physician Needs to Know

• Is the appearance consistent with the diagnosis of adrenal hemorrhage?

• Following these lesions with sequential US examinations is the accepted standard of care if there are no other mitigating factors, such as evidence for adrenal cortical hormonal effects or positive urine screening tests for neuroblastomas (catecholamines and vanillylmandelic acid [VMA]).

Answers

1. Neonatal adrenal hemorrhage is often discovered incidentally during examinations performed for other reasons, as in this case. Flank mass, anemia, prolonged jaundice, and hypovolemic shock have been reported as infrequent manifestations.

2. US is typically the first imaging examination used, and is also used for sequential follow-up examinations. If further investigation is warranted, MRI is helpful in demonstrating the presence of blood products.

3. Adrenal insufficiency is a rare complication.

REFERENCES

1. Kawashima A, Sandler CM, Ernst RD, et al. Imaging of nontraumatic hemorrhage of the adrenal gland. *Radiographics.* 1999;19(4):949–963.

2. Westra SJ, Zaninovic AC, Hall TR, et al. Imaging of the adrenal gland in children. *Radiographics.* 1994;14(6):1323–1340.

3. Mittelstaedt CA, Volberg FM, Merten DF, et al. The sonographic diagnosis of neonatal adrenal hemorrhage. *Radiology.* 1979;131(2):453–457.

CLINICAL HISTORY *A 16-year-old female with multisystem failure and dehydration*

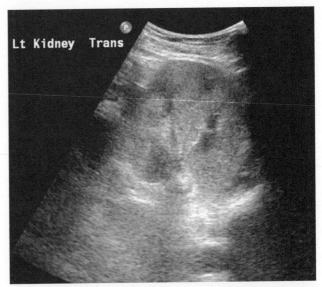

FIGURE 4.19A

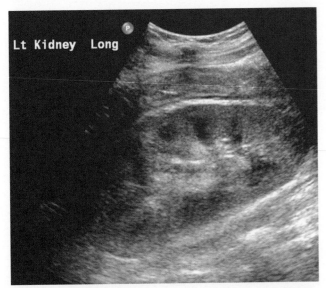

FIGURE 4.19B

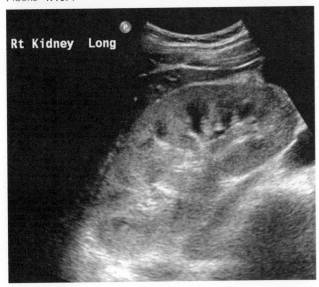

FIGURE 4.19C

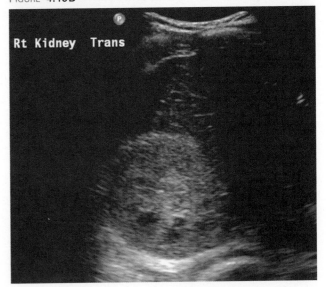

FIGURE 4.19D

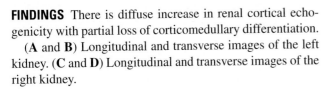

FINDINGS There is diffuse increase in renal cortical echogenicity with partial loss of corticomedullary differentiation.

(**A** and **B**) Longitudinal and transverse images of the left kidney. (**C** and **D**) Longitudinal and transverse images of the right kidney.

DIFFERENTIAL DIAGNOSIS Acute tubular necrosis (ATN), glomerulonephritis, storage diseases, sickle cell anemia

DIAGNOSIS ATN

DISCUSSION ATN is one of the most common causes of acute renal failure. Renal tubular cells have a high metabolic rate, rendering them susceptible to ischemia and toxins, such as free hemoglobin or myoglobin, antibiotics, chemotherapeutic agents, ethylene glycol, and heavy metals. As the basement membrane remains intact, and tubular cells are continuously renewed, the prognosis is good if the offending etiology is removed.

Typically, the renal cortex is diffusely echogenic in comparison to the adjacent liver and spleen, although this finding is fairly nonspecific. In addition, in the neonatal period, normal cortical hyperechogenicity can complicate the diagnosis. Corticomedullary differentiation is variably preserved, dependent upon any associated medullary injury. Renal Doppler studies may demonstrate decreased or reversed diastolic flow.

Questions for Further Thought

1. What laboratory findings can help to confirm the diagnosis of ATN?

2. What are some of the potential contributors to tubular ischemia?

Reporting Responsibilities

- Recognition of the diffuse increase in cortical echotexture, which may be subtle given the diffuse nature of the condition, and the subjective assessment compared to the adjacent liver.

- Renal Doppler US may be helpful, although various renal conditions may also result in increased renal arterial resistance.

What the Treating Physician Needs to Know

- The US appearance is nonspecific, and correlation with history and laboratory studies is needed in narrowing the differential diagnosis.

- ATN is self-limiting if the offending agents are removed.

Answers

1. Fractional excretion of sodium (FENa) >3 and the presence of muddy casts on urinalysis

2. Perinatal asphyxia, sepsis, surfactant deficiency, congenital heart disease, prostaglandin therapy, neuromuscular blocking agents, positive pressure ventilation, iodinated contrast agents, and umbilical catheters

REFERENCES

1. Mercado-Deane MG, Beeson JE, John SD. US of renal insufficiency in neonates. *Radiographics.* 2002;22(6):1429–1438.

2. Krensky AM, Reddish JM, Teele RL. Causes of increased renal echogenicity in pediatric patients. *Pediatrics.* 1983;72(6):840–846.

3. Hayden CK Jr, Santa-Cruz FR, Amparo EG, et al. Ultrasonographic evaluation of the renal parenchyma in infancy and childhood. *Radiology.* 1984;152(2):413–417.

CLINICAL HISTORY *A 14-year-old female with cardiac transplant and infraumbilical abdominal pain*

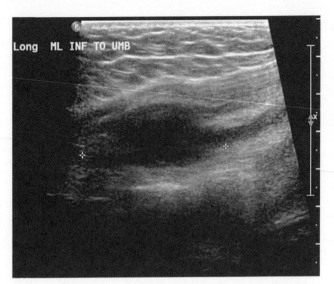

FIGURE 4.20A

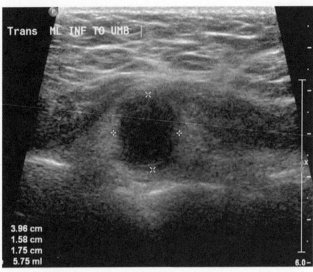

FIGURE 4.20B

FINDINGS There is a midline infraumbilical supravesicular cystic structure beneath the anterior abdominal wall with indistinct thickened walls suggestive of inflammation or infection.

(**A**) Longitudinal and (**B**) transverse sonographic images of the abdomen below the level of the umbilicus.

DIFFERENTIAL DIAGNOSIS Bladder diverticulum, urachal cyst, vitelline cyst, mesenteric cyst, enteric duplication, Meckel diverticulum

DIAGNOSIS Infected urachal cyst

DISCUSSION The urachus is an embryonic structure that develops from the superior portion of the urogenital sinus, extending from the bladder dome to the fetal allantoic duct. Typically, the urachus involutes prenatally, resulting in the medial umbilical ligament within the space of Retzius.

The urachus may persist as a patent urachus (50%) or urachal diverticulum (3% to 5%), urachal cyst (30%), or urachal sinus (15%), with anomalies twice as common in males. These vestigial structures can present with a urine leak at the umbilicus, infection, bleeding, or be incidentally discovered during imaging for other indications. Stone formation and carcinoma are later complications of urachal remnants.

Questions for Further Thought

1. What imaging tests are most appropriate in the setting of suspected urachal remnants?
2. What conditions are associated with an increased incidence of persistent urachal anomalies?

Reporting Responsibilities

• Characterize the type of urachal remnant
• Suggest further imaging: CT, VCU

What the Treating Physician Needs to Know

- Type of urachal anomaly
- Presence of complications and associated conditions

Answers

1. US is the initial imaging modality of choice. CT can be quite helpful in confirming the diagnosis and in the setting of suspected suprainfection.
2. Prune belly syndrome and lower urinary tract obstruction.

REFERENCES

1. Cacciarelli AA, Kass EJ, Yang SS. Urachal remnants: Sonographic demonstration in children. *Radiology.* 1990;174(2):473–475.
2. Yu JS, Kim KW, Lee HJ, et al. Urachal remnant diseases: Spectrum of CT and US findings. *Radiographics.* 2001;21(2): 451–461.
3. Berrocal T, López-Pereira P, Arjonilla A, et al. Anomalies of the distal ureter, bladder, and urethra in children: Embryologic, radiologic, and pathologic features. *Radiographics.* 2002; 22(5):1139–1164.

CASE 4.21

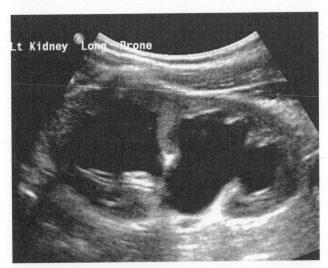

FIGURE **4.21A**

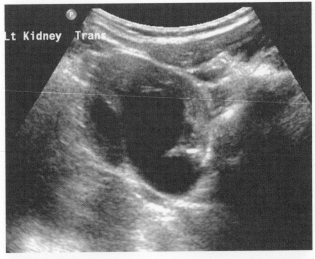

FIGURE **4.21B**

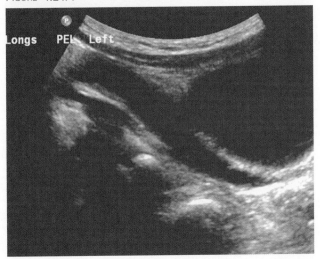

FIGURE **4.21C**

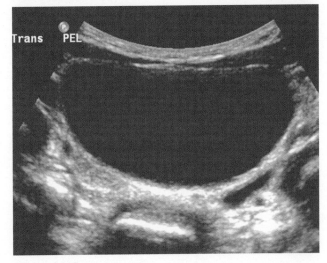

FIGURE **4.21D**

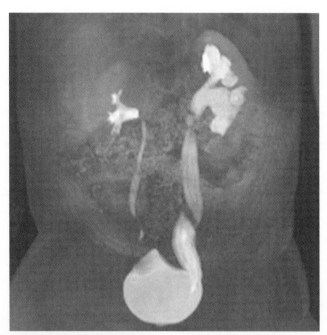

FIGURE **4.21E**

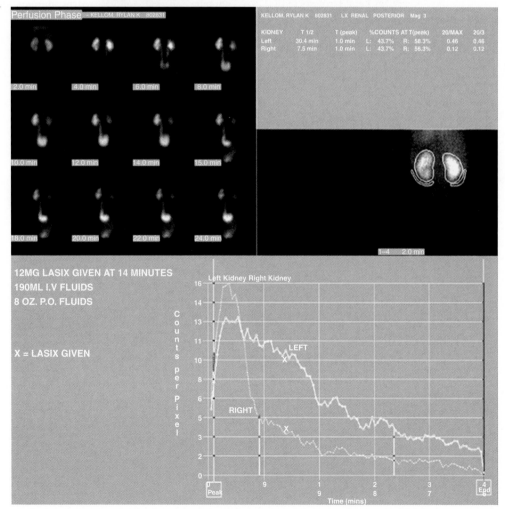

FIGURE **4.21F**

FINDINGS Renal sonography reveals moderate left pelvi-caliectasis and hydroureter, with mild associated renal cortical thinning. This is confirmed with MRU, with MAG-3 renography disclosing decreased left renal function with prolonged intrarenal transit. A VCU showed no evidence for VUR.

Longitudinal (**A**) and transverse (**B**) sonographic images of the left kidney. Longitudinal (**C**) and transverse (**D**) images of the pelvis. (**E**) Diuretic MAG-3 renal scintigraphy. (**F**) MRU MIP 10 minutes post-contrast administration.

DIFFERENTIAL DIAGNOSIS Megaureter with hydronephrosis, moderate left hydroureteronephrosis, obstructive versus non-obstructive dilating uropathy

DIAGNOSIS Megaureter with hydronephrosis, eventually requiring ureteral reimplantation as left renal function declined over time

DISCUSSION Evaluation of hydronephrosis is one of the most common indications for evaluation of the pediatric urinary tract. Hydronephrosis reflects a balance between urinary excretion and some degree of urinary tract obstruction which can become unbalanced due to developmental or extrinsic factors. Evaluation of hydronephrosis detected in utero has become very common, and awareness of the grading system proposed by the Society for Fetal Urology (SFU) can be very helpful in standardized reporting.

While US remains the initial examination of choice, with diuretic MAG-3 renal scintigraphy commonly utilized for assessing the degree of differential renal function and obstruction, MRU has demonstrated potential in replacing both of these examinations with a single study capable of morphologic and functional assessment without radiation, albeit generally requiring sedation and relatively higher cost.

US and MRU can demonstrate the presence of uropathic renal parenchymal changes, such as architectural disorganization, small subcortical cysts, and loss of T2 signal on MRU. This information, combined with functional analysis via MAG-3 renal scintigraphy or MRU, is quite helpful for urologic management.

Questions for Further Thought

1. How are hydronephrosis and obstructive uropathy related?
2. What are helpful findings on MRU suggestive of decompensated hydronephrosis?

Reporting Responsibilities

- Discern the level of obstruction
- Describe any etiology for the obstruction—that is, crossing vessels, calyceal stenosis, valves, duplication, or extrinsic etiology

- Note any associated evidence of renal dysplasia, uropathic changes, or parenchymal loss
- Comparison with prior examinations crucial to assessing severity and progression of obstruction

What the Treating Physician Needs to Know

- Level and nature of the obstruction
- Interval morphologic stability or progression
- Evidence suggesting compensated or decompensated hydronephrosis

Answers

1. Obstructive uropathy is a subset of hydronephrosis, resulting in renal damage due to an obstruction to urine flow, compounded by various vasoactive factors and cytokines, resulting in altered glomerular and tubular function.

2. Edematous renal parenchyma on T2 imaging, delayed and dense MR nephrogram, and delayed calyceal transit time, renal transit time, and increased vDRF-pDRF.

REFERENCES

1. Grattan-Smith and Jones Grattan-Smith JD, Jones RA. Magnetic resonance urography in children. *Magn Reson Imaging Clin N Am.* 2008;16(3):515–531.

2. Riccabona M. Obstructive diseases of the urinary tract in children: Lessons from the last 15 years. *Pediatr Radiol.* 2010;40(6): 947–955.

3. Conway JJ, Maizels M. The "well tempered" diuretic renogram: A standard method to examine the asymptomatic neonate with hydronephrosis or hydroureteronephrosis. A report from combined meetings of The Society for Fetal Urology and members of The Pediatric Nuclear Medicine Council–The Society of Nuclear Medicine. *J Nucl Med.* 1992;33(11): 2047–2051.

CLINICAL HISTORY *A 14-month-old child with poor weight gain and abdominal distension*

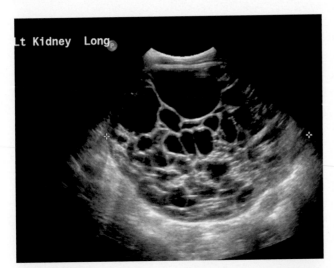

FIGURE **4.22A**

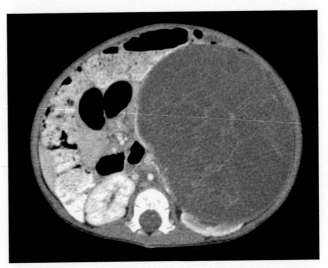

FIGURE **4.22B**

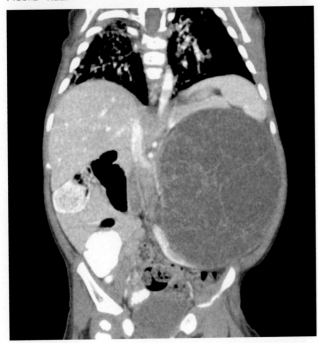

FIGURE **4.22C**

FINDINGS There is a large left-sided multilocular cystic mass. Splaying of the left renal parenchyma (claw sign) suggests a renal origin. Numerous thin internal septations without significant solid tissue component are present. No involvement of the IVC.

(**A**) Longitudinal sonographic image of the left flank. (**B**) Axial and (**C**) coronal images from contrast-enhanced volumetric CT of the abdomen.

DIFFERENTIAL DIAGNOSIS Multilocular cystic nephroma, cystic Wilms' tumor, cystic RCC, clear cell sarcoma, mesoblastic nephroma, MCDK

DIAGNOSIS Multilocular cystic nephroma

DISCUSSION Multilocular cystic nephroma is a rare benign renal neoplasm, one part of a spectrum of multilocular cystic renal tumors (MCRTs) that includes cystic partially differentiated nephroblastoma (CPDN). These tumors are indistinguishable from one another by imaging or gross pathology.

This tumor typically presents in boys between 3 months and 4 years of age, with another peak incidence in adult women between 40 and 60 years, possibly representing a distinct entity called mixed epithelial and stromal tumor of the kidney. Bilateral tumors have been described. In children, the tumor usually presents as a painless mass, with hematuria or UTI occasionally precipitating the diagnosis.

Questions for Further Thought

1. How can one distinguish multilocular cystic nephroma from a cystic Wilms' tumor?
2. Does the presence of solid tissue components suggest an alternative diagnosis?

Reporting Responsibilities

- Tumor description, including the presence of internal septations, solid tissue components, and calcifications
- Any evidence for caval involvement, pulmonary metastases, or lymphadenopathy

What the Treating Physician Needs to Know

- Multilocular cystic nephroma cannot be reliably distinguished from a CPDN and, therefore, these tumors are all surgically resected.

Answers

1. Multilocular cystic nephroma is a benign cystic tumor with fibrous septa containing mature tubules and an epithelial lining. It is indistinguishable from a CPDN that contains blastemal cells within the septa.
2. Yes. Solid components are not a characteristic imaging feature of multilocular cystic nephroma.

REFERENCES

1. Silver IM, Boag AH, Soboleski DA. Best cases from the AFIP: Multilocular cystic renal tumor: cystic nephroma. *Radiographics.* 2008;28(4):1221–1225; discussion 1225–1226.
2. Hopkins JK, Giles HW Jr, Wyatt-Ashmead J, et al. Best cases from the AFIP: Cystic nephroma. *Radiographics.* 2004;24(2): 589–593.
3. Lee EY. CT imaging of mass-like renal lesions in children. *Pediatr Radiol.* 2007;37(9):896–907.

CLINICAL HISTORY *An 8-year-old female with the acute onset of lower abdominal pain*

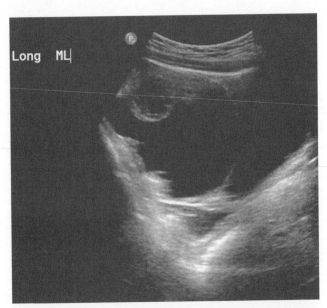

FIGURE 4.23A

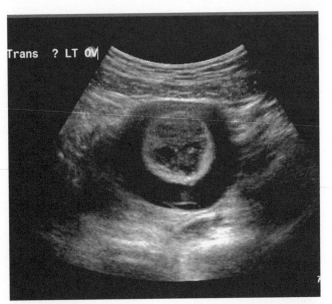

FIGURE 4.23B

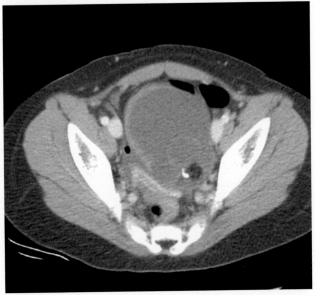

FIGURE 4.23C

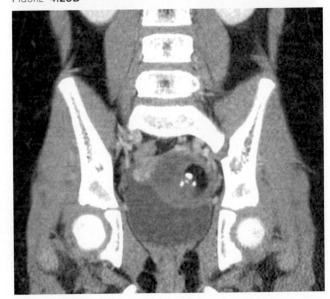

FIGURE 4.23D

FINDINGS There is a large complex cystic left adnexal mass containing a mural nodule with small calcifications and fatty component. A small amount of free pelvic fluid is also noted.

(**A**) Longitudinal and (**B**) transverse sonographic images of the pelvis. (**C**) Axial and (**D**) coronal images from contrast-enhanced CT of the abdomen and pelvis.

DIFFERENTIAL DIAGNOSIS Ovarian dermoid cyst. Immature teratoma, monodermal teratoma. Hemorrhagic ovarian cyst, perforated appendix containing appendicoliths, or cystadenofibroma is unlikely, given the presence of fat within the mass.

DIAGNOSIS Mature cystic teratoma (dermoid cyst) complicated by ovarian torsion

DISCUSSION Mature cystic teratomas (also known as dermoid cysts) account for 50% of pediatric ovarian tumors, and contain components of endodermal, mesodermal, and ectodermal origin. Typically, these are cystic tumors with a mural nodule (Rokitansky nodule) where hair and teeth typically develop.

Immature teratomas are relatively rare (<1%), affect younger patients, and exhibit malignant behavior. Typically, immature teratomas are larger and more often solid.

Monodermal teratomas are predominantly composed of one tissue type. The main variants include struma ovarii, ovarian carcinoid, and those exhibiting neural differentiation.

Complications of mature ovarian teratomas include torsion (16%), rupture (1% to 4%), malignant transformation (1% to 2%), infection (1%), and autoimmune hemolytic anemia (<1%).

Questions for Further Thought

1. What is the significance of teratoma growth in an otherwise asymptomatic patient?
2. What MR techniques can reliably detect the presence of fat within the tumor?
3. What findings are most helpful in determining malignant transformation?
4. What is the most common form of malignant degeneration arising from a mature cystic teratoma?

Reporting Responsibilities

- Detection of fat with the mass is diagnostic for teratoma
- Detection of complications which will require surgical management

What the Treating Physician Needs to Know

- Diagnostic certainty for mature cystic teratoma
- Findings suggesting any of the above complications

Answers

1. Mature cystic teratomas grow at an average rate of 1.8 mm/year, and nonsurgical management of smaller (<6 cm) tumors has been suggested.
2. Frequency selective fat suppression is probably the most common technique currently in use. Chemical shift artifact and in and out of phase gradient echo techniques are also helpful for detection of fat and differentiating fat from hemorrhage.
3. The presence of an enhancing soft tissue component and an obtuse angle between the soft tissue mass and inner cyst wall.
4. Squamous cell carcinoma (80%).

REFERENCES

1. Outwater EK, Siegelman ES, Hunt JL. Ovarian teratomas: Tumor types and imaging characteristics. *Radiographics.* 2001; 21(2):475–490.
2. Park SB, Kim JK, Kim KR, et al. Imaging findings of complications and unusual manifestations of ovarian teratomas. *Radiographics.* 2008;28(4):969–983.
3. Sisler CL, Siegel MJ. Ovarian teratomas: A comparison of the sonographic appearance in prepubertal and postpubertal girls. *AJR Am J Roentgenol.* 1990;154(1):139–141.

CASE 4.24

CLINICAL HISTORY *An 8-month-old male with recurrent UTIs*

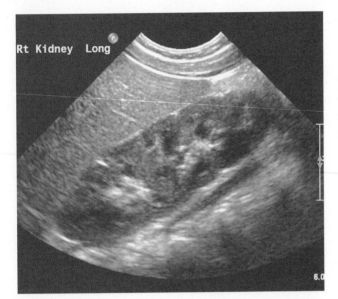

FIGURE **4.24A**

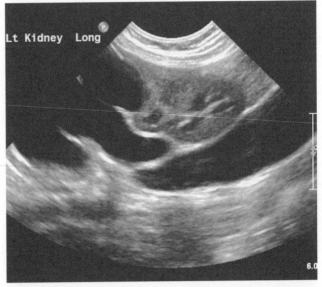

FIGURE **4.24B**

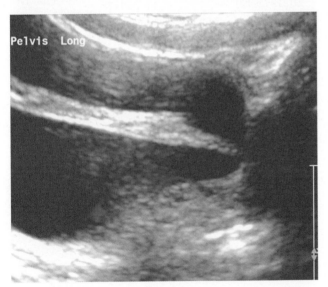

FIGURE **4.24C**

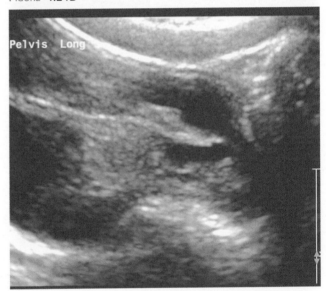

FIGURE **4.24D**

FINDINGS There is marked dilation of the left upper pole renal collecting system, with a moderately dilated tortuous ureter extending to the midline below the bladder base. An image from a cystoscopic retrograde ureterogram demonstrates the ectopic tortuous dilated ureter and dilated upper pole renal collecting system, with the ectopic ureteral orifice identified within the prostatic urethra.

(**A** and **B**) Longitudinal sonographic images of the right and left kidneys. (**C** and **D**) Longitudinal sonographic images of the left pelvis. (**E**) Anteroposterior (AP) spot image from intraoperative retrograde urography.

DIFFERENTIAL DIAGNOSIS None

DIAGNOSIS Duplex left renal collecting system with ectopic obstructed upper pole ureter draining to the prostatic urethra

DISCUSSION Renal collecting system duplication is the most common congenital abnormality of the kidneys, seen in 0.7% of the population. However, the prevalence is higher (8% with UTI; 15% with parenchymal scarring) in patients with urinary tract disease. Renal collecting system duplication is slightly more common on the left, and is frequently bilateral (17% to 23%). It is also more common in girls, and frequently associated with VUR (45% in the presence of UTI, compared to 25% in those patients without duplication)

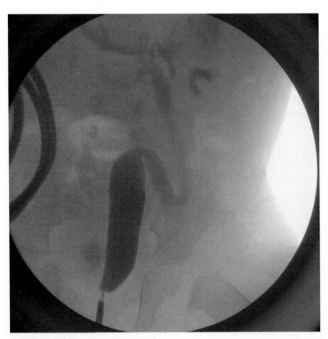

FIGURE 4.24E

and renal parenchymal damage at DMSA (36% of those with duplication, compared to 26% without duplication).

Ectopic ureteral insertion of the upper pole collecting system moiety is common, and follows the Weigert–Meyer rule, which states that the upper pole moiety ureter will insert inferomedial to the lower pole moiety. In males, this ectopic insertion typically occurs above the level of the urethral sphincter, whereas in females the insertion can be below the level of the sphincter, leading to a characteristic pattern of continence with continual dribbling.

Questions for Further Thought

1. What is the sensitivity of the various imaging modalities in detecting renal collecting system duplication?
2. What modality is currently the methodology of choice when evaluating a complicated duplex collecting system?

Reporting Responsibilities

• Identification of a duplex collecting system and degree of certainty

• Identification of associated ectopic ureteral insertion and the presence of a ureterocele, if possible
• Assessment of the renal parenchyma of both upper and lower poles

What the Treating Physician Needs to Know

• Is there evidence for a complicated duplex renal collecting system (obstruction, ureterocele, reflux, associated renal dysplasia, or parenchymal loss)? These entities often require surgical management.

Answers

1. Renal sonography is the initial modality used when urinary tract abnormalities are suspected. While detection of a dilated collecting system duplication is straightforward, this diagnosis may be missed without dilatation. Diuretic MAG-3 scintigraphy is currently the preferred functional assessment, but is not generally recommended below 3 months of age due to renal physiologic immaturity. While the sensitivity of contrast-enhanced CT is quite good, this modality is generally deferred given the radiation dose. Intravenous urography has relatively little place in today's imaging arsenal, given the superior anatomic depiction and lesser radiation of other modalities, particularly MRU.

2. MRU currently provides the most comprehensive morphologic assessment of the kidneys, ureters, bladder, and associated anomalies. It is the optimal modality for detection and assessment of ectopic ureteral insertion.

REFERENCES

1. Avni FE, Nicaise N, Hall M, et al. The role of MR imaging for the assessment of complicated duplex kidneys in children: Preliminary report. *Pediatr Radiol.* 2001;31(4):215–223.
2. Siomou E, Papadopoulou F, Kollios KD, et al. Duplex collecting system diagnosed during the first 6 years of life after a first urinary tract infection: A study of 63 children. *J Urol.* 2006;175(2):678–681; discussion 681–682.
3. Stokland E, Jodal U, Sixt R, et al. Uncomplicated duplex kidney and DMSA scintigraphy in children with urinary tract infection. *Pediatr Radiol.* 2007;37(8):826–828.

CASE 4.25

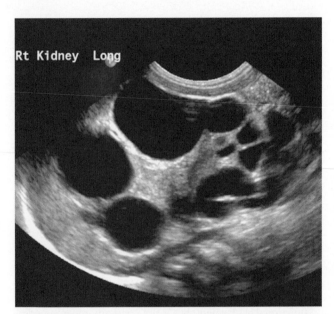

FIGURE **4.25A**

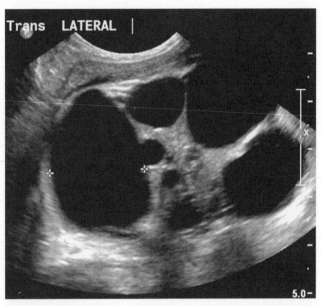

FIGURE **4.25B**

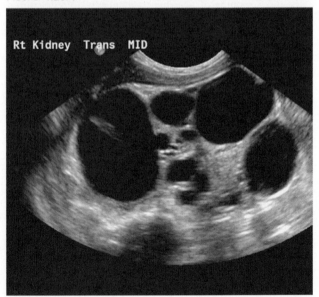

FIGURE **4.25C**

FINDINGS The right kidney is enlarged and contains numerous, variably sized noncommunicating cysts with visualized parenchyma echogenic and disordered.

(**A**) Longitudinal and (**B** and **C**) transverse sonographic images of the right kidney.

DIFFERENTIAL DIAGNOSIS MCDK, UPJ obstruction

DIAGNOSIS MCDK

DISCUSSION MCDK is the second most common cause of an abdominal mass in a newborn (after hydronephrosis), although approximately 50% are not clinically detectable. Generally it is unilateral, as bilateral involvement is incompatible with life. It is slightly more common in males and involving the left kidney.

It is a developmental abnormality thought to be related to atresia of the ureter and renal pelvis (infundibulopelvic variant) or upper ureter (less common hydronephrotic variant). Rarely, an MCDK may be related to an obstructed ureterocele. MCDK may rarely involve only one portion of a duplex kidney, often simulating a multicystic renal mass.

Diagnosis is generally made with antenatal or postnatal US. Typically, there are numerous variably sized noncommunicating renal cysts without normal renal parenchyma, although in the less common hydronephrotic variant the cysts do communicate. Excretory renal scintigraphy is helpful in excluding the presence of any functioning renal tissue.

Questions for Further Thought

1. What other renal conditions are associated with MCDK?
2. What are current recommendations for management?
3. Are large MCDKs more likely to persist at follow-up examination?

Reporting Responsibilities

- Description including cyst characterization, renal size, and any contralateral anomalies

- Suggest excretory renal scintigraphy to exclude functional renal tissue

What the Treating Physician Needs to Know

- Spontaneous involution will occur in 20% by 1 year and in 60% by 6 years.
- Typical US appearance is diagnostic. Excretory renal scintigraphy helpful in excluding the possibility of UPJ obstruction. VCU generally not recommended, as VUR is typically low grade in the absence of a dilated contralateral ureter.

Answers

1. The contralateral kidney may exhibit abnormalities (20% to 30%), including UPJ or ureteral obstruction. VUR is commonly present, either ipsilateral or bilateral. Historically, an increased incidence of hypertension, malignant degeneration, and infection were described, but more recent investigation have not supported these perceptions.
2. Routine nephrectomy is no longer the standard approach, now reserved for symptomatic patients or those kidneys that fail to demonstrate involution.
3. The initial size of an MCDK has been found to be a poor predictor of eventual persistence or involution.

REFERENCES

1. Chakraborty S, McHugh K. Cystic diseases of the kidney in children. *Imaging.* 2005;17:69–75.
2. Kaneko K, Suzuki Y, Fukuda Y, et al. Abnormal contralateral kidney in unilateral multicystic dysplastic kidney disease. *Pediatr Radiol.* 1995;25(4):275–277.
3. Greenbaum LA. Renal dysplasia and MRI: A clinician's perspective. *Pediatr Radiol.* 2008;38(Suppl 1):S70–S75.

CLINICAL HISTORY *A 6-month-old asymptomatic female with right-sided abdominal mass detected on physical examination*

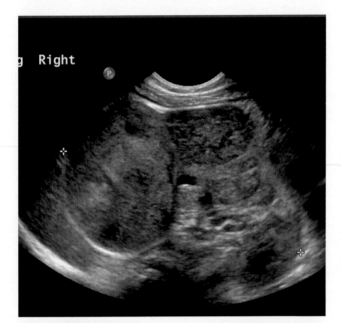

FIGURE 4.26A

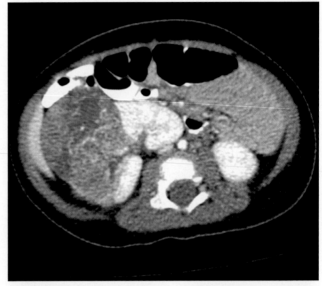

FIGURE 4.26B

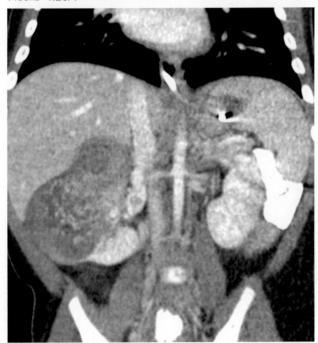

FIGURE 4.26C

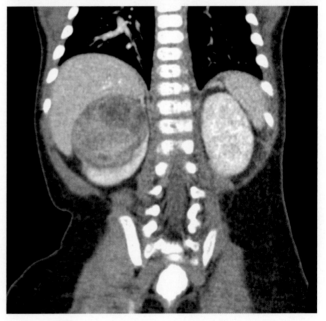

FIGURE 4.26D

DIAGNOSIS Mesoblastic nephroma, cellular variant

FINDINGS US and CT images demonstrate a larger heterogeneous mass involving the upper portion of the right kidney.

(A) Longitudinal sonographic image of the right kidney. (B–D) Axial and coronal images from contrast-enhanced volumetric CT of the abdomen.

DIFFERENTIAL DIAGNOSIS Mesoblastic nephroma, primarily Wilms' tumor and multilocular cystic nephroma, rarely rhabdoid tumor and clear cell sarcoma

DISCUSSION Mesoblastic nephroma is the most common renal tumor in the first year of life. There are two main variants. The classic type presents in the neonatal period, whereas the more aggressive cellular variant presents at several months of age, with local invasion and recurrence following resection more common. No sex predilection.

The classic variant more commonly exhibits a uniform soft tissue mass with concentric peripheral hypervascular hyperechoic and hypoechoic rings on US, although these findings can also be found in the cellular variant. The cellular variant more commonly shows regions of hemorrhage and cystic necrosis, making distinction from Wilms' tumor problematic.

Questions for Further Thought

1. How common is Wilms' tumor in the neonatal period?
2. What findings and conditions are associated with the prenatal diagnosis of mesoblastic nephroma?

Reporting Responsibilities

Imaging features of the mass: Solid, cystic, hemorrhage, invasion of surrounding structure

What the Treating Physician Needs to Know

- Cannot reliably make a specific diagnosis of mesoblastic nephroma, but appearance and young age will favor this possibility

- Imaging features suggestive of the cellular variant will be helpful during surgical planning

Answers

1. Only 2% of Wilms' tumors occur under 3 months of age.
2. Renal mass, polyhydramnios, and premature labor.

REFERENCES

1. Chaudry G, Perez-Atayde AR, Ngan BY, et al. Imaging of congenital mesoblastic nephroma with pathological correlation. *Pediatr Radiol.* 2009;39(10):1080–1086.
2. Bayindir P, Guillerman RP, Hicks MJ, et al. Cellular mesoblastic nephroma (infantile renal fibrosarcoma): Institutional review of the clinical, diagnostic imaging, and pathologic features of a distinctive neoplasm of infancy. *Pediatr Radiol.* 2009;39(10):1066–1074.
3. Fuchs IB, Henrich W, Brauer M, et al. Prenatal diagnosis of congenital mesoblastic nephroma in 2 siblings. *J Ultrasound Med.* 2003;22(8):823–827.

Randalph K. Otto

CASE 4.27

CLINICAL HISTORY *A 4-year-old child with 2 days of left scrotal pain*

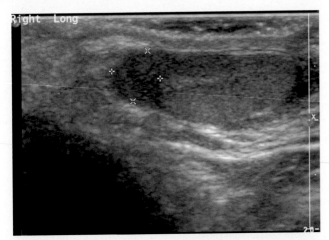

FIGURE 4.27A

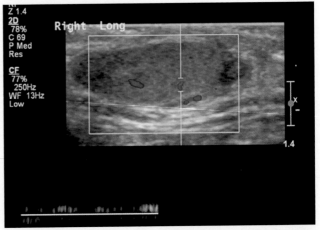

FIGURE 4.27B

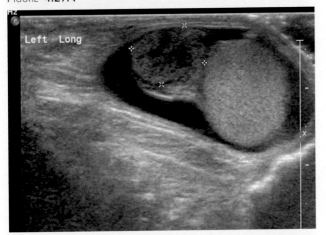

FIGURE 4.27C

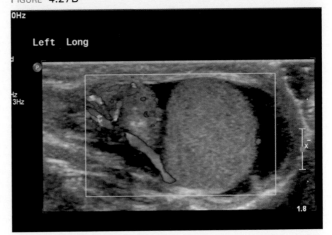

FIGURE 4.27D

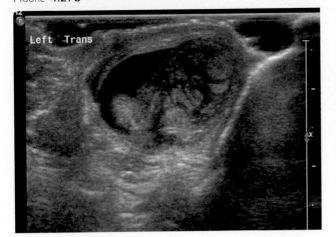

FIGURE 4.27E

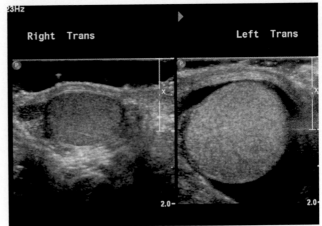

FIGURE 4.27F

FINDINGS There is a moderate left hydrocele with an enlarged echogenic left testicle and enlarged heterogeneous epididymis. There is moderate epididymal and lesser testicular hypervascularity. Mild overlying skin thickening and echogenicity.

(**A** and **B**) Longitudinal sonographic images of the right hemiscrotum. (**C** and **D**) Longitudinal sonographic images of the left hemiscrotum. (**E**) Transverse sonographic images of the left superior hemiscrotum. (**F**) Representative transverse sonographic images of the scrotum.

DIFFERENTIAL DIAGNOSIS Epididymo-orchitis, or chronic granulomatous epididymo-orchitis, as well as recent detorsion or partial torsion of the testicle. Leukemia and lymphoma can diffusely infiltrate the testicle with enlargement and heterogeneous echotexture mimicking orchitis. Torsed testicular appendages can mimic the clinical presentation.

DIAGNOSIS Epididymo-orchitis

DISCUSSION Acute epididymo-orchitis is one of the most common causes of acute acrotal pain in children. Typically, scrotal pain, swelling, and tenderness develop over a few days, in contrast to the more acute time course of testicular torsion.

Most commonly, it occurs without underlying pathology, but it may occur with UTI, trauma, autoimmune disease, and vasculitis.

On US, typical findings include an enlarged hyperemic epididymis (particularly the head), variable testicular enlargement, echogenicity, and hyperemia. Associated hydrocele and skin thickening are common findings. Epididymal and testicular arterial waveforms may show decreased diastolic resistance, although this can also be a feature of recent testicular de-torsion or partial torsion.

Associated abnormalities of the genitourinary tract that may predispose to epididymo-orchitis and potentially require surgical intervention include imperforate anus or rectourethral fistula, hypospadias, müllerian duct cyst, ectopic ureter draining to the seminal vesicle, PUVs, bladder extrophy, neurogenic bladder, and dysfunctional voiding syndromes.

Questions for Further Thought

1. Given that partial or recent testicular de-torsion may mimic epididymo-orchitis, what clinical and imaging details can be helpful in differentiating acute epididymo-orchitis from testicular torsion?
2. What are findings on physical examination that suggest testicular torsion?

Reporting Responsibilities

- Characterization of US findings within scrotum and spermatic cord.
- Description of any associated genitourinary tract pathology. Renal sonography and potentially VCU may be helpful in further evaluation.

What the Treating Physician Needs to Know

- Degree of certainty for epididymo-orchitis versus other etiologies
- Indications for surgical intervention, generally due to one of the associated abnormalities listed above

Answers

1. The typical clinical time course of testicular torsion is generally shorter than that of epididymo-orchitis. While some testicular blood flow may still persist in cases of partial torsion, examination of the spermatic cord for a spiral twist can be the most reliable sign of testicular torsion, regardless of testicular findings.
2. Diffuse tenderness, abnormal testicular position, and absence of the cremasteric reflex.

REFERENCES

1. Aso C, Enríquez G, Fité M, et al. Gray-scale and color Doppler sonography of scrotal disorders in children: An update. *Radiographics.* 2005;25(5):1197–1214.
2. Vijayaraghavan SB. Sonographic differential diagnosis of acute scrotum: Real-time whirlpool sign, a key sign of torsion. *J Ultrasound Med.* 2006;25(5):563–574.
3. Karmazyn B, Kaefer M, Kauffman S, et al. Ultrasonography and clinical findings in children with epididymitis, with and without associated lower urinary tract abnormalities. *Pediatr Radiol.* 2009;39(10):1054–1058.

CLINICAL HISTORY *Blunt abdominal trauma and hematuria*

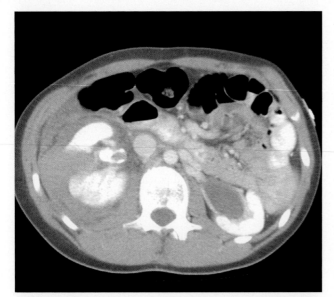

FIGURE 4.28A

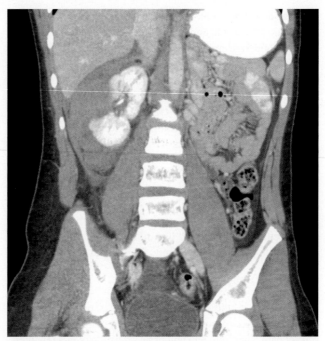

FIGURE 4.28B

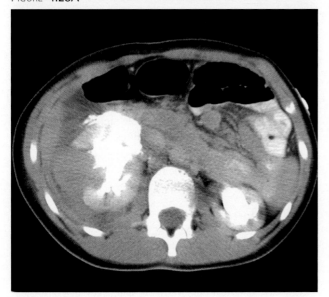

FIGURE 4.28C

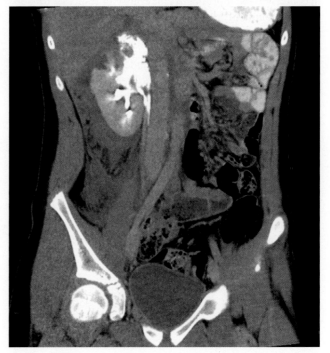

FIGURE 4.28D

FINDINGS On the nephrogram phase, an extensive right renal laceration is apparent with perinephric hematoma and filling defect within the renal pelvis representing blood clot. On the delayed images, contrast extravasation is apparent, consistent with collecting system involvement.

Axial and coronal images from the nephrogram (**A** and **B**) and delayed (**C** and **D**) phases of contrast-enhanced CT of the abdomen and pelvis.

DIFFERENTIAL DIAGNOSIS None

DIAGNOSIS Right grade IV renal injury with ureteropelvic injury

DISCUSSION Renal Injury occurs in 8% to 10% of blunt or less commonly penetrating abdominal trauma, serious injuries are usually associated with injuries to other organs. Most isolated renal injuries are minor.

Radiologic Classification:

Category I minor cortical contusions, subcapsular hematoma (75% to 80%)

Category II renal lacerations <1 cm deep, extending to the medulla, without collecting system involvement or segmental infarction (10%)

Category III are characterized by a nonexpanding perinephric hematoma and lacerations >1-cm deep. The collecting system is not involved (5%)

Category IV injuries involve injury to the UPJ and main renal vessels, with resulting segmental infarctions

Category V injuries are characterized by a shattered kidney or extensive devascularization

Questions for Further Thought

1. What is the significance of hematuria in the setting of blunt abdominal trauma?

2. What is the utility of ultrasonography in the setting of suspected renal injury?

Reporting Responsibilities

• Description and classification of any renal injuries
• Description of any associated renal anomalies

What the Treating Physician Needs to Know

• Classification of renal injury as above.
• Any underlying abnormalities that may affect management. Trauma to abnormal kidneys is much more common in children than adults due to the relative renal size and relative decrease in surrounding protective tissue. Hydronephrosis, cystic disease, tumors, horseshoe kidney, and renal ectopia are not uncommon findings.

Answers

1. All children with any degree of hematuria and history of blunt traumas should undergo renal imaging. However, renal artery thrombosis and ureteropelvic injuries may not have any hematuria.

2. Renal US has limited value in the evaluation of trauma relative to CT. Various renal injuries may be missed or underestimated with US alone.

REFERENCES

1. Harris AC, Zwirewich CV, Lyburn ID, et al. Ct findings in blunt renal trauma. *Radiographics.* 2001;21(Spec No):S201–S214.

2. Kawashima A, Sandler CM, Corl FM, et al. Imaging of renal trauma: A comprehensive review. *Radiographics.* 2001;21(3): 557–574.

3. Park SJ, Kim JK, Kim KW, et al. MDCT findings of renal trauma. *AJR Am J Roentgenol.* 2006;187(2):541–547.

4. Donnelly LF. Imaging issues in CT of blunt trauma to the chest and abdomen. *Pediatr Radiol.* 2009;39(Suppl 3):406–413.

CLINICAL HISTORY *A 3-month-old asymptomatic male with an abnormal prenatal US*

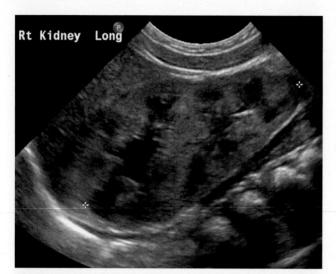

FIGURE **4.29A**

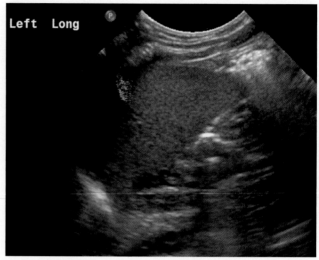

FIGURE **4.29B**

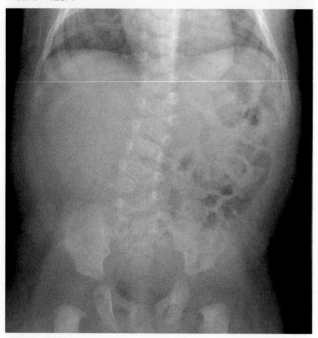

FIGURE **4.29C**

FINDINGS The abdominal radiograph demonstrates balanced lumbar hemivertebral anomalies, as well as a prominent right renal outline, absent renal outline on the left, with bowel gas filling much of the left abdomen.

Renal sonography discloses a prominent size of the right kidney with absent left kidney, the left renal fossa filled with bowel.

MAG-3 diuretic renal scintigraphy confirms the absence of the left kidney with normal function on the right.

Sonographic images of (**A**) the right and (**B**) the left flank. (**C**) AP radiograph of the abdomen. (**D**) Diuretic MAG-3 renal scintigraphy.

DIFFERENTIAL DIAGNOSIS Considerations for an empty renal fossa on US include an ectopic kidney, involuted MCDK, or congenital renal agenesis

DIAGNOSIS Unilateral renal agenesis with associated vertebral anomalies

DISCUSSION Renal agenesis is currently thought to result from a vascular insult to the ureteral bud during the fifth week of gestation. Incidence of unilateral agenesis is estimated at 1/500 to 1/3,200. Bilateral renal agenesis is a lethal abnormality with incidence approximately 1/10,000. There is a male predominance of 3:1, and 20% to 36% has a familial association.

An empty renal fossa by US suggests renal agenesis (47%) or renal ectopia (42%). An involuted MCDK is another consideration.

Renal agenesis is often associated with other abnormalities. Urologic abnormalities are most common, and include VUR, hydronephrosis, UVJ and UPJ obstruction, primary megaureter, contralateral MCDK, PUVs, mesoblastic nephroma, and genital anomalies (cloacal extrophy and seminal vesicle cysts).

Other associations most commonly include congenital heart disease, congenital diaphragmatic hernia, and VACTERL syndrome (as in this case).

Questions for Further Thought

1. What is the status of the adrenal gland in renal agenesis?
2. Where is the typical location of ectopic kidneys?

Reporting Responsibilities

- Documentation of empty renal fossa and no evidence for an ectopic kidney, with examination directed along the ipsilateral psoas muscle
- Suggest confirmation of renal agenesis with renal scintigraphy, CT, or MRU
- Documentation of associated anomalies

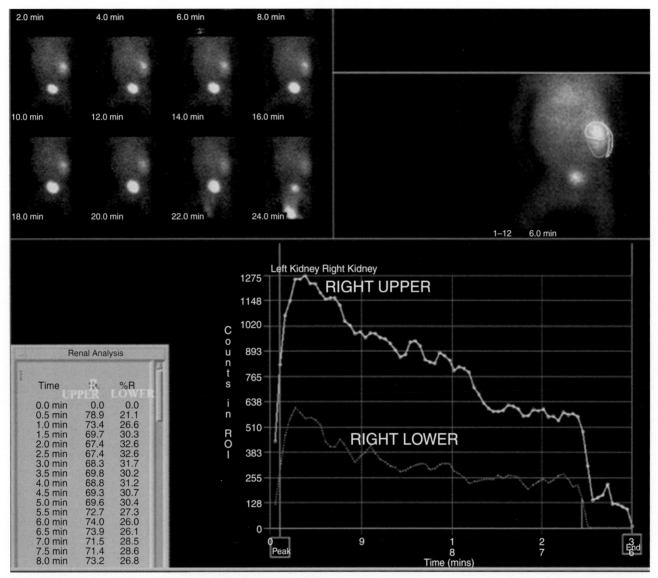

Figure **4.29D**

What the Treating Physician Needs to Know

- It is necessary to exclude renal ectopia, given that this is a frequent explanation for an empty renal fossa.
- Any associated contralateral urologic abnormality which may threaten function of the remaining kidney.
- Documentation of any associated abnormalities.

Answers

1. Ipsilateral adrenal agenesis occurs in 8% to 10% of renal agenesis.

2. Ipsilateral pelvis (87%), crossed fused ectopia (8%), horseshoe kidney (2%), and intrathoracic (2%, especially with associated congenital diaphragmatic hernia (CDH).

REFERENCES

1. Chow JS, Benson CB, Lebowitz RL. The clinical significance of an empty renal fossa on prenatal sonography. *J Ultrasound Med.* 2005;24(8):1049–1054; quiz 1055–1057.

2. Mishra A. Renal agenesis: Report of an interesting case. *Br J Radiol.* 2007;80(956):e167–e169.

3. Mercado-Deane MG, Beeson JE, John SD. US of renal insufficiency in neonates. *Radiographics.* 2002;22(6):1429–1438.

CASE 4.30

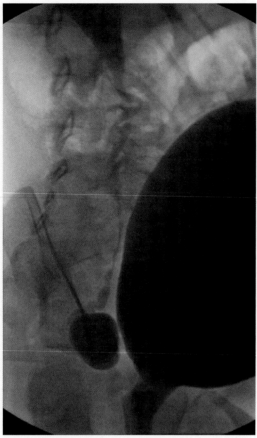

FIGURE **4.30A**

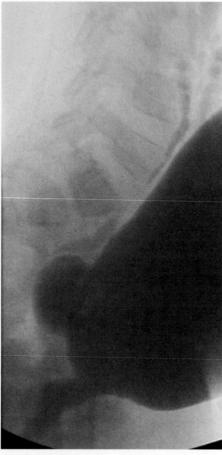

FIGURE **4.30B**

FINDINGS Fluroscopic images (**A** and **B**) demonstrate a bladder diverticulum at the UVJ with the ureter feeding directly into the diverticulum and tortuosity of the ureter with grade IV VUR also noted.

DIFFERENTIAL DIAGNOSIS None

DIAGNOSIS Bladder diverticulum

DISCUSSION A bladder diverticulum is a protrusion of the mucosa through a defect in the detrusor musculature. There are acquired diverticula that are associated with increased intravesical pressure secondary to obstruction and in cases of neurogenic bladder associated with detrusor–sphincter dyssynergia. These diverticula are usually multiple and associated with saccules and severe bladder wall trabecula- tion. There are also acquired diverticula due to postsurgical

etiologies. Congenital bladder diverticula are more common in boys, typically occur on the posterolateral wall above the ureteric hiatus, can be unilateral or bilateral, and often present without evidence for bladder outlet obstruction. There are also congenital paraureteric diverticula often encountered in children and associated with primary VUR, termed Hutch diverticula. These Hutch diverticula appear to be associated with muscular deficiency near the ureteric insertion. Finally, the last group of bladder diverticula is those associated with specific syndromes such as Prune belly syndrome, Menkes syndrome, and Ehlers–Danlos syndrome (EDS).

Questions for Further Thought

1. In any child with a bladder diverticulum, what are the most important steps in a VCUG?
2. What differentiates a saccule from a diverticulum? Are saccules clinically significant?

Reporting Responsibilities

- Describe the location, specifically with regard to the ureteral orifice, size, and number of diverticula present on the examination
- Describe any evidence for VUR or bladder outlet obstruction

What the Treating Physician Needs to Know

- Multiple bladder diverticula are very suspicious for an underlying disorder or bladder outlet obstruction. Surgical treatment is indicated in all symptomatic cases of congenital bladder diverticulum.
- If there is significant VUR noted, a nuclear medicine study could be obtained to evaluate renal function.

Answers

1. The most important steps to a VCUG in a child with an identified bladder diverticulum are appropriate evaluation of the urethra to rule out any evidence of obstruction and postvoid residuals to demonstrate any pooling of contrast within the diverticula that can lead to urinary retention from obstruction of the urethra or recurrent UTIs from accumulation of residual urine.

2. Saccules are considered to be any out pouching measuring <2 cm in diameter and diverticula are considered to measure more than 2 cm in diameter. Saccules can be clinically significant along with diverticula since either can produce significant functional changes at the ureterovesical angle.

REFERENCES

1. Blane C, Zerin J, Bloom D. Bladder diverticula in children. *Radiology.* 1994;190:695–697.
2. Barrett DM, Malek RS, Kelalis PP. Observations on vesical diverticulum in children. *J Urol.* 1976;116:234–236.
3. Pieretti R, Pieretti-Vanmarcke R. Congenital bladder diverticula in children. *J Pediatr Surg.* 1976;34:468–473.

Deborah Conway

CASE 4.31

CLINICAL HISTORY *Abdominal pain*

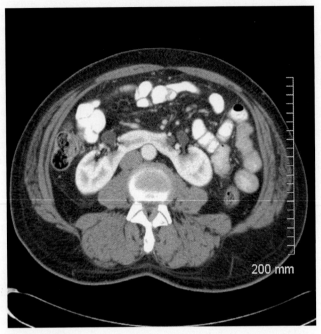

FIGURE **4.31**

FINDINGS CT contrasted axial image of the abdomen and pelvis demonstrates fusion of the lower poles of both kidneys by a parenchymal isthmus. The isthmus is caudal to the origin of the inferior mesenteric artery.

DIFFERENTIAL DIAGNOSIS Horseshoe kidney, crossed-fused renal ectopia, malrotated kidney, disc or pancake kidney, cake or lump kidney

DIAGNOSIS Horseshoe kidney

DISCUSSION Horseshoe kidney represents the most common type of renal fusion anomaly and results from a failure of separation of the embryologic metanephric ridges such that the lower poles of both kidneys are fused by an isthmus and directed medially.[1] In rare instances, the upper poles may be the site of fusion. The isthmus may be composed of renal or fibrous tissue. It prevents normal renal rotation so that the renal axes are abnormally oriented and also prevents cephalic migration of the horseshoe kidney above the level of the inferior mesenteric artery.[2] Specifically, the lower poles lie more medial than the upper poles. Therefore, a horseshoe kidney is actually an anomaly of renal fusion, malrotation, and ectopia.[1] The horseshoe kidney obtains its blood supply from several sources during its incomplete ascent including the inferior mesenteric artery, aorta, renal arteries, and iliac arteries. Multiple aberrant arteries can cross the UPJs and proximal ureters. These crossing vessels result in obstruction and urinary stasis that lead to infection and calculus formation.

Questions for Further Thought

1. What are some of the complications of horseshoe kidney?
2. What genetic syndromes are horseshoe kidneys frequently associated with?

Reporting Responsibilities
- Offer the most likely alternative diagnosis if not horseshoe kidney
- Evaluate for potential complications of horseshoe kidney, including calculi, infection, trauma, and malignancy

Answers
1. Although most cases of horseshoe kidneys are found incidentally and are asymptomatic, they are prone to a number of complications including hydronephrosis, nephrolithiasis, infection, and increased susceptibility to trauma.[3] Furthermore, there is an increased incidence of renal and transitional cell carcinoma as well as Wilms' tumor in a horseshoe kidney.[2]

2. Horseshoe kidneys are found in approximately 1 in 400 to 500 adults and are more frequently encountered in males by 2:1. Although most cases are sporadic, horseshoe kidneys are associated with genetic syndromes. These include Turner syndrome, Edward syndrome (Trisomy 18), and Patau syndrome (Trisomy 13) to name a few. Horseshoe kidney is also found in conjunction with VACTERL association.[1]

REFERENCES
1. Davidson AJ, Hartman DS. *Radiology of the Kidney and Urinary Tract.* 2nd ed. Philadelphia, PA: Saunders; 1994:81, 84.
2. Donnelly LF. *Fundamentals of Pediatric Radiology.* 1st ed. Philadelphia, PA: Saunders; 2001:149–150.
3. Alonso RC, Nacenta SB, Martinez PD, et al. Kidney in danger: CT findings of blunt and penetrating renal trauma. *Radiographics.* 2009;29:2033–2054.

CASE 4.32

Deborah Conway

CLINICAL HISTORY *A 10-month-old female with distended abdomen and palpable mass*

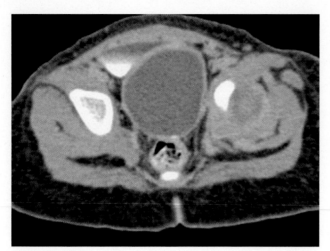

FIGURE **4.32A**

FINDINGS (**A**) Axial CT image of pelvis demonstrating fluid-filled dilated peripherally enhancing structure anterior to the rectum and displacing the urinary bladder anteriorly and to the right (structure containing contrast/fluid level). (**B**) Lateral fluoroscopic image of uterus after instillation of contrast via surgically constructed mucus fistula demonstrating uterine distension. Forceps are present anteriorly and inferiorly in region of vaginal atresia.

DIFFERENTIAL DIAGNOSIS Hydrometrocolpos, pelvis abscess, ovarian cyst/tumor, pelvic rhabdomyosarcoma

DIAGNOSIS Hydrometrocolpos

DISCUSSION Hydrometrocolpos is defined as a collection of fluid within the vagina and uterus (metro = uterus, colpos = vagina) in an infant. After menarche, this is more commonly hematometrocolpos due to the blood content of menstruation. Prenatally, this is usually diagnosed by US as echogenic layering debris within a well-defined cavity between the rectum and urinary bladder. No internal blood flow should be seen. CT findings are as above, demonstrating a fluid-filled peripherally enhancing structure between the urinary bladder and rectum that displaces pelvic structures. MR findings are similar to CT findings, and MR is generally used when complex abnormalities are not clearly defined on other modalities. Fluoroscopy is usually reserved for evaluation of uterine morphology during convalescent phase, as seen in our

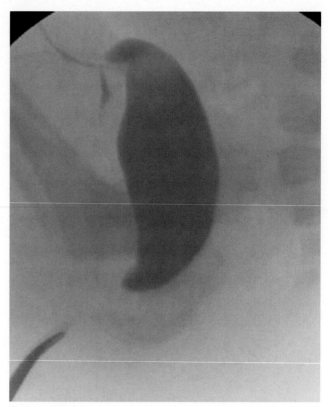

FIGURE **4.32B**

clinical scenario. Common causes include imperforate hymen (most common), vaginal stenosis or atresia, cervical stenosis or atresia, mass effect from uterine/vaginal duplications, or transverse vaginal septa. Hydrometrocolpos is associated with multiple other urogenital abnormalities, including intestinal aganglionosis, imperforate anus, urogenital sinus, cloacal anomalies, renal agenesis, and müllerian fusion abnormalities.[1] The disease can be seen as part of multiple syndromes, including McKusick–Kaufman syndrome and Bardet–Biedl syndrome.[2] Treatment depends on the cause. Imperforate hymen and low transverse vaginal septa can be treated with simple incision and drainage. Higher vaginal septa and more complex etiologies require more complex surgical intervention.[3]

Questions for Further Thought

1. What is McKusick–Kaufman syndrome?
2. What is Bardet–Biedl syndrome?

Reporting Responsibilities

- Describe whether dilatation involves vagina, uterus, or both
- Evaluate for and describe other associated abnormalities

What the Treating Physician Needs to Know

- Whether or not there are any associated abnormalities.
- Define specific etiology if possible to guide corrective/surgical approach.

Answers

1. McKusick–Kaufman is a genetic syndrome consisting of hydrometrocolpos, postaxial polydactyly, and congenital heart malformations. It is inherited in an autosomal recessive pattern. If seen in males, abnormalities include hypospadias, chordee (downward curving of penis), and cryptorchidism.

2. Bardet–Biedl syndrome is also a genetic syndrome with significant overlap with McKusick–Kaufman syndrome. It consists of hydrometrocolpos, postaxial polydactyly, retinitis pigmentosa, truncal obesity, and learning disabilities. It is also inherited in an autosomal recessive pattern.

REFERENCES

1. Donnelly LF, Jones BV, O'hara SM, et al., eds. *Diagnostic Imaging: Pediatrics.* 1st ed. Altona, Manitoba, Canada: Friesens; 2005.
2. David A, Bitoun P, Lacombe D, et al. Hydrometrocolpos and polydactyly: A common neonatal presentation of Bardet-Biedl and McKusick-Kaufman syndromes. *J Med Genet.* 1999;154 (3):545–548.
3. Ameh EA, Mshelbwala PM, Ameh N. Congenital vaginal obstruction in neonates and infants: Recognition and management. *J Pediatr Adolesc Gynecol.* 2011;24(2):74-8. Epub January 22, 2011.

Deborah Conway

CLINICAL HISTORY *A 17-month-old male with hematuria and UTI*

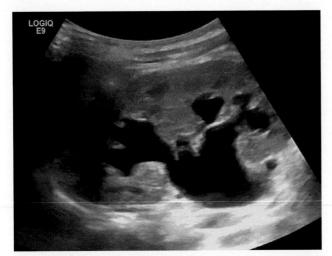

FIGURE **4.33A**

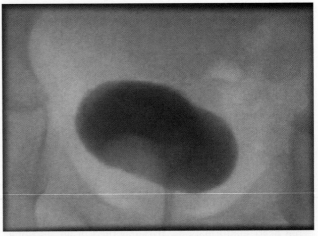

FIGURE **4.33B**

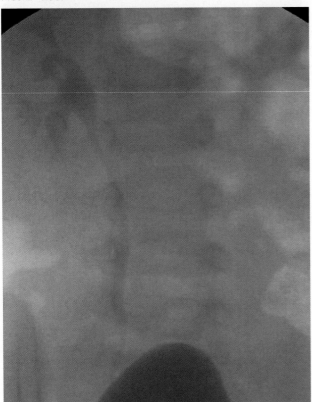

FIGURE **4.33C**

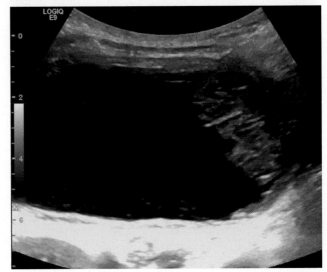

FIGURE **4.33D**

DIFFERENTIAL DIAGNOSIS Rhabdomyosarcoma pseudotumoral cystitis, hematoma, polyp, ureterocele

DIAGNOSIS Rhabdomyosarcoma

FINDINGS VCUG (**A**) reveals a smooth filling defect at the base of the bladder on early filling that persists on later imaging. There is also grade III reflux noted on the right (**B**). Sagittal image of the bladder (**C**) reveals a heterogeneous lobulated lesion adherent to the bladder wall without appreciable Doppler flow measuring 4.5 × 3 × 5.1 cm as well as debris within the bladder. US of the left kidney (**D**) reveals hydronephrosis.

DISCUSSION Rhabdomyosarcoma is the most common lower genitourinary tumor in children during the first two decades of life. Genitourinary rhabdomyosarcoma accounts for 15% to 30% of all rhabdomyosarcoma cases in children, which is the second most common location behind the head and neck. Most children with rhabdomyosarcoma of the bladder are male and present in the first 3 years of life. A common presentation for rhabdomyosarcoma of the bladder is urinary retention, dysuria, hematuria, and UTI. Genitourinary rhabdomyosarcoma is a relatively favorable anatomic site for staging, with approximately 43% of patients having stage 1 disease. Local recurrence is common following treatment. Metastatic disease is most commonly found in the lungs, cortical bone, and lymph nodes.[1]

CT and MR are superior imaging modalities for determining local invasion and lymphadenopathy. Rhabdomyosarcoma demonstrates low signal intensity on T1-weighted imaging and high signal intensity on T2-weighted MRI. Botryoid rhabdomyosarcoma appears as multiple grapelike intraluminal masses.[2]

Questions for Further Thought

1. Is the lack of Doppler flow on US a useful differentiating factor when deriving a differential diagnosis for a bladder lesion?
2. Is frontline therapy usually chemotherapy or surgical resection?

Reporting Responsibilities

- Describe the degree of hydronephrosis on the affected side
- Describe the origin of the mass and what adjacent structures are involved

What the Treating Physician Needs to Know

- Is the tumor locally invasive? Is there lymphadenopathy?

Answers

1. No. Rhabdomyosarcoma does not always demonstrate Doppler flow as seen in this case. Contrast enhancement is a better differentiating factor.
2. Chemotherapy is used more often as a first-line therapy. This has decreased the need for radial surgery and has actually increased survival rate.[2]

REFERENCES

1. Agrons G, Wagner B, Lonerman G, et al. Genitourinary rhabdomyosarcoma in children: Radiologic-pathologic correlation. *Radiographics*. 1997;17:919–937.
2. Wong-You-Cheong J, Woodward P, Manning MA, et al. Neoplasms of the urinary bladder: Radiologic-pathologic correlation. *Radiographics*. 2006;26:553–580.

CHAPTER 5

Airway, Neck, Chest, and Cardiac Imaging

CASE 5.1

Paritosh C. Khanna

CLINICAL HISTORY *A 2-year-old male who presents with high fever, sore throat, and odynophagia*

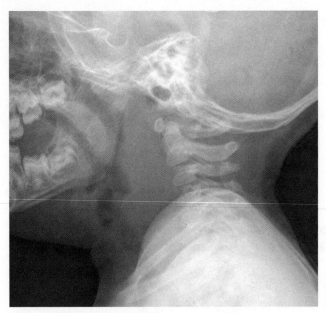

FIGURE **5.1A**

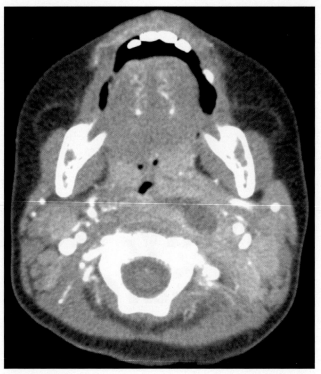

FIGURE **5.1B**

FINDINGS Lateral soft-tissue neck radiograph (**A**) demonstrates significant retropharyngeal and prevertebral soft-tissue thickening, measuring considerably more than the anteroposterior (AP) dimension of the adjacent cervical vertebral bodies, without foci of gas. Axial contrast-enhanced computed tomography (CT) (**B**) demonstrates a rim-enhancing, low-attenuation area in the left retropharyngeal and parapharyngeal spaces, which medially effaces and causes narrowing of the airway.

DIFFERENTIAL DIAGNOSIS Retropharyngeal abscess, pseudothickening, vascular and lymphatic malformations, croup, epiglottitis

DIAGNOSIS Retropharyngeal abscess

DISCUSSION Much reduced in incidence in the post-antibiotic era, retropharyngeal infections usually follow upper respiratory infections or pyogenic infections of the palatine tonsils. Infection may present as retropharyngeal cellulitis or progress through phases of phlegmon and abscess. Abscess may be amenable to drainage. Radiographs demonstrate retropharyngeal soft-tissue thickening when imaged with adequate neck extension. In young children, true thickening usually exceeds adjacent cervical vertebrae in AP dimension. In a patient older than about 10 years, true thickening should exceed approximately 6 mm in AP dimension at the C2 vertebral level and 20 mm at the C6 vertebral level. Contrast-enhanced CT demonstrates enhancing soft tissue in the cellulitis phase, an ill-defined near-fluid attenuation area in the phlegmon phase, and a walled-off, hypoattenuating, rim-enhancing abscess in the final phase. Gas may be seen within nondependent portions of the abscess. Reactive adenopathy is often associated. Airway narrowing and neck vascular thromboses are important complications. Infection may track inferiorly into the superior mediastinum along intermuscular or other fascial planes.[1,2]

DIFFERENTIAL DIAGNOSTIC CONSIDERATIONS

"Pseudothickening" in infants: See Answer 2, below.

Vascular and lymphatic malformations: CT with contrast or magnetic resonance imaging (MRI) demonstrates a vascular component with or without phleboliths with vascular malformation and a multiseptated, fluid-filled insinuating lesion with lymphatic malformation.

Croup: Croup may show edema of retropharyngeal tissues but there is also subglottic edema. Look for airway narrowing with the "steeple" sign on frontal radiograph. There may also be distension of the supraglottic airway.

Epiglottitis: Epiglottitis may show edema of retropharyngeal tissues but also swollen/enlarged epiglottis and aryepiglottic folds.

Questions for Further Thought

1. What is the common age group for retropharyngeal abscess?
2. What is "pseudothickening"?

Reporting Responsibilities

Extent of inflammation; presence, if any, of drainable abscess; complications such as jugular vein thrombosis.

What the Treating Physician Needs to Know

Extent of abnormality; whether drainable; complications.

Answers

1. Within the first few years of life.
2. "Pseudothickening," which may simulate pathologic thickening of prevertebral tissues, is commonly seen in infants who normally have a large proportion of fat in the retropharyngeal space, particularly if the radiograph is not obtained with adequate neck extension. This finding is frequently seen in children under age of 6 months and repeat radiograph in extension may be helpful to show a more normal appearance. Presence of anterior convexity of retropharyngeal soft tissues increases suspicion that the finding represents a true pathologic process.

REFERENCES

1. Craig FW, Schunk JE. Retropharyngeal abscess in children: Clinical presentation, utility of imaging, and current management. *Pediatrics.* 2003;111(6 Pt 1):1394–1398.
2. Swischuk LE. Stiff and sore neck. *Pediatr Emerg Care.* 2003; 19(4):282–284.

CLINICAL HISTORY *An 8-year-old child with mild exercise limitation due to dyspnea*

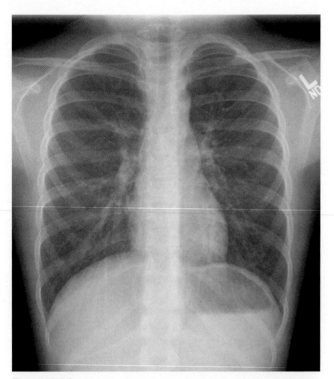

FIGURE **5.2A**

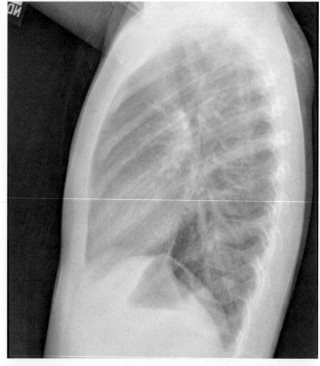

FIGURE **5.2B**

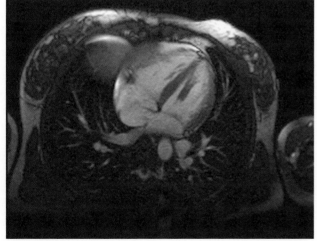

FIGURE **5.2C**

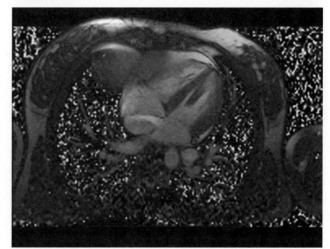

FIGURE **5.2D**

FINDINGS Frontal (**A**) and lateral (**B**) radiographs of the chest are normal. Four-chamber MRI view with bright-blood technique (**C**) shows a defect within the central aspect of the atrial septum. Four-chamber view fused with phase-contrast blood flow data (**D**) shows a jet of blood (brightest signal) coursing from the left atrium into the right atrium through the septal defect.

DIFFERENTIAL DIAGNOSIS

• Chest radiograph: Normal.
• MRI: Atrial septal defect (ASD).

DIAGNOSIS ASD

DISCUSSION Patients with an ASD can have a normal radiograph or one that shows increased pulmonary vasculature as well as cardiomegaly (typically right-sided) and an enlarged pulmonary artery. The left atrium typically does not enlarge unless there are additional complications such as mitral valve regurgitation or right heart failure.[1] The diagnosis of ASD is usually first made with echocardiography. Some ASDs may close spontaneously whereas others, if left untreated, may ultimately lead to pulmonary hypertension.

There are four major types of ASDs[2]:

1. Ostium primum defect: Located within the inferior aspect of the atrial septum; may be associated with atrioventricular (AV) defects (which are associated with trisomy 21).

2. Ostium secundum defect: Most common form of ASD, located in the central septum at the site of the fossa ovalis.

3. Sinus venosus defect: Located high in the atrial septum near the junction with the superior vena cava (SVC); almost always associated with partial anomalous pulmonary venous connection (PAPVC) which is typically right upper lobe drainage into the SVC or right atrium directly.

4. Coronary sinus septal defect: Least common; a portion of the coronary sinus roof is missing allowing for blood to travel from the left atrium to the coronary sinus and ultimately to the right atrium. This can be seen with a left-sided SVC.

Questions for Further Thought

1. What is a common repair method for ostium secundum defects?
2. What is the foramen ovale?

Reporting Responsibilities

- If conventional radiographs show mild prominence of the pulmonary vasculature and heart size but without left atrial enlargement, one must consider the presence of an ASD. However, a concomitant ventricular septal defect (VSD) cannot be excluded. Recommend further imaging.
- If a highly positioned ASD is identified during an MRI exam, one must complete a thorough evaluation for PAPVC.

What the Treating Physician Needs to Know

A normal chest radiograph does not exclude an ASD, but typically the larger symptomatic defects show at least some subtle abnormality.

Answers

1. Percutaneous, transvenous placement of a septal occluder device.
2. The foramen ovale is an interatrial communication that in utero allows flow from inferior vena cava (IVC) into left atrium. Typically, the foramen ovale functionally closes in the first few weeks of life. The foramen ovale may remain patent for various reasons, including elevated right atrial pressures, such as in tricuspid atresia, with resultant right to left shunt.

REFERENCES
1. Kellenberger CJ. Lesions with left-to-right shunts. In: Yoo SJ, MacDonald C, Babyn P, eds. *Chest Radiographic Interpretation in Pediatric Cardiac Patients.* New York: Thieme Medical Publishers; 2010:177–184.
2. Driscoll DJ. Left-to-right shunt lesions. *Pediatr Clin North Am.* 1999;46(2):355–368.

Mark R. Ferguson

CLINICAL HISTORY *A 16-month-old child with chronic cough for 1 year*

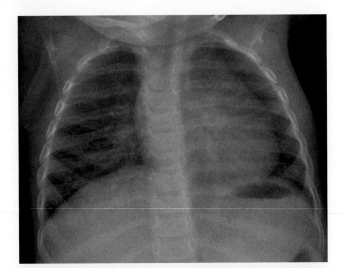

FIGURE **5.3A**

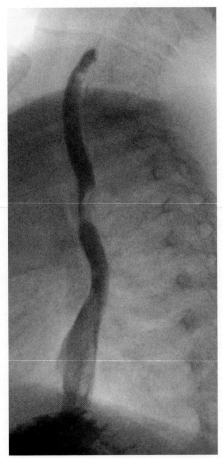

FIGURE **5.3B**

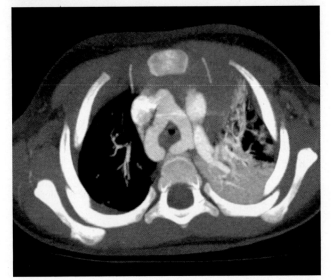

FIGURE **5.3C**

FINDINGS Frontal chest radiograph (**A**) shows minimal perihilar opacities but no definite abnormality of pulmonary blood flow. The side of aortic arch is not clearly demonstrated. There is suggestion of subtle narrowing of the airway just superior to the carina. Lateral view from esophagram (**B**) shows posterior impression upon the esophagus. Axial (**C**) and coronal (**D**) CT maximum intensity projection (MIP) images demonstrate double aortic arch with the right arch slightly larger than the left. There is some left lung atelectasis.

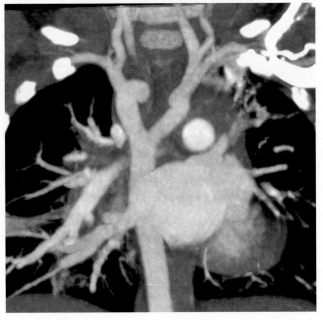

FIGURE **5.3D**

DIFFERENTIAL DIAGNOSIS

• Chest radiograph and esophagram: Vascular etiologies (double aortic arch, right arch with an aberrant left subclavian artery, left arch with an aberrant right subclavian artery), foregut duplication cyst, lymphadenopathy, other mass
• CT: Double aortic arch

DIAGNOSIS Double aortic arch

DISCUSSION A double aortic arch is a true vascular ring encircling the trachea and esophagus. During fetal development, there are six pairs of pharyngeal arch arteries. These normally progress through a sequence of partial regression. However, with a double aortic arch, there is abnormal persistence of complete bilateral fourth arches. Double aortic arches can have patent bilateral arches or there can be atretic segments. About 75% of the time, the right arch is dominant in size compared to the left.[1]

Patients can present with feeding difficulties, stridor, cough, aspiration, or recurrent pneumonia. The chest radiograph may show evidence for a right arch and possibly some narrowing of the airway, but the radiograph may certainly be inconclusive.[2] Although esophagram may be performed next for further evaluation, some clinicians will elect to go straight to MRI or CT as these modalities provide additional cross-sectional information. Surgical repair involves a thoracotomy and ligation of the smaller aortic arch to deconstruct the ring.[2]

Questions for Further Thought

1. What is another form of a complete vascular ring?
2. In patients with a double aortic arch, what is an associated chromosomal abnormality?

Reporting Responsibilities

• If suspicious, by radiograph, of a double aortic arch or right-sided arch with aberrant left subclavian artery in a patient presenting with a compatible history, an esophagram may demonstrate the posterior impression on the esophagus. However, cross-sectional imaging (CT, MRI) is better to more fully delineate the anatomy.
• When evaluating a double arch by cross-sectional imaging, describe which is the dominant arch by size and whether there is a high coursing arch (cervical arch). Also, comment upon any narrowing of the airway at the level of the vascular ring.

What the Treating Physician Needs to Know

Which arch is dominant and on which side is the descending aorta located. These findings are important to assist in surgical planning.

Answers

1. A right aortic arch with an aberrant left subclavian artery can form a vascular ring with the ligament of the ductus arteriosus completing the ring. On the other hand, a left arch with an aberrant right subclavian artery is rarely symptomatic.
2. Patients with a double aortic arch have an increased risk for a chromosomal band 22q11 deletion which is associated with DiGeorge, velocardiofacial, and conotruncal anomaly face syndromes.

REFERENCES

1. Hernanz-Schulman M. Vascular rings: A practical approach to imaging diagnosis. *Pediatr Radiol.* 2005;35(10):961–979.
2. Alsenaidi K, Gurofsky R, Karamlou T, et al. Management and outcomes of double aortic arch in 81 patients. *Pediatrics.* 2006; 118(5):e1336–e1341.

Mark R. Ferguson

CASE 5.4

CLINICAL HISTORY *A 15-year-old teenager with dyspnea on exertion*

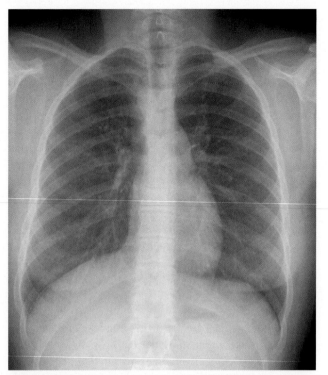

FIGURE **5.4A**

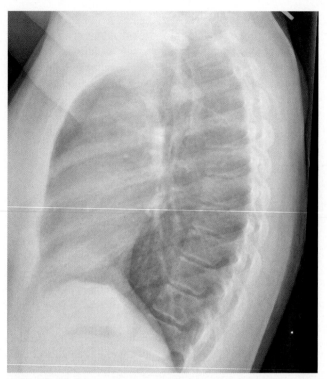

FIGURE **5.4B**

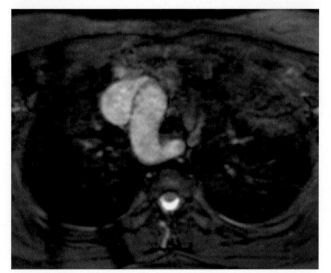

FIGURE **5.4C**

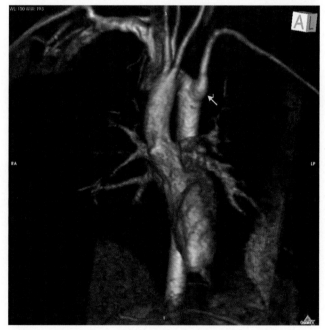

FIGURE **5.4D**

FINDINGS Frontal chest radiograph (**A**) shows slight leftward deviation of the trachea with a soft-tissue density to the right of the trachea suggesting a right aortic arch. Lateral view (**B**) shows subtle ovoid density posterior to the trachea near the level of the aortic arch. Lungs are clear. Axial contrast-enhanced MRI image (**C**) and MRI 3D oblique reconstruction (**D**) demonstrate a right arch with an aberrant left subclavian artery coursing posterior to the trachea with a dilated origin of the artery consistent with a diverticulum of Kommerell (*arrow,* **D**).

DIFFERENTIAL DIAGNOSIS

- Chest radiograph: Right aortic arch with aberrant left subclavian artery, right aortic arch with mirror-image branching, double aortic arch
- MRI: Right aortic arch with aberrant left subclavian artery originating from a diverticulum of Kommerell

DIAGNOSIS Right aortic arch with an aberrant left subclavian artery

DISCUSSION Recognition of right aortic arch on the pediatric chest film is important as it may have significant implications for patient care. For example, the patient who has a right aortic arch with mirror-image branching almost always has associated congenital heart disease whereas the patient with right aortic arch and an aberrant left subclavian artery usually has vascular ring anatomy (similar to double aortic arch) with a left-sided ligamentum arteriosum completing the ring.

A right aortic arch with an aberrant left subclavian artery is secondary to an interruption of the developing left fourth aortic arch between the left common carotid and left subclavian arteries. Bulbous enlargement of/at the origin of the left subclavian artery may occur, known as a diverticulum of Kommerell. A left ligamentum arteriosum often completes the vascular ring. However, only about 5% of these patients have associated airway symptoms. Typically, these patients have an associated large diverticulum of Kommerell or "tight" ligamentum arteriosum. In addition, patients with a midline descending aorta can have lower tracheal or main bronchi compression.[1]

Patients who have a right aortic arch with an aberrant left subclavian artery can present with feeding difficulties, stridor, cough, aspiration, or recurrent pneumonia. The chest radiograph may show the right arch, and possibly a soft-tissue density posterior to the trachea resulting in anterior bowing of the airway at the level of the arch, representing the aberrant left subclavian artery; however, the radiograph may certainly be inconclusive. An esophagram would show a posterior impression upon the esophagus; however, MRI or CT is more definitive in making the diagnosis. Surgical repair involves a thoracotomy and ligation of the left ligamentum arteriosum to deconstruct the ring.[1]

Questions for Further Thought

1. Patients with a right arch and aberrant left subclavian artery will not always have a vascular ring. What is the anatomy in these cases?
2. What percentage of patients with a right arch with an aberrant left subclavian artery have associated congenital heart disease and what is the most common lesion?

Reporting Responsibilities

- Based on chest radiographs, one needs to comment on a right-sided aortic arch and the possibility of a vascular ring or possible congenital heart disease. Recommend further imaging where indicated.
- Based on cross-sectional imaging, one needs to clearly describe the aortic arch anatomy, presence of a diverticulum of Kommerell, and position of the descending aorta. Also, comment upon any airway compromise.

What the Treating Physician Needs to Know

A right arch with an aberrant left subclavian artery can often represent a true vascular ring.

Answers

1. Approximately 10% of patients with a right arch and aberrant left subclavian artery have a right-sided ligamentum arteriosum and no resultant vascular ring.[2]
2. Less than 10% of patients with a right aortic arch and an aberrant left subclavian artery will have associated congenital heart disease with the most common form being tetralogy of Fallot (TOF).[3] On the other hand, it should be noted that patients with a right arch and mirror-image branching almost always have associated congenital heart disease.

REFERENCES

1. Donnelly LF, Fleck RJ, Pacharn P, et al. Aberrant subclavian arteries: Cross-sectional imaging findings in infants and children referred for evaluation of extrinsic airway compression. *AJR Am J Roentgenol.* 2002;178(5):1269–1274.
2. Hernanz-Schulman M. Vascular rings: a practical approach to imaging diagnosis. *Pediatr Radiol.* 2005;35(10):961–979.
3. Smith A, McKay R. Anomalies of the thoracic aorta. In: Smith A, McKay R, eds. *A Practical Atlas of Congenital Heart Disease.* London: Springer; 2004:11–34.

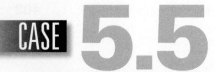

Mark R. Ferguson

CLINICAL HISTORY *A newborn with dyspnea and cyanosis*

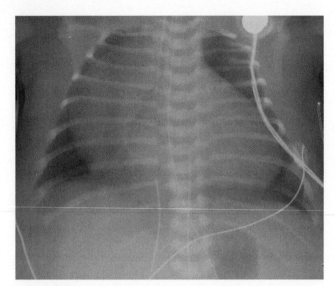

FIGURE **5.5A**

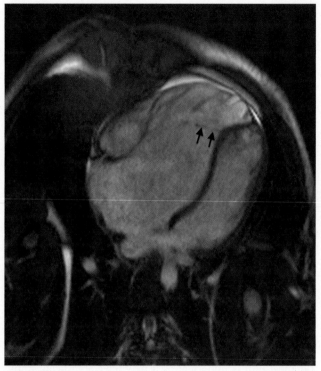

FIGURE **5.5B**

FINDINGS Frontal chest radiograph (**A**) shows a markedly enlarged heart with decreased pulmonary vasculature. Note presence of umbilical arterial and venous catheters. MRI four-chamber view of the heart (**B**) shows apical displacement of the hinge point of the tricuspid valve septal leaflet (*arrows*) with marked enlargement of the right heart. An ASD is also present.

DIFFERENTIAL DIAGNOSIS

- Chest radiograph: Ebstein anomaly, critical pulmonary stenosis, pulmonary atresia, tricuspid atresia
- MRI: Ebstein anomaly

DIAGNOSIS Ebstein anomaly

DISCUSSION Ebstein anomaly accounts for 0.5% to 0.7% of cases of congenital heart disease. This entity has a wide age range of presentation (some patients are even asymp-

tomatic) depending on extent of anatomic abnormality. The principal feature in Ebstein anomaly is apical displacement of the hinge points of the septal and posterior leaflets of the tricuspid valve combined with dilatation of the tricuspid annulus. This results in atrialization of the right ventricle (RV) with poor coaptation of the valve leaflets, and subsequent tricuspid regurgitation and marked right heart enlargement. Most patients will also have a patent foramen ovale or other type of ASD. Additionally, there are relatively small aortic and pulmonary trunks that combine with the marked cardiomegaly to create a "box-shaped" heart.[1]

Questions for Further Thought

1. What other organ malformation may be present secondary to a massively enlarged, "box-shaped" heart?
2. What is a common classification system for Ebstein anomaly?

Reporting Responsibilities

- Alert the physician about the likelihood of congenital heart disease based on radiographic findings so that more detailed follow-up imaging can be performed.
- With regard to MRI, the degree of leaflet apical displacement as well as the relative degree of tricuspid regurgitation should be conveyed. Any additional congenital heart lesions need to be described.

What the Treating Physician Needs to Know

Ebstein anomaly can be associated with other congenital structural abnormalities of the heart. Identifying these lesions is important for the treating cardiac surgeon to allow for proper presurgical planning. Therefore, cross-sectional imaging (MRI) is warranted.

Answers

1. Pulmonary underdevelopment.[2]
2. Carpentier classification (**A** through **D**) which categorizes on basis of progressive degree of anterior septal leaflet dysfunction.[3]

REFERENCES

1. Ferguson EC, Krishnamurthy R, Oldham SA. Classic imaging signs of congenital cardiovascular abnormalities. *Radiographics.* 2007;27(5):1323–1334.

2. Kellenberger CJ. Ebstein's malformation and other forms of congenital tricuspid regurgitation. In: Yoo SJ, MacDonald C, Babyn P, eds. *Chest Radiographic Interpretation in Pediatric Cardiac Patients.* New York, NY: Thieme Medical Publishers, Inc.; 2010:189–192.

3. Carpentier A, Chauvaud S, Macé L, et al. A new reconstructive operation for Ebstein's anomaly of the tricuspid valve. *J Thorac Cardiovasc Surg.* 1988;96(1):92–101.

Mark R. Ferguson

CASE 5.6

CLINICAL HISTORY *A 3-year-old child with stridor*

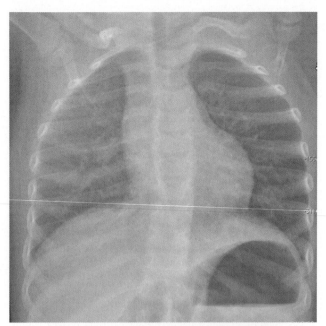

FIGURE **5.6A**

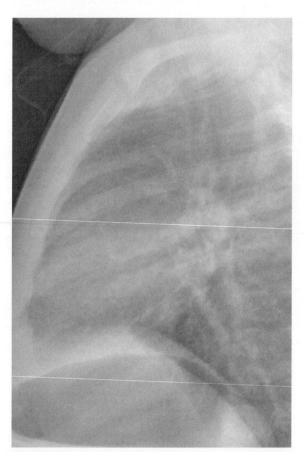

FIGURE **5.6B**

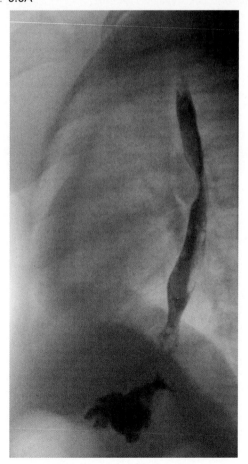

FIGURE **5.6C**

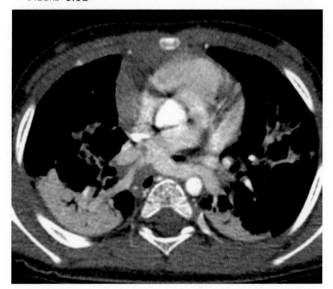

FIGURE **5.6D**

FINDINGS Frontal (**A**) and lateral (**B**) views of the chest show clear lungs with normal pulmonary vascularity. On frontal view, the distal tracheal and proximal mainstem bronchi are not well seen. On lateral view, there is a focal ovoid density just anterior to the spine at the level of the pulmonary hila. Lateral view from esophagram (**C**) suggests a space occupying structure causing an anterior impression upon the esophagus and posterior impression upon the trachea. Axial CT (**D**) shows anomalous origin of the left pulmonary artery, arising from the right pulmonary artery with a subsequent course between the esophagus and trachea. Low-density tissue anterior and to right of heart is normal thymus. There is some bilateral atelectasis.

DIFFERENTIAL DIAGNOSIS

- Chest radiograph/esophagram: Left pulmonary artery sling, foregut duplication cyst, lymphadenopathy, other mass
- CT: Left pulmonary artery sling

DIAGNOSIS Left pulmonary artery sling

DISCUSSION The term "pulmonary sling" typically refers to an anomalous origin of the left pulmonary artery which arises from the right pulmonary artery and then takes a subsequent course in-between the esophagus and trachea. This is secondary to failure of normal development of the left sixth aortic arch and collateral formation off the right pulmonary artery to supply the left lung. This configuration results in an anterior impression upon the esophagus which may not be appreciated on a chest radiograph but is usually quite evident on an esophagram. Cross-sectional imaging better demonstrates the anomalous vessel course. Hyperinflation or atelectasis, depending on the degree of airway compression, can be seen on radiographs involving either the right or left lower lungs. In addition to direct airway compression, pulmonary artery sling is frequently associated with hypoplasia/dysplasia/stenosis of the distal trachea and proximal bronchi. Patients with pulmonary artery sling typically present in the neonatal period with symptoms referable to the airways, such as stridor.

Two major types of pulmonary artery sling have been described. Type I lesions demonstrate a normal position of the carina at approximately the level of T4 or T5, and can result in compression of the right mainstem bronchus. Surgical reimplantation of the anomalous vessel is usually a sufficient repair. Type II lesions demonstrate a low position of the carina which sometimes is associated with a tracheal bronchus supplying the right upper lobe and a bridging bronchus, which originates from the left mainstem bronchus and crosses back to the right to supply the right lower or right middle and lower lobes. Type II lesions are often associated with tracheal stenosis secondary to complete cartilaginous rings.[1]

Question for Further Thought

1. What forms of congenital heart disease are most commonly seen with a pulmonary sling?

Reporting Responsibilities

- If there is concern for pulmonary artery sling on esophagram, recommend CT or MRI to evaluate type.
- If found or confirmed on CT or MRI, describe anomalous vessel course but also pay particular attention to the airway to evaluate for tracheal stenosis and/or a bridging bronchus.

What the Treating Physician Needs to Know

The type II lesion can have a long segment of tracheal stenosis. If so, reimplantation of the anomalous vessel alone may be insufficient to correct a patient's potential respiratory difficulties. Rather a tracheoplasty/bronchoplasty may be necessary.[2]

Answer

1. ASD, VSD, patent ductus arteriosus (PDA), and left SVC.

REFERENCES

1. Berdon WE. Rings, slings, and other things: vascular compression of the infant trachea updated from the midcentury to the millennium – the legacy of Robert E. Gross, MD, and Edward B.D. Neuhauser, MD. *Radiology.* 2000;216(3):624–632.
2. Rutter MJ, Willging JP, Cotton RT. Nonoperative management of complete tracheal rings. *Arch Otolaryngol Head Neck Surg.* 2004;130(4):450–452.

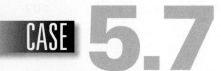

CASE 5.7

CLINICAL HISTORY *A 2-year-old child with dyspnea and cyanosis*

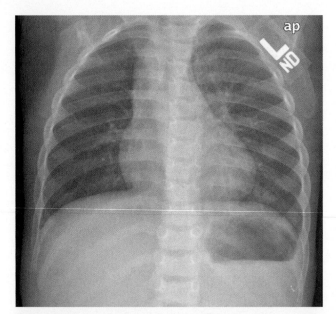

FIGURE **5.7A**

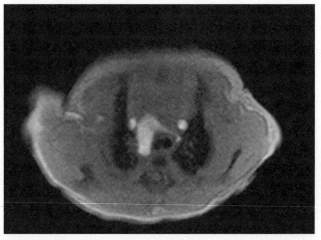

FIGURE **5.7B**

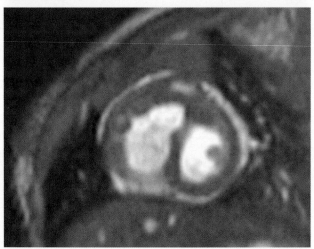

FIGURE **5.7C**

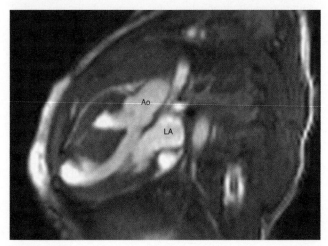

FIGURE **5.7D**

FINDINGS Frontal chest radiograph (**A**) shows a right aortic arch with normal heart size and normal pulmonary vascularity. No definite left apical density to suggest an aberrant left subclavian artery. Axial contrast-enhanced MRI (**B**) shows a right aortic arch with the left brachiocephalic artery seen coursing obliquely anterior to the trachea with incidental note of a persistent left SVC. Short-axis bright-blood MRI image (**C**) shows right ventricular hypertrophy. Three chamber view (**D**) shows a VSD with an overriding aorta (Ao, aorta; LA, left atrium).

DIFFERENTIAL DIAGNOSIS

• Chest radiograph: Right aortic arch
• MRI: TOF

DIAGNOSIS TOF

DISCUSSION A right-sided aortic arch with mirror-image branching is associated with congenital heart disease 95% to 97% of the time. Of these patients, 90% have TOF. TOF is the most common form of cyanotic congenital heart disease, accounting for 10% to 11% of cases of congenital heart disease.[1] TOF is secondary to a conoventricular defect with anterosuperior displacement resulting in an overriding aorta and pulmonary infundibular stenosis associated with a VSD and resultant right ventricular hypertrophy.[2] A classic radiographic appearance is the "boot-shaped" heart related to right ventricular hypertrophy. However, many patients will present with a normal chest radiograph. Pulmonary vasculature is usually decreased or normal. Cardiomegaly, if present, tends to be associated with TOF variants or ventricular dysfunction.[3]

Patients with TOF may have a spectrum of findings, ranging from pulmonary valve atresia to complete absence of the pulmonary arteries. Those with pulmonary valve atresia rely on a PDA for pulmonary arterial flow, while those with absence of the pulmonary arteries will have numerous aorticopulmonary collaterals.[4] TOF with an absent pulmonary valve is another noteworthy variation. These patients develop enlarged central pulmonary arteries that can produce mass effect upon the adjacent airways resulting in air trapping. These patients should be screened for DiGeorge syndrome as this association is present about 25% of the time.

The essence of surgical repair revolves around the VSD and right ventricular outflow tract (RVOT) obstruction. The VSD repair can be performed through a right atrial or ventricular approach. The RVOT obstruction can be treated with a simple valvotomy with or without a transannular incision with patch placement. Previously, large pulmonary valvectomies were routinely performed which left patients with large dyskinetic outflow tracts and free pulmonary regurgitation. This ultimately led to numerous patients requiring subsequent pulmonary valve replacement.[3]

Questions for Further Thought

1. What is the pentalogy of Fallot?
2. A right-sided aortic arch is present in 25% to 30% of patients with TOF. Which congenital heart lesion has the highest association with a right-sided arch?

Reporting Responsibilities

• Note right aortic arch on chest radiograph that is highly associated with congenital heart disease if there is mirror-image branching. On the other hand, the patient who has a right aortic arch with aberrant left subclavian artery is likely to have vascular ring anatomy with a left-sided ligamentum arteriosum usually completing the ring.
• On cross-sectional imaging, one needs to catalog all findings and quantify function if applicable.

What the Treating Physician Needs to Know

Surgeons will need to know if there is an anomalous left anterior descending coronary artery which arises from the right coronary artery and crosses the RVOT, as a right ventricular incision for repair of the RVOT obstruction and/or VSD could be detrimental.

Answers

1. The features of TOF as well as an ASD.
2. Truncus arteriosus; patients have right-sided arch 30% to 35% of the time.

REFERENCES

1. Ferguson EC, Krishnamurthy R, Oldham SA. Classic imaging signs of congenital cardiovascular abnormalities. *Radiographics.* 2007;27(5):1323–1334.
2. Hastreiter AR, D'Cruz IA, Cantez T, et al. Right-sided aorta. I. Occurrence of right aortic arch in various types of congenital heart disease. II. Right aortic arch, right descending aorta, and associated anomalies. *Br Heart J.* 1966;28(6):722–739.
3. Kellenberger CJ. Tetralogy of Fallot and related conditions. In: Yoo SJ, MacDonald C, Babyn P, eds. *Chest Radiographic Interpretation in Pediatric Cardiac Patients.* New York: Thieme Medical Publishers; 2010:193–199.
4. Gaca AM, Jaggers JJ, Dudley LT, et al. Repair of congenital heart disease: A primer–Part 2. *Radiology.* 2008;248(1):44–60.

Mark R. Ferguson

CLINICAL HISTORY *An 8-year-old child with clinical concern for heart failure*

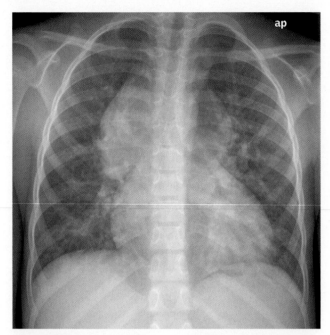

FIGURE **5.8A**

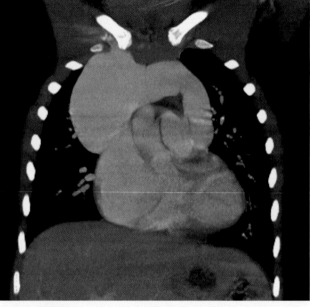

FIGURE **5.8B**

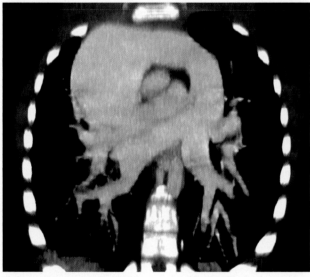

FIGURE **5.8C**

FINDINGS Frontal radiograph of the chest (**A**) shows a lobular density projecting over the superior mediastinum and suprahilar regions creating a "snowman" appearance of the cardiomediastinal borders. Coronal CT reconstruction (**B**) demonstrates a large caliber left brachiocephalic vein coursing superior to the heart, crossing left to right, and contributing to an enlarged SVC. Coronal oblique CT reconstruction (**C**) shows bilateral pulmonary veins joining into a vertical pulmonary vein which then drains into the large left brachiocephalic vein.

DIFFERENTIAL DIAGNOSIS

- Chest radiograph: Total anomalous pulmonary venous connection (TAPVC), lymphadenopathy, other soft-tissue mass
- CT: TAPVC.

DIAGNOSIS Supracardiac TAPVC

DISCUSSION With TAPVC, all of the pulmonary venous blood flow returns to the right atrium either directly or through a venous channel. These lesions account for approximately 2% of cardiac malformations. There are four major types: Type I, supracardiac, is the most common. As in the presented case, the venous connection is via a common vertical pulmonary vein into a dilated left brachiocephalic vein creating the "snowman" appearance, and is typically associated with cardiomegaly. Obstruction of the venous course is uncommon with type I connections. Type II, cardiac, is the second most common. Here, the anomalous venous drainage is either via the coronary sinus or directly to the right atrium. Type III, infracardiac, involves pulmonary drainage coursing below the diaphragm with connection to portal vein, IVC, ductus venosus, or hepatic veins. This type is nearly always associated with some relative obstruction at the level of the diaphragm, resulting in pulmonary venous congestion. Type IV is a mixed pattern often with drainage of the left lung through the left brachiocephalic vein and drainage of the right lung through the coronary sinus and directly to the right atrium. Type IV is often associated with other major cardiac lesions. The presenting radiographic appearance will vary by anomaly type and degree of obstruction.[1]

If some of the pulmonary blood flow returns normally to the left atrium, the term PAPVC is used. This is most commonly seen in the setting of an anomalous connection of a right upper lobe pulmonary vein to the SVC.

Questions for Further Thought

1. What other cardiac lesion is present with TAPVC to allow for survival?

2. What is the classic chest radiograph appearance for a newborn with type III TAPVC (infracardiac)?

Reporting Responsibilities

Provide clear delineation of anatomy including distinction between partial and total anomalous venous connection to allow for surgical planning. In addition, patients with TAPVC have a higher likelihood of having other congenital cardiac abnormalities as well as heterotaxy syndrome.[1]

What the Treating Physician Needs to Know

- Patients with TAPVC may have other cardiac anomalies as well as heterotaxy.
- Patients with TAPVC often have recurrent pulmonary vein stenosis following repair.[2]

Answers

1. ASD or patent foramen ovale.
2. Pulmonary venous congestion and a normal sized heart.

REFERENCES

1. Ferguson EC, Krishnamurthy R, Oldham SA. Classic imaging signs of congenital cardiovascular abnormalities. *Radiographics.* 2007;27(5):1323–1334.
2. Douglas YL, Jongbloed MR, den Hartog WC, et al. Pulmonary vein and atrial wall pathology in human total anomalous pulmonary venous connection. *Int J Cardiol.* 2009;134(3):302–312.

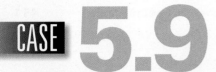

Mark R. Ferguson

CLINICAL HISTORY *Abnormal prenatal ultrasound (Fig. 5.9A)*

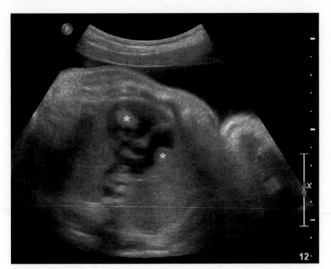

FIGURE **5.9A**

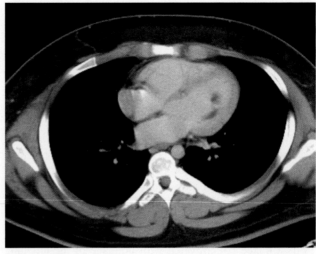

FIGURE **5.9B**

FINDINGS Prenatal ultrasound four-chamber view of heart (**A**) shows at least two echogenic mass lesions within the ventricles (one lesion in each, denoted by *). Axial contrast-enhanced CT (**B**) from a different patient shows two hypodense foci with the left ventricle (LV).

DIFFERENTIAL DIAGNOSIS

- Ultrasound: Cardiac rhabdomyomas, multiple fibromas
- CT: Cardiac rhabdomyomas, multiple fibromas

DIAGNOSIS Cardiac rhabdomyomas

DISCUSSION Rhabdomyoma is the most common cardiac tumor in children.[1] A rhabdomyoma is a hamartoma that, in about 50% of cases, is associated with tuberous sclerosis. These lesions originate in myocardium and are typically multiple, up to 90% of the time.[1] Usually, patients are asymptomatic with regard to the cardiac lesions; however, occasionally, the masses can be large enough or located in such a way as to cause obstruction or arrhythmia.

Rhabdomyomas appear as echogenic masses on ultrasound and may be hyper- or hypoattenuating compared to normal myocardium on contrast-enhanced CT.[2] MRI typically reveals lesions which are iso- to slightly hyperintense on T1-weighted and hyperintense on T2-weighted imaging relative to normal myocardium. The lesions may become hypointense to myocardium following contrast administration.[1] In contradistinction, cardiac fibromas are usually solitary, iso- to hyperintense on T1-weighted and hypointense on T2-weighted imaging relative to normal myocardium. Post-contrast images of fibromas may show heterogeneous enhancement with nonenhancing areas that may correlate with fibrous tissue.

Questions for Further Thought

1. What is the typical management of these patients?
2. Besides the intracranial manifestations of the associated condition of tuberous sclerosis, what other abdominal lesions are often present?

Reporting Responsibilities

- If intracardiac masses are noted on ultrasound, suggest MRI for further evaluation, although this can typically be delayed until the patient is in a stable postnatal period.
- Based on MRI, describe size and location of masses as well as quantify heart function to determine if impaired by mass.

What the Treating Physician Needs to Know

If multiple cardiac lesions suggestive of rhabdomyomas are identified on ultrasound or otherwise, there is a high association with tuberous sclerosis; screening the brain for cortical/subcortical tubers with MRI should be considered.

Answers

1. The natural history of rhabdomyomas is regression; therefore, conservative management is typical unless there is associated significant obstruction or refractory arrhythmia.
2. Renal angiomyolipomas.

REFERENCES

1. Sparrow PJ, Kurian JB, Jones TR, et al. MR imaging of cardiac tumors. *Radiographics.* 2005;25(5):1255–1276.
2. Burke A, Jeudy J Jr, Virmani R. Cardiac tumours: An update. *Heart.* 2008;94(1):117–123.

CASE 5.10

Marla Sammer

CLINICAL HISTORY *A 10-year-old female with 1 week history of cough and high fever acutely complicated by sore throat and air hunger*

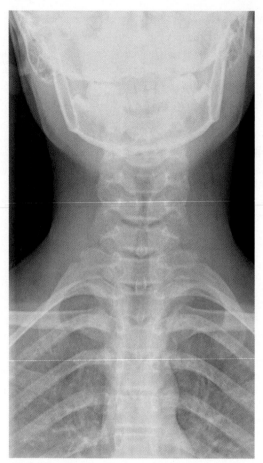

FIGURE **5.10A**

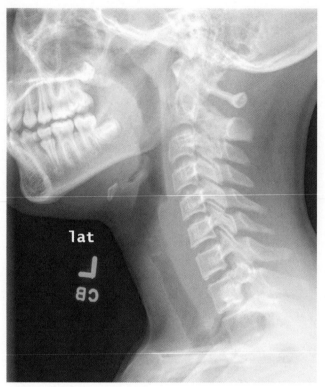

FIGURE **5.10B**

FINDINGS Frontal (**A**) and lateral (**B**) soft-tissue neck radiographs demonstrate narrowing of the subglottic airway with loss of normal shouldering on the frontal view and several linear soft-tissue densities (membranes) projecting within the upper trachea on the lateral view.

DIFFERENTIAL DIAGNOSIS Exudative tracheitis, airway foreign body

DIAGNOSIS Exudative tracheitis

DISCUSSION Exudative tracheitis, also known as bacterial tracheitis and membranous croup, is an uncommon but severe upper airway infection often caused by invasive bacterial infection of the trachea.[1] Patients with exudative tracheitis may have a history of antecedent or concurrent viral illness. Symptomatology mainly results from infectious inflammation of the trachea with production of purulent exudates which have the appearance of membranes.[2] The hypopharynx, larynx, and bronchi may also be involved. The typical age of presentation is 6 to 10 years (although patients can be younger or older), usually older than those patients who present with croup.[3] Radiographically, the diagnosis should be suspected in older pediatric patients presenting with croup-like subglottic narrowing and tracheal irregularity (classically with linear membranes). Tracheal membranes may mimic airway foreign bodies, but clinical history and symptomatology should be helpful in differentiating these two entities.

Questions for Further Thought

1. How may patient demographics help differentiate exudative tracheitis from croup?
2. How may clinical picture help differentiate from epiglottitis?

Reporting Responsibilities

- Patients often require emergent airway management; prompt diagnosis and direct physician communication is highly recommended.

- Reporting signs of accompanying bronchitis/pneumonia (seen in the imaged lung apices or chest radiograph if available) may be helpful for clinical management.

What the Treating Physician Needs to Know

- Endoscopy is usually necessary for definitive diagnosis (and sometimes for airway management).
- Laboratory findings are not specific for confirming the diagnosis.

Answers

1. Patients with exudative tracheitis are typically older (6- to 10-year old) than patients with croup (6 months to 3 years).

2. Patients with exudative tracheitis are typically able to tolerate lying flat as they are able to handle their oral secretions. Patients with epiglottitis are classically in the "tripod position" – sitting up with jaw thrust forward.

REFERENCES

1. Hedlund GL, Wiatrak BJ, Pranikoff T. Pneumomediastinum as an early radiographic sign in membranous croup. *AJR Am J Roentgenol.* 1998;170(1):55–56.
2. Salamone FN, Bobbitt DB, Myer CM, et al. Bacterial tracheitis reexamined: Is there a less severe manifestation? *Otolaryngol Head Neck Surg.* 2004;131(6):871–876.
3. Donnelly LF. Exudative tracheitis. In: Donnelly LF, ed. *Diagnostic Imaging: Pediatrics.* 2nd ed. Salt Lake City, Utah: Amirsys; 2012;1:12–15.

Jonathan O. Swanson

CLINICAL HISTORY *A 2-year-old girl with fever and productive cough*

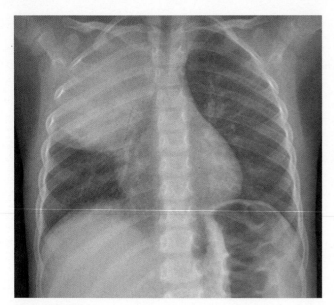

FIGURE **5.11A**

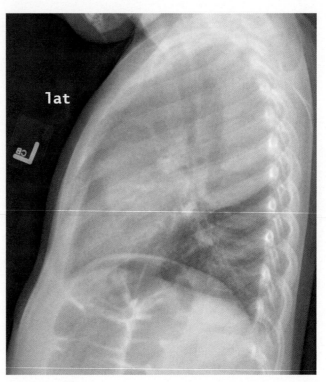

FIGURE **5.11B**

FINDINGS Frontal (**A**) and lateral (**B**) radiographs of the chest demonstrate consolidation of the right upper lobe. There is no evidence of volume loss. There is no evidence of central lucency to suggest cavitation.

DIFFERENTIAL DIAGNOSIS Lobar pneumonia, atelectasis, hemorrhage, pulmonary mass

DIAGNOSIS Lobar pneumonia

DISCUSSION The clinical scenario of fever and cough in the young pediatric patient along with a radiograph of airspace disease found predominantly in a lobar distribution is highly suggestive of lobar pneumonia. The prime bacterial etiology in the pediatric population is *Streptococcus pneumoniae.* Complete lobar consolidation is uncommon in infants and children; in most cases, some portion of the affected lobe still contains air.[1] The differential includes atelectasis, but in this case, there is no evidence of volume loss. The adjacent ribs are normal, which decrease the likelihood of an atypical mass, such as neuroblastoma.

Questions for Further Thought

1. In an uncomplicated pneumonia, how long after the initiation of therapy should follow-up radiographs be obtained?

2. What role does CT play in the diagnosis of uncomplicated pneumonia in an immune-competent child?

Reporting Responsibilities

Exclude other processes such as malignancy and foreign body. Evaluate for complications of pneumonia, such as parapneumonic effusion, loculated empyema, cavitation, or abscess.[2]

What the Treating Physician Needs to Know

As discussed above, the treating physician needs to know if there are complications of the pneumonia. Also, if radiographic comparisons show that there have been recurrent pneumonias in a similar location, the treating physician should be informed of additional imaging options to exclude the possibility of missed foreign body, endobronchial lesion, or underlying congenital pulmonary lesion.

Answers

1. The radiographic findings in a child with pneumonia can persist for 2 to 4 weeks after initiation of treatment,

even if there is rapid clinical improvement.[2] Nonetheless, follow-up imaging is rarely indicated if the patient clinically improves. In some pediatric patients, bacterial pneumonia may have a round appearance on chest films, and this is termed round pneumonia. As round pneumonia may simulate a mass lesion, this is one instance where one should consider follow-up imaging to assess for resolution. Timing of this follow-up imaging would depend on clinical course; if the patient, on a course of antibiotic therapy, is improving as expected, the imaging can be obtained several weeks after the course of therapy.

2. There is no role for CT in uncomplicated lobar pneumonia. CT imaging should be reserved for complications (persistent fever, concern for empyema, cavitation) and recurrent pneumonia in the same location. CT can also be used in the case of large areas of consolidation when there is clinical concern for underlying mass.

REFERENCES

1. Adler B, Effmann EL. Pneumonia and pulmonary infection. In: Slovis TL, ed. *Caffey's Pediatric Diagnostic Imaging.* 11th ed. Philadelphia, PA: Mosby; 2008:1184–1228.
2. Donnelly LF. Practical issues concerning imaging of pulmonary infection in children. *J Thorac Imaging.* 2001;16(4):238–250.

Jonathan O. Swanson

CLINICAL HISTORY *A 9-month-old child with inspiratory stridor and barking cough*

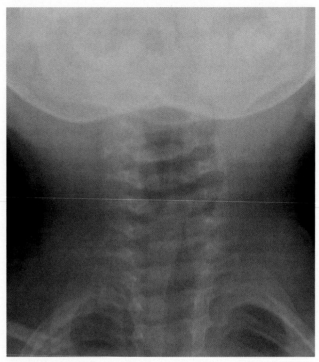

FIGURE 5.12A

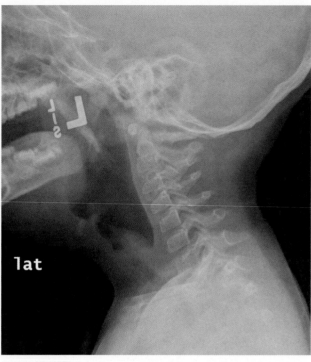

FIGURE 5.12B

FINDINGS Frontal radiograph of the neck (**A**) demonstrates smooth, symmetric, subglottic narrowing. The lateral film (**B**) demonstrates hyperinflation of the hypopharynx with normal epiglottis and normal width of the prevertebral soft tissues. There is loss of clear delineation of the subglottic air column at the level of narrowing seen on the frontal radiograph.

DIFFERENTIAL DIAGNOSIS Croup, epiglottitis, retropharyngeal abscess, foreign body, subglottic stenosis, hemangioma, acute bacterial tracheitis

DIAGNOSIS Croup

DISCUSSION Croup, also known as acute laryngotracheobronchitis, is a common upper respiratory infection typically affecting children aged 6 months to 3 years. The most common cause of croup is parainfluenza, but other viral and bacterial agents can also cause croup, including *Mycoplasma* and respiratory syncytial virus (RSV).[1] The diagnosis can usually be made clinically in those patients who present with barking coughs. Radiography is used to exclude other possible diagnoses including foreign body and epiglottitis.[2] On the frontal neck radiograph of a patient with croup, one can see the upward tapering of the subglottic airway which is symmetric and smooth (steeple sign). On the lateral view, this subglottic edema usually results in loss of clear delineation of the upper tracheal air column.

Questions for Further Thought

1. What is the most common cause of tracheal stenosis?
2. What is exudative tracheitis?

Reporting Responsibilities

In excluding other causes of subglottic narrowing, evaluate the airway contour. Irregular or asymmetric narrowing can be associated with subglottic hemangioma and acute bacterial tracheitis.

What the Treating Physician Needs to Know

Croup is a clinical diagnosis. The radiograph is used to exclude other causes of upper airway obstruction, such as foreign body or epiglottitis.

Answers

1. Acquired subglottic stenosis secondary to prolonged endotracheal intubation is the most common cause of tracheal stenosis.
2. Exudative tracheitis, also known as acute bacterial tracheitis or membranous croup, is a purulent infection of the airway.[2] The presence of exudative membranes on the neck radiographs can suggest this diagnosis.

REFERENCES

1. Klassen TP. Croup. A current perspective. *Pediatr Clin North Am.* 1999;46(6):1167–1178.
2. Cohen RA, Kuhn JP. Larynx and cervical trachea. In: Slovis TL, ed. *Caffey's Pediatric Diagnostic Imaging.* 11th ed. Philadelphia, PA: Mosby; 2008:1068–1077.

Jonathan O. Swanson

CLINICAL HISTORY *A 2-week-old infant in respiratory distress (Fig. 5.13A)*

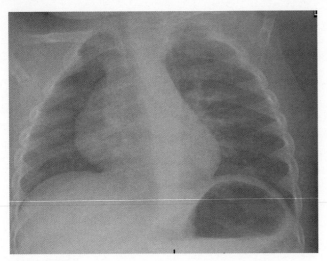

FIGURE **5.13A**

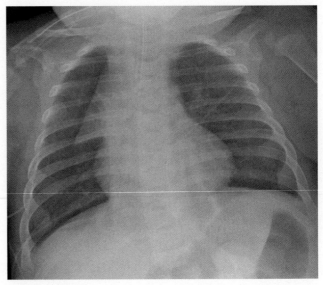

FIGURE **5.13B**

FINDINGS Frontal radiograph of the chest (**A**) shows prominence of the right side of cardiomediastinal border with subtle undulation along the right lung/mediastinal interface. A radiograph from a different patient (**B**) demonstrates a "sail"-like appearance along the right aspect of the mediastinum with a sharp horizontal interface at the level of the minor fissure.

DIFFERENTIAL DIAGNOSIS Normal thymus, mediastinal mass, cardiomegaly, right upper lobe atelectasis

DIAGNOSIS Normal thymus

DISCUSSION On conventional radiographs, a normal thymus should have smooth contours. It is most prominent in infants and young children, often border-forming, obscuring the normal superior cardiac margin until the age of approximately 3 years.[1] With age, the normal thymus regresses and becomes less and less apparent. The "normal" thymic appearance is somewhat of a misnomer given the vast variability of this soft organ depending on age, phase of respiration, and health of the patient. Two common appearances consistent with a normal thymus are the thymic wave (seen in **A**), which describes the smooth indentations from the overlying ribs and costal cartilages, and the sail sign (seen in **B**), which describes the sharp, horizontal margin of the right inferior aspect of the thymus at the level of the minor fissure. The thymus can mimic cardiomegaly in young children. A normal posterior margin of the cardiac silhouette on the lateral radiograph can be a useful discriminating feature.[2] In general, a prominent thymus in the infant is normal and illustrative of good health and nutrition.

Questions for Further Thought

1. What malignancies most commonly affect the thymus in children?
2. What are the imaging features of the normal pediatric thymus on CT and MRI?

Reporting Responsibilities

It is important to be familiar with the various appearances of a normal thymus so as not to subject a patient to unnecessary additional imaging.

What the Treating Physician Needs to Know

No additional testing is needed as this is the normal appearance of thymus.

Answers

1. In children, lymphoma and germ cell tumors are the most likely to affect the thymus. Thymomas are rare in children.

2. On both CT and MRI, the normal pediatric thymus should have homogeneous appearance. In general, normal thymic tissue should not compress or displace vessels and airway. However, as a normal variant, thymic tissue can sometimes extend posterior to the SVC and in these cases some displacement of vessels and airways may be seen.[3]

REFERENCES

1. Nasseri F, Eftekhari F. Clinical and radiologic review of the normal and abnormal thymus: Pearls and pitfalls. *Radiographics.* 2010;30(2):413–428.

2. Binkovitz L, Binkovitz I, Kuhn JP. The mediastinum. In: Slovis TL, ed. *Caffey's Pediatric Diagnostic Imaging.* 11th ed. Philadelphia, PA: Mosby; 2008:1324–1388.

3. Donnelly LF. Normal thymus. In: Donnelly LF, ed. *Diagnostic Imaging: Pediatrics.* 2nd ed. Salt Lake City, Utah: Amirsys; 2012; 2:84–87.

CASE 5.14

Jonathan O. Swanson

CLINICAL HISTORY *A 3-day-old premature neonate with respiratory distress*

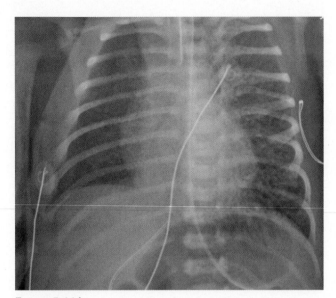

FIGURE **5.14A**

FINDINGS Initial frontal chest radiograph (**A**) demonstrates an intubated premature neonate with multiple dark distinct rounded and linear lucencies, predominantly left sided. No focal consolidation. No evidence of pneumothorax or pneumomediastinum. A follow-up radiograph (**B**) obtained 1 day later demonstrates an accentuation of this pattern, now bilateral and with increased hyperinflation of the lungs. Again, no evidence of pneumothorax or pneumomediastinum.

DIFFERENTIAL DIAGNOSIS Pulmonary interstitial emphysema (PIE)

DIAGNOSIS PIE

DISCUSSION PIE is most common in low-birth-weight neonates receiving mechanical ventilatory support. This form of air leak begins with the rupture of an alveolus with air that then escapes into the perivascular tissues of the lung. This exacerbates the respiratory distress by decreasing lung compliance and increasing overinflation of the lung.[1] PIE can be

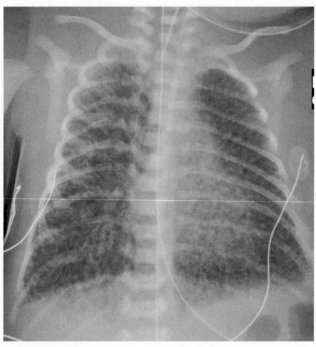

FIGURE **5.14B**

unilateral or bilateral. The characteristic radiographic findings are rounded or linear radiolucencies. The rounded lucencies, if focal, can be confused with congenital pulmonary airway malformation (CPAM). However, the cysts associated with CPAM are typically present at birth, and are usually larger and more variable in size than those seen in PIE.

Questions for Further Thought

1. What would be the therapeutic positioning of a patient with unilateral PIE? Why?
2. When is PIE most likely to present in the mechanically ventilated, low-birth-weight neonate?

Reporting Responsibilities

PIE represents one of the air leak complications seen with intubated premature infants. Pneumothorax, pneumopericardium, pneumomediastinum, and lung parenchymal cyst are additional air leak complications.

What the Treating Physician Needs to Know

The neonatologist needs to know if there are any additional forms of air leak that must be treated, such as pneumothorax.

Answers

1. Placing the neonate in the lateral decubitus position with the affected side down improves ventilation to the unaffected lung and decreases aeration of the side with PIE.[2] PIE is usually a transient process but some patients can progress to a persistent form that may require surgical management.

2. The first few days of life.

REFERENCES

1. Slovis TL, Bulas DI. Congenital and acquired lesions (most causing respiratory distress) of the neonatal lung and thorax. In: Slovis TL, ed. *Caffey's Pediatric Diagnostic Imaging.* 11th ed. Philadelphia, PA: Mosby; 2008:93–133.

2. Swingle HM, Eggert LD, Bucciarelli RL. New approach to management of unilateral tension pulmonary interstitial emphysema in premature infants. *Pediatrics.* 1984;74(3):354–357.

CLINICAL HISTORY *Newborn (postdates) who presents with respiratory distress*

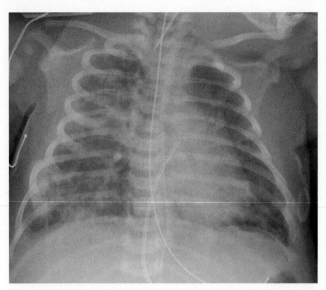

FIGURE 5.15A

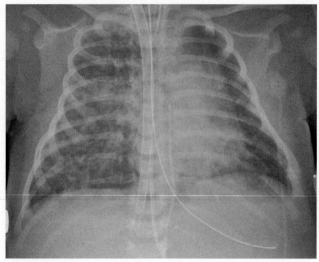

FIGURE 5.15B

FINDINGS Frontal chest radiograph (**A**) demonstrates an asymmetric coarse reticular pattern with hyperinflation of the lungs. The heart size is normal. There is no pleural effusion and no pneumothorax. Of note, the umbilical venous catheter (UVC) is malpositioned with tip crossing a patent foramen ovale into the left atrium. Follow-up radiograph obtained later the same day (**B**) demonstrates similar reticular opacities in the lungs but also the presence of an extracorporeal membrane oxygenation (ECMO) catheter suggesting a worsening of clinical state.

DIFFERENTIAL DIAGNOSIS Meconium aspiration syndrome, pneumonia

DIAGNOSIS Meconium aspiration syndrome

DISCUSSION Meconium aspiration syndrome refers to neonatal respiratory distress that occurs secondary to intrapartum/intrauterine aspiration of meconium, the thick material found in neonatal bowel.

A pattern of coarse pulmonary opacities which may be associated with hyperinflation on the newborn chest is most frequently seen in the setting of meconium aspiration and pneumonia. The useful discriminating clinical information is whether or not the amniotic fluid was stained with meconium and if there was meconium on initial suction of the airway. The presence of pleural effusion is more often seen in the setting of pneumonia. The pulmonary complications associated with meconium aspiration are secondary to a combination of airway obstruction, chemical inflammation, and surfactant dysfunction.[1] Clinically, this combination may lead to pulmonary hypertension with resultant persistent fetal circulation and hypoxemia. Radiographically, coarse pulmonary opacities and hyperinflation of the lungs may be seen. Meconium also provides an excellent medium for bacteria to grow and thus patients with meconium aspiration are at risk for pneumonia. Although some patients with meconium aspiration may recover within days, others may develop complications such as air leak or require ECMO if there is pulmonary hypertension.

Questions for Further Thought

1. What patients are at risk for meconium aspiration?
2. What percent of neonates who are born through meconium-stained amniotic fluid actually aspirate?

Reporting Responsibilities

Air leaks (pneumothorax, PIE, pneumomediastinum) are common in this population and evidence of air leak should be reported promptly.

What the Treating Physician Needs to Know

As mentioned above, detection of concomitant air leak is vital. Determining whether or not there is concomitant infection is less important because these patients are usually treated with antibiotics.

Answers

1. Meconium aspiration occurs in term and postdates infants who are exposed to in utero or intrapartum hypoxia/stress.
2. Approximately 5% of neonates with meconium-stained amniotic fluid aspirate meconium.[2]

REFERENCES

1. Slovis TL, Bulas DI. Congenital and acquired lesions (most causing respiratory distress) of the neonatal lung and thorax. In: Slovis TL, ed. *Caffey's Pediatric Diagnostic Imaging.* 11th ed. Philadelphia, PA: Mosby; 2008:93–133.
2. Wiswell TE. Delivery room management of the meconium-stained newborn. *J Perinatol.* 2008;28(Suppl 3):S19–S26.

CLINICAL HISTORY *A 9-month-old child in respiratory distress*

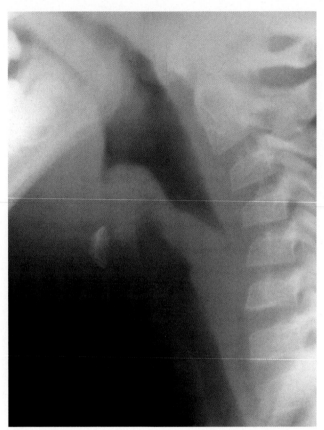

FIGURE 5.16A

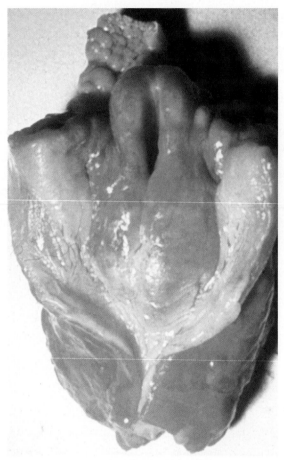

FIGURE 5.16B

FINDINGS Lateral radiograph of the neck (**A**) shows thickening of the epiglottis and the aryepiglottic folds. No prevertebral soft-tissue swelling. There is mild distension of the hypopharynx. The gross specimen (**B**) shows pathologic correlation with thickening of the epiglottis and aryepiglottic folds.

DIFFERENTIAL DIAGNOSIS Epiglottitis, croup

DIAGNOSIS Epiglottitis

DISCUSSION The incidence of epiglottitis has decreased substantially since the introduction of the *Haemophilus influenzae* type B (Hib) vaccine which became available in 1985. However, due to a combination of other pathogens that cause epiglottitis and due to a growing population of unvaccinated children, acute epiglottitis remains a real threat.[1] Like croup, epiglottitis is often a clinical diagnosis. When the diagnosis is in question, a lateral radiograph of the neck should be obtained. Enlargement of the epiglottis and aryepiglottic folds is diagnostic. Of note, approximately 25% of children with epiglottitis also have subglottic edema that is similar to that seen in croup.[2] The typical child with croup tends to be younger than the mean age of epiglottitis, which has increased from 3.5 to 14.6 years since the introduction of the Hib vaccine.[3]

Questions for Further Thought
1. What is an omega epiglottis and how can you differentiate an omega epiglottis from epiglottitis?
2. Besides infectious acute epiglottitis, what other entities can cause enlargement of the epiglottitis?

Reporting Responsibilities
If there is strong clinical suspicion of epiglottitis, the radiograph should be obtained in the upright position to avoid exacerbating the airway obstruction.

What the Treating Physician Needs to Know

If there is any suspicion of epiglottitis raised by the radiographs, the ordering provider must immediately be made aware of this possibility as epiglottitis is a life-threatening emergency that requires the patient to be in close proximity to rapid respiratory support in case the airway becomes compromised.

Answers

1. The omega epiglottis is an imaging normal variant where the left and right sides of the curved epiglottis project next to each other (as in when the epiglottis is imaged obliquely), giving the appearance of a thickened epiglottis. However, in an omega epiglottis, there is no thickening of the aryepiglottic folds.

2. Hemophilia, thermal injury, angioedema.

REFERENCES

1. Slovis TL, Bulas DI. Congenital and acquired lesions (most causing respiratory distress) of the neonatal lung and thorax. In: Slovis TL, ed. *Caffey's Pediatric Diagnostic Imaging.* 11th ed. Philadelphia, PA: Mosby; 2008:93–133.

2. Rogers DJ, Sie KC, Manning SC. Epiglottitis due to nontypeable Haemophilus influenzae in a vaccinated child. *Int J Pediatr Otorhinolaryngol.* 2010;74(2):218–220.

3. Donnelly LF. Epiglottitis. In: Donnelly LF, ed. *Diagnostic Imaging: Pediatrics.* 2nd ed. Salt Lake City, Utah: Amirsys; 2012;1:4–7.

CASE 5.17

CLINICAL HISTORY *A 5-week-old infant with persistent respiratory distress who had history of respiratory distress syndrome (surfactant deficiency disorder)*

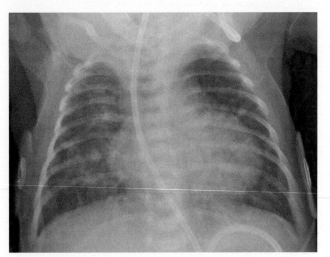

FIGURE **5.17A**

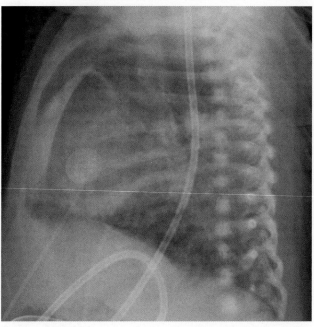

FIGURE **5.17B**

FINDINGS Frontal chest radiograph (**A**) demonstrates bilateral coarse reticular opacities. Lateral radiograph (**B**) demonstrates hyperinflation of the lungs with flattening of the hemidiaphragms. No pleural effusion.

DIFFERENTIAL DIAGNOSIS Bronchopulmonary dysplasia (BPD), PIE, meconium aspiration, neonatal pneumonia

DIAGNOSIS BPD

DISCUSSION BPD is also referred to as chronic lung disease of prematurity. Thought to be the result of a combination of mechanical ventilation and oxygen toxicity, BPD is most common in premature infants but can also be seen in near-term and term infants with underlying conditions that required prolonged mechanical ventilation (for example, meconium aspiration).[1] On chest radiographs, BPD changes in appearance over time. In the first weeks of life, the films on a patient who goes on to develop BPD may be normal or can have a diffuse, homogeneous bilateral opacity that overlaps with the appearance of respiratory distress syndrome or edema. Over the course of weeks to months, this changes to a heterogeneous pattern with coarse reticular opacities mixed with focal lucencies, and the lungs may also be hyperinflated. This pattern usually normalizes with age but some patients will have longer lasting sequelae such as abnormal pulmonary function tests.

Focal lucencies and coarse reticular opacities can also be seen in the setting of PIE and meconium aspiration. Age of the patient is helpful in differentiating these entities, as BPD presents later on in the neonatal period than PIE or meconium aspiration. Differentiating BPD from neonatal pneumonia is more difficult. Pleural effusion is more likely to be seen with pneumonia than BPD.

Questions for Further Thought

1. What are important risk factors for BPD?
2. What is Wilson–Mikity syndrome?

Reporting Responsibilities

Evaluate for pleural effusion to help determine if there may be pneumonia superimposed upon a pattern of BPD.

What the Treating Physician Needs to Know

Patients with a history of BPD have an increased rate of infection over the first 2 years of life.

Answers

1. Prematurity and low birth weight.[2]

2. Wilson–Mikity syndrome describes a patient population composed of premature neonates who do not require early ventilatory support but go on to develop BPD.[1]

REFERENCES

1. Slovis TL, Bulas DI. Congenital and acquired lesions (most causing respiratory distress) of the neonatal lung and thorax. In: Slovis TL, ed. *Caffey's Pediatric Diagnostic Imaging.* 11th ed. Philadelphia, PA: Mosby; 2008:93–133.

2. Lemons JA, Bauer CR, Oh W, et al. Very low birth weight outcomes of the National Institute of Child health and human development neonatal research network, January 1995 through December 1996. NICHD Neonatal Research Network. *Pediatrics.* 2001;107(1):E1.

Puneet Bhargava

CASE 5.18

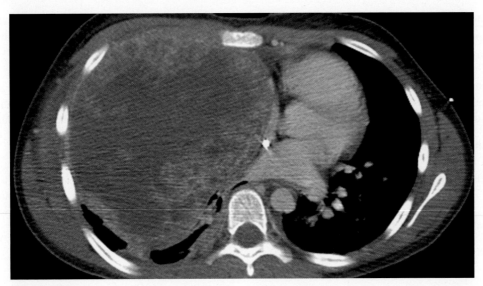

FIGURE 5.18

FINDINGS Axial contrast-enhanced CT image shows a large heterogeneous pleuropulmonary mass with mass-effect but without definite mediastinal or chest wall invasion.

DIFFERENTIAL DIAGNOSIS Pleuropulmonary blastoma (PPB), rhabdomyosarcoma, undifferentiated sarcoma, Ewing sarcoma, primitive neuroectodermal tumor (PNET), pulmonary inflammatory pseudotumor, parapneumonic effusion/empyema, lung cysts, neuroblastoma

DIAGNOSIS PPB

DISCUSSION PPB is a rare aggressive malignant primary pleuroparenchymal mesenchymal neoplasm occurring in children younger than 6 years associated with a poor prognosis.[1] Patients usually present late with nonspecific respiratory distress and an opacified hemithorax on chest radiograph. The diagnosis should be suspected if there is cardiomediastinal shift and absence of chest wall invasion. Pleural effusion may be present. PPB may have both cystic and solid components and may be classified depending on whether they are purely cystic (type I), purely solid (type III), or mixed (type II). It should be noted that a purely cystic PPB (type I) may be radiographically indistinguishable from a benign lung cyst and type 4 CPAM.[2,3]

DIFFERENTIAL DIAGNOSTIC CONSIDERATIONS

Rhabdomyosarcoma, undifferentiated sarcoma, Ewing sarcoma, and PNET may invade the chest wall. All of these are solid masses and may be indistinguishable from a PPB.

Pulmonary inflammatory pseudotumor often contains calcifications and is typically smaller than PPB.

Parapneumonic effusion/empyema usually presents with an opacified hemithorax; clinical symptomatology is helpful in making this diagnosis and the abnormalities should resolve with antibiotics and pleural fluid drainage.

Lung cysts, including bronchogenic cyst, and as seen in certain types of CPAM and pulmonary sequestration, may be indistinguishable from a type I PPB. Presence of systemic arterial supply to the abnormal lung helps to make the diagnosis of pulmonary sequestration.

Neuroblastoma typically occurs in the posterior mediastinum and calcifications are frequently seen on CT. Presence of rib erosion as well as extension into widened neural foramina and spinal canal helps to make this diagnosis.

Questions for Further Thought

1. What is the imaging study of choice to evaluate initial extent of disease in PPB?

2. What imaging finding argues against the diagnosis of PPB?

Reporting Responsibilities

- Describe location and extent of the abnormalities.
- Suspect the diagnosis of PPB if there is a large pleural-based mass in a child younger than 6 years of age.

What the Treating Physician Needs to Know

- A type I PPB may be radiologically indistinguishable from a benign lung cyst.
- Twenty-five percent of PPBs occur in association with neoplasms in family members.

Answers

1. Contrast-enhanced CT is usually sufficient to evaluate the extent of disease in PPB.

2. Evaluate for chest wall invasion. PPB rarely invades the chest wall, unlike other solid pediatric chest tumors.

REFERENCES

1. Priest JR, McDermott MB, Bhatia S, et al. Pleuropulmonary blastoma: A clinicopathologic study of 50 cases. *Cancer.* 1997; 80(1):147–161.
2. Naffaa LN, Donnelly LF. Imaging findings in pleuropulmonary blastoma. *Pediatr Radiol.* 2005;35(4):387–391.
3. Towbin AJ. Pleuropulmonary blastoma. In: Donnelly LF, ed. *Diagnostic Imaging: Pediatrics.* 2nd ed. Salt Lake City, Utah: Amirsys; 2012;2:102–105.

Mark R. Ferguson

CLINICAL HISTORY *A 3-year-old child with a cardiac murmer (Figs. 5.19A and B)*

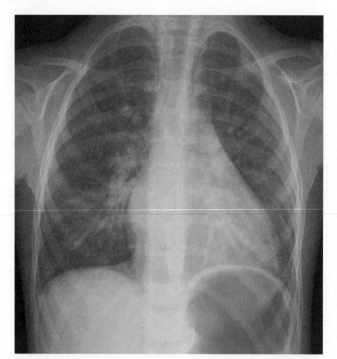

FIGURE **5.19A**

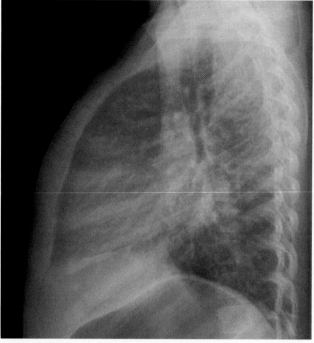

FIGURE **5.19B**

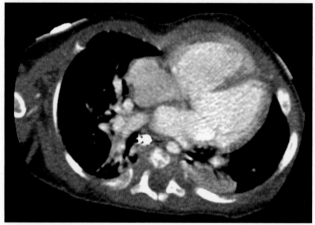

FIGURE **5.19C**

FINDINGS Frontal (**A**) and lateral (**B**) chest radiographs show prominence of pulmonary vessels and slightly large heart. There is evidence for an enlarged left atrium with mild widening of the carinal angle and perhaps posterior displacement of the left mainstem bronchus as well as a double density overlapping the right heart. The aorta is left sided and grossly normal in size. Axial CT image (**C**), from a different patient, demonstrates diffuse cardiomegaly and a defect within the membranous portion of the ventricular septum. There is also some posterior atelectasis.

DIFFERENTIAL DIAGNOSIS

- Chest radiograph: VSD, PDA, ASD, PAPVC
- CT: VSD

DIAGNOSIS VSD

DISCUSSION The differential diagnosis for an acyanotic patient with increased pulmonary blood flow includes VSD, PDA, ASD, and PAPVC. To narrow this differential, the next step is to evaluate for left atrial enlargement, typically seen in patients with VSD and PDA. Signs for left atrial enlargement include widening of the carinal angle beyond 90°, posterior displacement of the left mainstem bronchus, and double density near the right heart margin secondary to the enlarged left atrium extending downward and rightward. The older child with PDA may also show aortic enlargement.[1] In both ASD and PAPVC, cardiac enlargement, if any, should be right sided. Plain films, however, are often inconclusive and echocardiography has become the modality of choice for initial evaluation of suspected congenital heart disease.

VSD can be classified into four subtypes[2]:

1. Outlet, supracristal, subpulmonary, infundibular, or conoseptal defects: Located in the outlet portion of the left and RVs with the joined annulus of the aortic and pulmonary valves forming the superior margin of the VSD. Five percent of all VSDs.

2. Perimembranous, paramembranous, infracristal, or subaortic defects: Located around the membranous septum but with a component of a muscular defect. Seventy-five percent of all VSDs.

3. AV canal, AV septal, or inlet defects: Located in the posterior region of the septum below the tricuspid valve. Ten percent of all VSDs.

4. Muscular defects: Located in the muscular septum, commonly in the apical trabecular portion; may be single but commonly multiple. Ten percent of all VSDs.

Questions for Further Thought

1. When will a larger VSD typically become symptomatic and what is the reason for this time frame?

2. Which type of VSD has the greatest chance of spontaneous closure?

Reporting Responsibilities

- On the basis of radiographic findings, the referring physician should be alerted to the possibility of congenital heart disease. The patient with congenital heart disease may need follow-up imaging with echocardiography or possibly cardiac MRI.

- On the basis of MRI, the location of the VSD needs to be described as repair techniques vary by lesion location and size. Reporting the ratio of pulmonary to systemic blood flow (Qp/Qs) can also be helpful to the surgeons as a larger shunt, greater than 1.5 to 2, can influence timing of surgical management.

What the Treating Physician Needs to Know

- Spontaneous closure of a VSD after 10 years of age is unlikely.[3]

- VSD is the most common form of congenital heart disease that is associated with chromosomal abnormalities such as trisomy 13, 18, and 21, but the vast majority of patients with a VSD do not have a chromosomal abnormality.

Answers

1. Typically, patients with a larger VSD do not become symptomatic until 1 to 2 months of age. Newborn pulmonary arterial pressures are still high, reflecting the fetal circulation; however, as the pressures fall, left-to-right shunting can take place. Small VSDs often close spontaneously.

2. Muscular VSD.[3]

REFERENCES

1. Kellenberger CJ. Lesions with left-to-right shunt. In: Yoo SJ, MacDonald C, Babyn P, eds. *Chest Radiographic Interpretation in Pediatric Cardiac Patients.* New York: Thieme Medical Publishers; 2010:177–184.

2. Makaryus AN, Boxt LM. Ventricular septal defect. In: Ho VB, Reddy GP, eds. *Cardiovascular Imaging.* St. Louis, MO: Elsevier Saunders; 2011:572–582.

3. Turner SW, Hunter S, Wyllie JP. The natural history of ventricular septal defects. *Arch Dis Child.* 1999;81(5):413–416.

Mark R. Ferguson

CLINICAL HISTORY *A newborn with respiratory distress*

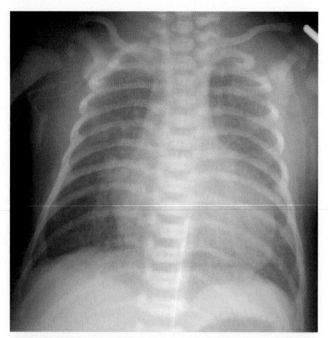

FIGURE **5.20A**

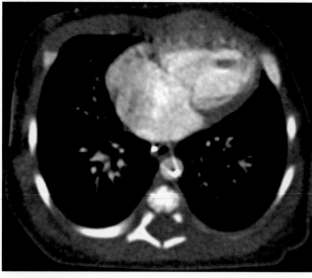

FIGURE **5.20B**

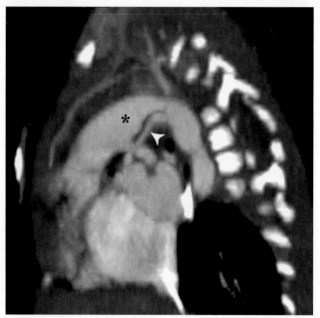

FIGURE **5.20C**

FINDINGS Frontal radiograph of the chest (**A**) shows cardiomegaly and diffuse pulmonary opacities consistent with pulmonary venous congestion. Axial CT (**B**) shows no interventricular septum, suggesting that there is a single domi-

nant ventricle. Sagittal CT reconstruction (**C**) shows a large PDA (*) connecting the pulmonary artery to the aortic arch with a markedly diminutive ascending aorta (*arrowhead*).

DIFFERENTIAL DIAGNOSIS

- Chest radiograph: Hypoplastic left heart (HLH) syndrome, tachyarrhythmia, high output extracardiac shunt (such as vein of Galen malformation), cardiomyopathy, critical aortic stenosis
- CT: HLH syndrome

DIAGNOSIS HLH syndrome

DISCUSSION HLH syndrome is not a single lesion but rather a constellation of abnormalities with a dominant finding of underdevelopment of the left heart. Typically, there is stenosis or even atresia of the aortic and mitral valves with a small left atrium, LV, and ascending aorta. An ASD or patent foramen ovale and a PDA are usually present.[1] The RV functions as both the pulmonary and systemic pump with blood reaching the aorta through the PDA. This results in partially oxygenated blood being delivered systemically.

Patients typically present as newborns with chest radiographs often showing cardiomegaly with pulmonary venous congestion. However, the clinical and radiographic presentations vary depending on the relative sizes of the PDA and ASD. An unrestrictive ASD can lead to increased pulmonary vascularity and heart enlargement secondary to left-to-right shunting if the pulmonary vascular resistance has dropped. On the other hand, a restrictive ASD can result in pulmonary venous hypertension with edema and a normal sized heart. HLH syndrome is the most common cause of congestive heart failure in the first few days of life.[1] MRI and CT are often not performed before surgical repair if the diagnosis has already been confirmed by echocardiography.

Questions for Further Thought

1. What is the most common surgical repair for HLH syndrome?
2. What is a major long-term limitation of the surgical repair?

Reporting Responsibilities

If CT or MRI is performed, the radiologist needs to accurately catalog the abnormalities of HLH syndrome and describe the degree and extent of aortic narrowing to allow for surgical planning.

What the Treating Physician Needs to Know

A newborn with cardiomegaly, cyanosis, and signs of failure has a high likelihood of having HLH syndrome. The diagnosis is usually made by echocardiography.

Answers

1. The Norwood procedure. This is a multistage surgical repair resulting in Fontan circulation where systemic venous return is routed directly to the pulmonary arteries and cardiac ventricular output is only systemic.[2]
2. The RV must function as a high-pressure systemic pump for which it is not suited, potentially resulting in failure.

REFERENCES

1. Epelman M. Hypoplastic left heart syndrome. In: Yoo SJ, MacDonald C, Babyn P, eds. *Chest Radiographic Interpretation in Pediatric Cardiac Patients.* New York, NY: Thieme Medical Publishers; 2010:225–228.
2. Gaca AM, Jaggers JJ, Dudley LT, et al. Repair of congenital heart disease: A primer–Part 1. *Radiology.* 2008;247(3): 617–631.

CLINICAL HISTORY *Newborn with cyanosis*

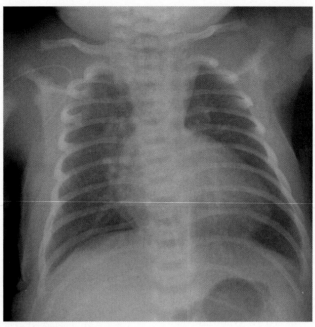

FIGURE **5.21**

FINDINGS Frontal view of the chest shows mild cardiomegaly and a narrow superior mediastinum. There is some prominence of the pulmonary vasculature. Incidental note made of malpositioned right upper extremity vascular catheter.

DIFFERENTIAL DIAGNOSIS Dextro-transposition of the great arteries (d-TGA), TAPVC, truncus arteriosus, tricuspid atresia, single ventricle

DIAGNOSIS d-TGA

DISCUSSION The differential diagnosis for a cyanotic patient with a radiograph showing cardiomegaly and increased pulmonary blood flow is provided above. However, in this case, the narrow vascular pedicle suggests d-TGA (egg-on-a-string appearance). Although the incidence of d-TGA is relatively low at 20 to 30 cases per 100,000 live births, it represents the most common etiology of cyanotic congenital heart disease in the newborn.[1]

Dextro-transposition anatomy results from ventriculoarterial discordance with the aorta arising from the RV and the pulmonary artery arising from the LV. The root of the aorta will be positioned anterior, superior, and rightward while the main pulmonary artery (MPA) will be posterior, inferior, and leftward. Sometimes this abnormal positioning will result in the vessels lying in nearly the same sagittal plane. This arrangement combined with stress-induced thymic atrophy results in the narrow appearance of the superior mediastinum.[2] Furthermore, this anatomy results in pulmonary and systemic vascular circuits coursing in parallel rather than in series. Patients often present as newborns with cyanosis, with admixture of blood between pulmonary and systemic vascular circuits necessary for patient survival. Most patients will have an ASD, PDA, or VSD; however, emergent atrial septostomy may be necessary to provide or augment mixing of blood prior to full corrective surgery.

A subset of patients with transposition of the great arteries (TGA) have levo-transposition (l-TGA) in which the aorta is also positioned anterior but leftward of the MPA. In addition to ventriculoarterial discordance, most of these patients also have AV discordance. This arrangement is "congenitally corrected" as the pulmonary and systemic circulations remain in series. However, this leaves the systemic circulation powered by a morphologic RV that is not designed to sustain such high pressures.

Questions for Further Thought

1. What is a long-term disadvantage of the Mustard or Senning surgical repairs of TGA?
2. What is now the preferred surgical repair technique?

Reporting Responsibilities

- Based on chest radiographs, alert the physician to the possibility of congenital heart disease and that further imaging may be warranted.
- Based on cross-sectional imaging, typically MRI, describe vessel anatomy and evaluate for the presence of any defect allowing for admixture of blood between pulmonary and systemic vascular circuits.

What the Treating Physician Needs to Know

With d-TGA, the LV can become deconditioned when facing the low-pressure pulmonary circulation. Therefore, if the patient presents later than about 2 months of life, it may be necessary to place a pulmonary artery band to increase the afterload of the LV, preparing it for the demands of systemic circulation following an arterial switch.

Answers

1. These repairs result in redirection of the systemic venous return into the embryologic LV and subsequently to the pulmonary artery. However, this anatomy also results in the morphologic RV acting as the systemic arterial pump for which it was not designed, and can lead to heart failure.[3]
2. The Jatene arterial switch procedure, as it restores ventriculoarterial concordance.[3]

REFERENCES

1. Rao PS. Diagnosis and management of cyanotic congenital heart disease: Part I. *Indian J Pediatr.* 2009;76(1):57–70.
2. Ferguson EC, Krishnamurthy R, Oldham SA. Classic imaging signs of congenital cardiovascular abnormalities. *Radiographics.* 2007;27(5):1323–1334.
3. Gaca AM, Jaggers JJ, Dudley LT, et al. Repair of congenital heart disease: A primer–Part 1. *Radiology.* 2008;247(3):617–631.

CLINICAL HISTORY *Acyanotic 2-month-old infant with abnormal prenatal ultrasound*

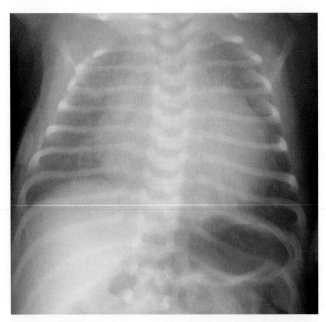

FIGURE **5.22A**

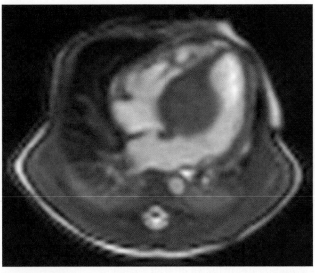

FIGURE **5.22B**

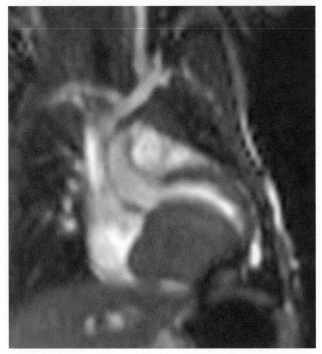

FIGURE **5.22C**

FINDINGS Frontal chest radiograph (**A**) shows cardiomegaly and diffuse slight pulmonary haziness. Four-chamber MRI bright-blood technique image (**B**) demonstrates a large mass originating from the interventricular septum that predominantly extends into the LV. The mass is also identified on the MRI left ventricular outflow tract image (**C**).

DIFFERENTIAL DIAGNOSIS

- Chest radiograph: Left-to-right shunt lesion, pericardial effusion, cardiac mass
- MRI: Cardiac fibroma, rhabdomyoma

DIAGNOSIS Cardiac fibroma

DISCUSSION Cardiac fibromas are the second most common pediatric cardiac neoplasm (rhabdomyoma is the most common), but are the most commonly resected pediatric cardiac tumors. Patients may present with heart failure, arrhythmias, or sudden death, although one-third of patients are asymptomatic.[1]

Radiographs will typically show cardiomegaly. Associated intratumoral calcification can be seen 25% of the time. MRI will show a discrete mural mass or focal wall thickening, which is usually iso- to hyperintense on T1-weighted and hypointense on T2-weighted imaging relative to normal myocardium. Post-contrast images may show heterogeneous enhancement with nonenhancing areas that may correlate with fibrous tissue.[1] In contradistinction, rhabdomyomas are typically multiple, iso- to slightly hyperintense on T1-weighted and hyperintense on T2-weighted imaging relative to normal myocardium, and may be hypointense relative to normal myocardium on post-contrast MRI.

Questions for Further Thought

1. What is the typical management of these patients?
2. What syndrome has an increased risk for cardiac fibromas?

Reporting Responsibilities

Based on MRI, describe size and location of mass as well as quantify heart function to determine if impaired by mass.

What the Treating Physician Needs to Know

Patients with cardiac fibromas are at increased risk for lethal arrhythmias.

Answers

1. Patients manifesting cardiac functional impairment due to obstruction or arrhythmias need surgical excision of the lesion. In cases with a particularly large mass, as the case presented, a heart transplant may be the only option.[2]
2. Nevoid basal cell carcinoma syndrome (Gorlin syndrome).[1]

REFERENCES

1. Grebenc ML, Rosado de Christenson ML, Burke AP, et al. Primary cardiac and pericardial neoplasms: Radiologic-pathologic correlation. *Radiographics.* 2000;20(4):1073–1103.
2. Stiller B, Hetzer R, Meyer R, et al. Primary cardiac tumours: When is surgery necessary? *Eur J Cardiothorac Surg.* 2001;20(5):1002–1006.

CLINICAL HISTORY *A 2-year-old child with sudden onset of persistent cough*

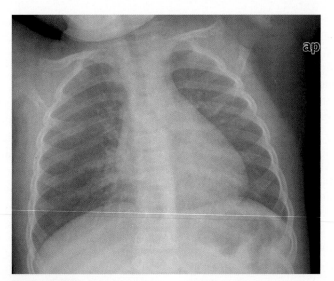

FIGURE **5.23A**

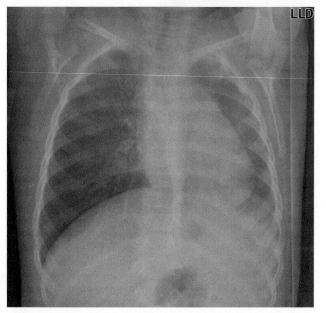

FIGURE **5.23B**

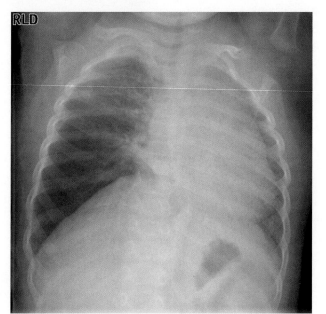

FIGURE **5.23C**

FINDINGS Frontal chest radiograph (**A**) demonstrates questionably more lucent right lower lobe as compared to rest of lungs. Left lateral decubitus radiograph (**B**) shows some decrease in aeration of the left lung. Right lateral decubitus radiograph (**C**) demonstrates no definite decrease in aeration of the right lung, especially the right middle lobe and right lower lobe.

DIFFERENTIAL DIAGNOSIS Foreign body aspiration, mucus plug, Swyer–James–MacLeod syndrome

DIAGNOSIS Foreign body aspiration

DISCUSSION Foreign body aspiration is most commonly seen in children from 6 months to 3 years of age. A less common at-risk age group is 9 to 13 years of age (for example, a 10-year-old boy throwing a peanut up in the air and catching it with his open mouth/airway). Most foreign bodies are non-radiopaque. Of the non-radiopaque foreign bodies, most are vegetable or food matter.[1] In bronchial aspirations, the majority of foreign bodies end up on the right side. Thus, the example of a peanut in the right mainstem bronchus is ubiquitous in medical education. Infants and toddlers can present with stridor, wheezing, cough, recurrent pneumonia, and hemoptysis. A high index of suspicion is helpful as the routine chest radiograph is often normal.

Helpful to making the diagnosis is obtaining an expiratory view. Given that a toddler may not be cooperative, the expiration view can be acquired via bilateral decubitus views or fluoroscopy of the hemidiaphragms. In both cases, we are looking for air trapping with relatively static lung volume of the affected side. The most common radiographic finding is a hyperlucent lung caused by the ball-valve effect of the foreign body. However, atelectasis distal to the obstruction can also be seen.

Swyer–James–MacLeod syndrome is a manifestation of postinfectious obliterative bronchiolitis in which a lung or portion of lung does not grow normally and there is hyperlucency of the affected lung. Unlike foreign body aspiration, the involved hyperlucent lung is typically smaller than the other lung.

Questions for Further Thought

1. How sensitive are chest radiographs for the diagnosis of intrabronchial foreign body?
2. When could CT be used for diagnosis of foreign body?

Reporting Responsibilities

Evaluate for radiopaque foreign body or filling defect in the airway. Evaluate for unilateral hyperlucent lung. Determine if there is a static volume between the inspiration and expiration views.

What the Treating Physician Needs to Know

Normal imaging studies do not absolutely exclude foreign body aspiration. If the imaging studies do not suggest the diagnosis and clinical concern is high, bronchoscopy may be needed for further evaluation.

Answers

1. The reported sensitivity of chest radiographs for foreign body detection range from 68% to 74%. The reported specificity of chest radiographs for foreign body detection range from 45% to 67%.[1] However, these studies did not evaluate the efficacy of expiration views.
2. CT is typically not indicated for the evaluation of suspected foreign body aspiration, but can be used to evaluate for other causes in the differential, such as Swyer–James–MacLeod syndrome (discussed above) and pulmonary artery sling that can show focal pulmonary hyperinflation.

REFERENCE

1. Long FR, Druhan SM, Kuhn JP. Diseases of the bronchi and pulmonary aeration. In: Slovis TL, ed. *Caffey's Pediatric Diagnostic Imaging.* 11th ed. Philadelphia, PA: Mosby; 2008:1121–1176.

Jonathan O. Swanson

CASE 5.24

CLINICAL HISTORY *Newborn who presents after cesarian section delivery with moderate respiratory distress*

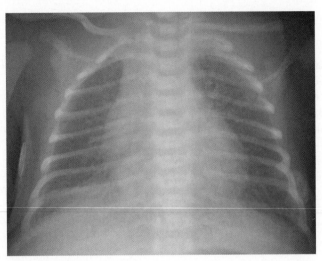

FIGURE **5.24**

FINDINGS Frontal chest radiograph demonstrates some prominence to interstitial markings with mild indistinctness of vessels. There is a small right pleural effusion. The cardiothymic silhouette is normal.

DIFFERENTIAL DIAGNOSIS Transient tachypnea of the newborn (TTN), cardiogenic edema, pneumonia

DIAGNOSIS TTN

DISCUSSION A fine interstitial pattern seen on the chest radiograph of a newborn is most frequently seen in the setting of TTN and edema. It is important to evaluate the heart on the radiograph. If the cause of the reticular pattern is cardiogenic edema, the heart may be enlarged. In TTN,

the heart size is typically normal. The lung volumes may be normal to slightly hyperinflated. Pleural effusion(s) may be present. The classic clinical presentation is that of a term or near-term infant status after a cesarian section without labor.

TTN represents a prolongation of the normal physiologic clearing of fluid from the lungs. In a normal infant, the fetal lung fluid clears within approximately three breaths. In TTN, this same fluid takes 1 to 3 days to clear. The infant with TTN may present with mild to moderate respiratory distress but this benign, self-limited condition, resolves with supportive measures.

Question for Further Thought

1. Besides cesarian section, what other maternal conditions predispose a newborn to TTN?

Reporting Responsibilities

If the clinical and radiographic appearance does not improve over a 24- to 48-hour period, an alternative diagnosis should be entertained such as congenital heart disease or pneumonia/sepsis, as it is rare for TTN to persist for more than 48 hours.

What the Treating Physician Needs to Know

TTN is a clinical diagnosis. The treating physician needs to be alerted if there are any suggestions on the radiograph that the patient may have another reason for respiratory distress.

Answer

1. Maternal asthma and maternal diabetes.[1]

REFERENCE

1. Slovis TL, Bulas DI. Congenital and acquired lesions (most causing respiratory distress) of the neonatal lung and thorax. In: Slovis TL, ed. *Caffey's Pediatric Diagnostic Imaging.* 11th ed. Philadelphia, PA: Mosby; 2008:93–133.

CASE 5.25

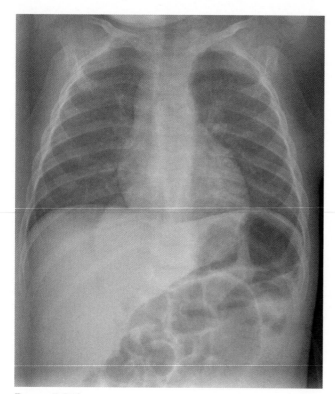

FIGURE 5.25A

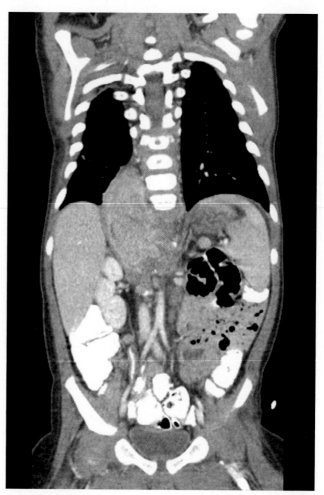

FIGURE 5.25B

FINDINGS Frontal radiograph (**A**) demonstrates a smoothly marginated oblong density along the right aspect of the lower thoracic spine with mild left convex curvature of the spine at this level. This density is centered at the level of the diaphragm. No calcification is identified. There may be slight widening of the space between ribs at the level of this density. Coronal CT image (**B**) demonstrates a heterogeneous mass with both abdominal and intrathoracic components. Some punctuate calcifications were present at the inferior aspect of the lesion.

DIFFERENTIAL DIAGNOSIS Neuroblastoma, round pneumonia, congenital foregut duplication cyst

DIAGNOSIS Abdominal neuroblastoma with intrathoracic extension

DISCUSSION Neuroblastoma is a malignant tumor derived from primitive neural crest tissue and is the third most common childhood cancer after leukemia and central nervous system tumors. The mean age at presentation is 14 months.[1] A younger age (<1 year) at presentation is usually associated with better prognosis. Neuroblastomas most often arise in the adrenal glands, but can arise from any tissue in the sympathetic nerve chains. Most patients have elevated catecholamine levels at time of diagnosis. Radiographically, neuroblastoma can be seen as a partially calcified mass with mass effect and invasion of adjacent structures. In this case, as in many cases of neuroblastoma with intrathoracic involvement, the only chest radiographic finding is widening of the lower thoracic paraspinal line secondary to thoracic extension of an abdominal mass. Round pneumonia and duplication foregut cysts should be in the differential of apparent posterior mediastinal masses. These two entities can sometimes be excluded radiographically when there is evidence of adjacent bony destruction and/or spreading apart of ribs. Otherwise, CT or MRI can be used to differentiate between the entities listed as differential diagnoses. Approximately 80% to 90% of neuroblastomas demonstrate internal calcifications on CT.[2] Other findings of neuroblastoma include a solid enhancing lesion that can invade the adjacent spinal neural foramina. If findings are equivocal, an iodine-123-metaiodobenzylguanidine (MIBG) study can be performed as the vast majority of neuroblastomas demonstrate MIBG avidity.

Questions for Further Thought

1. In the Evans anatomic staging for neuroblastoma, what is stage 4S and how is it treated?
2. How are ganglioneuromas and ganglioneuroblastomas related to neuroblastoma?

Reporting Responsibilities

On pediatric chest radiographs, special attention must be paid to the mediastinal and paraspinal contours. Abdominal neuroblastoma has a tendency to extend into the thorax along the spine.

What the Treating Physician Needs to Know

If neuroblastoma has been diagnosed by plain film or CT, the patient will often need an MRI of the spine to evaluate for the presence and extent of intraspinal disease. Both bone scan and I-123-MIBG should be performed at diagnosis to evaluate both primary soft-tissue mass and for the presence of osseous metastasis. If the patient is MIBG avid, this is the best test for serial follow-up.

Answers

1. Stage 4S represents metastatic disease to liver, skin, and bone marrow in patients less than 1 year of age. These patients have a near 100% survival. In some institutions, no chemotherapy will be initiated because of the high likelihood that these tumors will regress spontaneously.

2. The ganglioneuromas and ganglioneuroblastomas represent more differentiated forms of the neural crest tissue neoplasms, of which neuroblastoma is the most aggressive. The ganglioneuromas are the most differentiated in this spectrum, and are considered benign. The ganglioneuroblastomas are composed of mixed histology and represent an intermediate grade of tumor.

REFERENCES

1. Towbin AJ. Neuroblastoma. In: Donnelly LF, ed. *Diagnostic Imaging: Pediatrics*. 2nd ed. Salt Lake City, Utah: Amirsys; 2012; 2:96–99.
2. Lonergan GJ, Schwab CM, Suarez ES, et al. Neuroblastoma, ganglioneuroblastoma, and ganglioneuroma: Radiologic-pathologic correlation. *Radiographics*. 2002;22(4):911–934.

CLINICAL HISTORY *A 5-month-old immunocompromised child who had undergone bone marrow transplant, now with worsening respiratory distress*

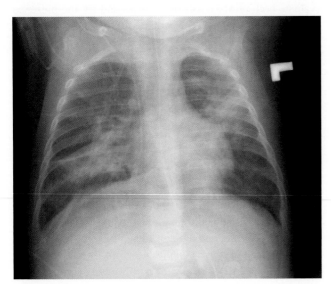

FIGURE 5.26A

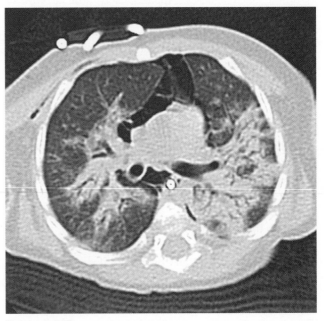

FIGURE 5.26B

FINDINGS Frontal chest radiograph (**A**) demonstrates bilateral fairly confluent areas of opacification. No definite pleural effusion or pneumothorax. A right-sided catheter has tip projecting in right atrium. On the single axial image from a CT performed 2 days later (**B**), there is a bat-wing pattern of perihilar consolidation with adjacent areas of ground-glass opacification. There is evidence of air leak in the form of pneumomediastinum.

DIFFERENTIAL DIAGNOSIS *Pneumocystis jirovecii* pneumonia (formally known as *Pneumocystis carinii* pneumonia), viral or atypical bacterial pneumonia, atypical pulmonary edema

DIAGNOSIS *Pneumocystis jirovecii* pneumonia

DISCUSSION Like adults, pediatric *P. jirovecii* is an infection that affects the immunocompromised population. *P. jirovecii* accounts for about half of the AIDS-defining illnesses diagnosed in the first year of life. It can also be seen as a pathogen in the setting of bone marrow transplant and other immunosuppressed states of childhood.[1] Like its adult counterpart, pediatric *P. jirovecii* has decreased in prevalence with the use of prophylactic antibiotics in susceptible populations.

The clinical presentation is often far worse than the imaging appearance. In fact, the chest radiograph may appear normal at initial presentation. The typical radiographic appearance is a perihilar haziness, which progresses to bilateral areas of airspace consolidation. In late-stage disease, the consolidation can become more confluent. On CT, scattered thin-walled cysts can develop.[2] Importantly, air leak is a common manifestation in *P. jirovecii* pneumonia.

Questions for Further Thought

1. What type of organism is *P. jirovecii*?
2. What nuclear medicine studies may be helpful in the diagnosis and management of patients with *Pneumocystis jirovecii* pneumonia?

Reporting Responsibilities

Air leaks are common in this population and evidence of air leak should be reported promptly.

What the Treating Physician Needs to Know

P. jirovecii pneumonia may have a fairly nonspecific appearance on chest radiographs. History and presentation are important as they may dictate further workup to evaluate for this possibility. The diagnosis of *P. jirovecii* pneumonia is made via tracheal washings or lung biopsy.

Answers

1. Originally thought to be protozoan, *P. jirovecii* is now considered a fungus.

2. Gallium-67 scanning demonstrates increased pulmonary uptake in patients with *Pneumocystis jirovecii* pneumonia with high sensitivity (but low specificity). The lung clearance of inhaled technetium-99m diethylenetriaminepentaacetate (Tc-99m DTPA) is decreased in patients with *Pneumocystis jirovecii* pneumonia and can be used to monitor response to therapy.

REFERENCES

1. Simonds RJ, Oxtoby MJ, Caldwell MB, et al. Pneumocystis carinii pneumonia among US children with perinatally acquired HIV infection. *JAMA* 1993;270(4):470–473.

2. Hansell DM, Lynch DA, McAdams HP, et al. The immunocompromised chest. In: Hansell DM, Lynch DA, McAdams HP, Bankier AA, eds. *Imaging of Diseases of the Chest.* 5th ed. Philadelphia: Mosby; 2010:295–384.

Puneet Bhargava

CLINICAL HISTORY *A 10-year-old child with chronic cough*

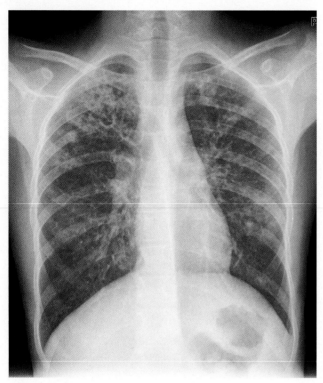

FIGURE 5.27A

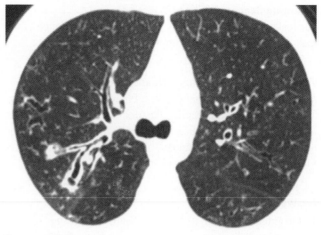

FIGURE 5.27B

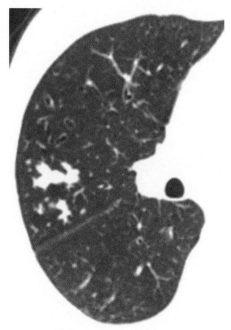

FIGURE 5.27C

FINDINGS Frontal chest radiograph (**A**) and axial CT (**B**) images show upper lobe predominant bronchiectasis with bronchial wall thickening. Axial CT image of right lung (**C**) also shows areas of mucous plugging.

DIFFERENTIAL DIAGNOSIS Cystic fibrosis, recurrent aspiration, asthma, BPD, primary ciliary dyskinesia, chronic granulomatous disease (CGD)

DIAGNOSIS Cystic fibrosis

DISCUSSION Cystic fibrosis is an autosomal recessive disorder of exocrine gland function which in the respiratory tract causes recurrent infection, mucoid impaction, bronchiectasis, and chronic sinusitis with nasal polyps. Chest radiograph in the early stages shows hyperinflation with increased perihilar marking with or without atelectasis. Later, upper lobe predominant bronchiectasis is seen. Disease progression may result in pulmonary arterial enlargement and cor pulmonale.

Predominantly upper lobe brochiectasis and mucuous plugging in hyperinflated lungs is the best diagnostic clue for cystic fibrosis. There is a predisposition to spontaneous pneumothorax and 10% of patients develop allergic bronchopulmonary aspergillosis (ABPA). There is a predisposition for recurrent pneumonias from *Pseudomonas aeruginosa, Staphylococcus aureus,* and *Haemophilus influenzae.* CT is the most sensitive study to detect early bronchial wall dilatation while chest radiographs are sufficient for long-term follow-up and most acute exacerbations. Expiratory high-resolution CT (HRCT) can demonstrate air trapping which may precede the development of bronchiectasis.[1,2]

DIFFERENTIAL DIAGNOSTIC CONSIDERATIONS

Recurrent aspiration should be suspected if there are changes of bronchiectasis in the lower lobes and posterior segments (dependent portions). Aspiration may be preceded by an episode of choking or gagging with feeds and patients with aspiration may have predisposing neuromuscular abnormalities.

Asthma, especially when complicated by ABPA, may appear similar to cystic fibrosis. However, asthma may be seasonal and there may be a history of allergies.

Patients with BPD usually have a history of prematurity and tend to improve over time.

Primary ciliary dyskinesia may present with bronchiectasis that is not upper lobe predominant. Situs inversus and associated cardiac anomalies are seen with this entity.

Patients with CGD may have lung abscesses as well as multi-organ involvement.

Questions for Further Thought

1. Which imaging study is recommended for long-term follow-up of cystic fibrosis and for most acute exacerbations?
2. What is the signet ring sign on CT imaging?

Reporting Responsibilities

- Describe location, extent, and complications, if any, in the lungs.
- Identify and describe stigmata of cystic fibrosis in the pancreas, liver, and the gastrointestinal tract.

What the Treating Physician Needs to Know

- Suspect the diagnosis if there is hyperinflation with upper lobe predominant bronchiectasis and mucous plugging.
- HRCT is the most sensitive study for detecting bronchiectasis.

Answers

1. Chest radiographs are usually sufficient for long-term follow-up and most acute exacerbations of cystic fibrosis.
2. The signet ring sign represents a dilated bronchus with an adjacent artery and is indicative of bronchiectasis. The ring represents the dilated bronchial wall.

REFERENCES

1. Crotty EJ. Cystic Fibrosis, Lung. In: Donnelly LF, ed. *Diagnostic Imaging: Pediatrics.* Salt Lake City: Amirsys; 2005;2: 110–113.
2. McGuinness G, Naidich DP. CT of airways disease and bronchiectasis. *Radiol Clin North Am.* 2002;40(1):1–19.

Puneet Bhargava

CLINICAL HISTORY *A 10-day-old neonate with respiratory distress*

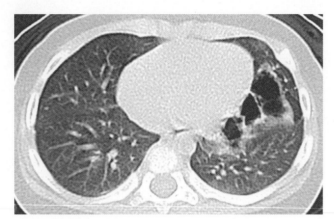

FIGURE **5.28A**

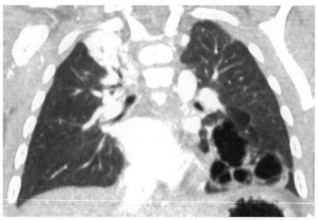

FIGURE **5.28B**

FINDINGS Axial (**A**) and coronal (**B**) images from a chest CT show multiple thin-walled cysts in the left lung. There is incidental right upper lobe atelectasis.

DIFFERENTIAL DIAGNOSIS CPAM, pulmonary sequestration, congenital diaphragmatic hernia (CDH), cavitary necrosis complicating pneumonia

DIAGNOSIS CPAM

DISCUSSION CPAM represents a mass of abnormal solid or cystic pulmonary tissue that may be due to an overgrowth of bronchial structures at the expense of alveolar development occurring at various stages of fetal lung development. CPAM most commonly presents with respiratory distress in the newborn. These lesions are now often diagnosed on prenatal ultrasound or MRI but may present later in life with recurrent infection or hemoptysis. Postnatal diagnosis is made with plain chest radiography. Imaging appearance varies from solid to multicystic mass with variable amounts of air and fluid. These lesions may cause local mass effect. CT shows a solid or multicystic mass with variable size of the cysts. The cysts may contain air–fluid levels. Variable amounts of enhancement may be seen in the cyst walls and solid component. Mediastinal shift or lung compression may be seen from mass effect.[1] Unlike congenital lobar emphysema, there is no lobar predilection. CT is useful for characterization of the lesions, evaluating extent, and surgical planning.[2]

CPAM was until recently known as congenital cystic adenomatoid malformation (CCAM) where a classification was made into three types depending on size of cysts: Type 1 CCAM, the most common, comprising one or more large, 2- to 10-cm cysts; type 2 with numerous small (0.5 to 2 cm)

cysts; and type 3 CCAM, a solid-appearing mass composed of bronchioalveolar microcysts. The more recent CPAM classification (types 0 to 4) also takes into account the fact that CPAMs are thought to originate at different levels of the tracheobronchial tree and at different stages of lung development: Type 0 arising principally from trachea or bronchi, with acinar dysgenesis or dysplasia, and having a solid appearance; type 1 bronchial or bronchiolar in origin; type 2 mainly bronchiolar in origin; type 3 bronchiolar or alveolar duct in origin; and type 4, appearing as large cysts, alveolar/acinar in origin.[3] Hybrid lesions, which have a systemic blood supply, have been described which have histologic and imaging features of both CPAM and pulmonary sequestration.[3] Some forms of CPAMs may represent the dysplastic consequences of airway obstruction in utero, which may explain the frequent imaging and pathologic overlap with other bronchopulmonary foregut malformations, including tracheal and bronchial atresia, pulmonary sequestration, and bronchogenic cyst.[4] Due to this overlap, there are those who suggest that it is more important to accurately describe the imaging findings rather than to insist on specific categorization.[4]

DIFFERENTIAL DIAGNOSTIC CONSIDERATIONS

Pulmonary sequestration is usually present in the left lower lobe, systemic arterial supply is present, and presence of air in sequestration suggests superimposed infection.

CDH presents as a multicystic air-containing mass and is less likely than CPAM to have an air–fluid level. There is paucity of gas in the abdomen and position of the nasogastric tube helps to diagnose this condition.

Patients with cavitary necrosis complicating pneumonia are usually quite ill and show temporal changes on radiographs. Surrounding consolidated lung is usually present.[1]

Questions for Further Thought

1. Is there a genetic predisposition to CPAM?
2. Which type of CPAM is most often associated with other congenital anomalies?

Reporting Responsibilities

- Describe location, size, and morphology of the cysts.
- Evaluate the aorta closely to exclude presence of systemic arterial supply.

What the Treating Physician Needs to Know

- Symptomatic CPAMs are managed with surgical resection.
- Surgical resection for asymptomatic CPAM is somewhat controversial but often performed due to risks of recurrent infection and malignancy.

Answers

1. CPAM can be associated with abnormalities of chromosome 18.

2. Type 2 lesions are associated with other congenital anomalies (such as esophageal atresia, renal dysgenesis, and other pulmonary malformations) in about 50% of the cases. The type 4 CPAM may be radiologically indistinguishable from cystic PPB.

REFERENCES

1. Larson D. Congenital pulmonary airway malformation. In: Donnelly LF, ed. *Diagnostic Imaging: Pediatrics.* 2nd ed. Salt Lake City, Utah: Amirsys; 2012;2:8–11.
2. Berrocal T, Madrid C, Novo S, et al. Congenital anomalies of the tracheobronchial tree, lung, and mediastinum: Embryology, radiology, and pathology. *Radiographics.* 2004;24(1):e17.
3. Biyyam DR, Chapman T, Ferguson MR, et al. Congenital lung abnormalities: Embryologic features, prenatal diagnosis, and postnatal radiologic-pathologic correlation. *Radiographics.* 2010; 30(6):1721–1738.
4. Newman B. Congenital bronchopulmonary foregut malformations: Concepts and controversies. *Pediatr Radiol.* 2006;36(8): 773–791.

Puneet Bhargava

CASE 5.29

CLINICAL HISTORY *A 5-month-old infant with an incidental mass in the left lower lobe*

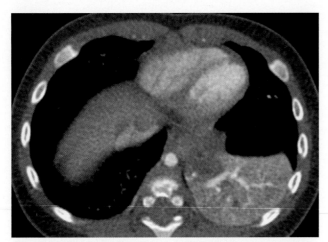

FIGURE **5.29A**

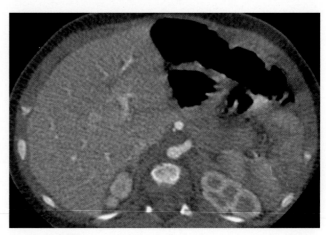

FIGURE **5.29B**

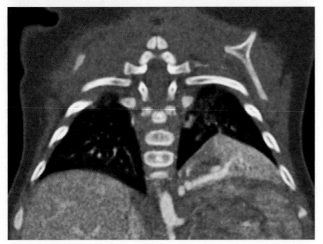

FIGURE **5.29C**

FINDINGS Axial (**A** and **B**) and coronal (**C**) CT images show a left lower lobe opacity with systemic arterial supply from descending thoracic aorta. No connection of the opacity to the bronchial tree was seen.

DIFFERENTIAL DIAGNOSIS Pulmonary sequestration, pneumonia, chronic bronchial obstruction, CPAM

DIAGNOSIS Pulmonary sequestration

DISCUSSION Pulmonary sequestration is a congenital area of dysplastic lung that does not connect to the bronchial tree and has anomalous systemic arterial supply, usually from the thoracic or abdominal aorta. Venous drainage is via the azygos system, pulmonary veins, or the IVC.[1] In extralobar sequestration, the mass is located outside normal lung (including below the hemidiaphragm) and has its own visceral pleura. Venous drainage is variable but often systemic. Intralobar sequestration is contained within lung and venous drainage is typically into inferior pulmonary veins. Patients with pulmonary sequestration may present with recurrent infection but the diagnosis may also be made as an incidental finding. The most common location is the left lower lobe. Imaging techniques such as CT, MRI, and sonography are used for diagnosis. Symptomatic lesions are treated with surgical resection.[2]

DIFFERENTIAL DIAGNOSTIC CONSIDERATIONS

Pneumonia and chronic bronchial obstruction do not have a systemic arterial supply. Patients with cavitary necrosis complicating pneumonia are typically quite ill and show temporal changes on chest x-rays. Presence of surrounding consolidated lung also helps to make this diagnosis. If chronic bronchial obstruction is suspected, a search for an aspirated foreign body or an endobronchial lesion such as a carcinoid should be performed. CPAM usually contains air. Air is typically not seen in sequestrated lung unless there is superimposed infection. However, sequestration may be present in conjunction with CPAM.[3]

Questions for Further Thought

1. Which are some imaging modalities that can be used to confirm the diagnosis of sequestration suspected on chest radiograph?
2. What are the management options for asymptomatic sequestration?

Reporting Responsibilities

- Describe the size and location of the sequestration.
- Describe the anatomy of the systemic arterial supply and try to define the venous return, to aid in surgical planning.

What the Treating Physician Needs to Know

- Consider sequestration in the differential diagnosis when there is recurrent left lower lobe pneumonia.
- Extralobar sequestration is associated with other congenital anomalies such as CPAM.

Answers

1. CT or MR angiography can be used to confirm the diagnosis of sequestration. Identification of the supplying systemic artery is the characteristic finding.
2. Management of asymptomatic cases can be either elective surgical resection or monitoring. However, it is easier to perform surgery prior to the lesion becoming infected.

REFERENCES

1. Berrocal T, Madrid C, Novo S, et al. Congenital anomalies of the tracheobronchial tree, lung, and mediastinum: Embryology, radiology, and pathology. *Radiographics.* 2004;24(1):e17.
2. Daltro P, Fricke BL, Kuroki I, et al. CT of congenital lung lesions in pediatric patients. *AJR Am J Roentgenol.* 2004;183(5): 1497–1506.
3. Larson D. Pulmonary sequestration. In: Donnelly LF, ed. *Diagnostic Imaging: Pediatrics.* 2nd ed. Salt Lake City, Utah: Amirsys; 2012;2:12–15.

CLINICAL HISTORY *A 14-year-old female with exercise intolerance*

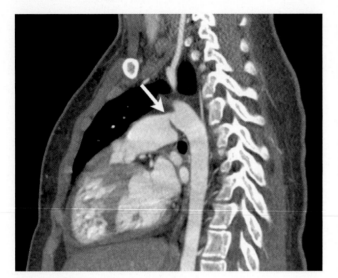

FIGURE **5.30A**

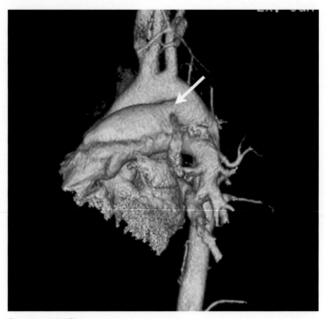

FIGURE **5.30B**

FINDINGS Parasagittal (**A**) and volume-rendered (**B**) images from a contrast-enhanced chest CT demonstrate an enhancing small tubular structure (*arrow*) extending from the superior aspect of the distal MPA to the proximal descending aorta, consistent with a PDA. Frontal and lateral chest radiographs (not shown) were normal.

DIFFERENTIAL DIAGNOSIS PDA

DIAGNOSIS PDA

DISCUSSION The ductus arteriosus embryologically derives from the sixth aortic arch. In fetal life, prostaglandins produced primarily within the placenta along with relatively low oxygen tension function to keep the ductus arteriosus open, allowing most (90%) of the right ventricular output to bypass the lungs. Upon birth, lung function is initiated, oxygen tension rises, and the placenta is removed, resulting in a marked drop in circulating prostaglandins. The ductus functionally closes at about 15 hours of life in a term infant, with true anatomic closure after several weeks. Premature infants have a higher incidence of ductal patency, thought to be related to the limited ability of the immature lung to metabolize prostaglandins, often compounded by hypoxia.

Overall, PDA represents approximately 10% to 12% of all congenital heart disease, most identified within the neonatal period.[1] A PDA can rarely persist later in life, and if accompanied by significant left to right shunting, the patient may develop congestive heart failure, with eventual development of pulmonary hypertension and Eisenmenger syndrome.

While an isolated patent ductus acts as a left to right shunt, the patent ductus is often seen in combination with, and is an essential feature of several types of complex congenital heart disease. For example, with pulmonary atresia, left to right flow through the ductus allows for oxygenation, while in d-TGA, a ductus helps with admixture. Reversed right to left shunting through a patent ductus is seen with HLH syndrome, preductal coarctation, and interrupted aortic arch, as a conduit for systemic perfusion.

With a left aortic arch, the ductus typically extends from the junction of the main and left pulmonary arteries to the proximal descending thoracic aorta just distal to the origin of the left subclavian artery. With a right aortic arch, the configuration is more varied, most commonly arising from the left pulmonary artery and inserting into the left innominate artery, and less commonly extending from the right pulmonary artery to the right subclavian artery. A right-sided ductus and bilateral ducti can occur, often associated with aortic arch or conotruncal anomalies.

PDAs have a wide range of age at presentation. In the premature infant with uncomplicated surfactant deficiency, radiographs typically stabilize or begin to improve by 3 to 5 days of life. If at this time there is a worsening pattern of perihilar hazy opacities, one should consider a PDA which is manifesting with the normal decline in perinatal pulmonary vascular resistance.[2] Older patients with PDA may show a prominent ascending aorta and left atrial enlargement. Later radiographic signs in older patients may also include visualization of the enlarged ductal outline at the level of the aorticopulmonary window, and peripheral eggshell calcifications. Enlarged pulmonary arteries related to the left to right shunt can eventually become "pruned" with the development of Eisenmenger physiology. If the patent ductus is small with minimal shunting, the radiographs may remain normal, as in the presented case. Echocardiography is often diagnostic for patent ductus.

Questions for Further Thought

1. Does the presence of ductal calcification have clinical implications?
2. What other imaging can be helpful in the management of a PDA?
3. What are some potential complications of surgical ductal ligation?

Reporting Responsibilities

- Recognition of this abnormality when present.
- Description of the ductal morphologic details.

What the Treating Physician Needs to Know

- Ductal morphology—length, diameter, anatomic connections. This will affect management options.
- Quantification of shunt (MRI).
- Secondary findings of long-standing pulmonary hypertension, such as right ventricular hypertrophy and pruning of pulmonary arterial vasculature.

Answers

1. Both CT and conventional radiographs may demonstrate incidental calcifications in the residual ligamentum arteriosum following normal ductal closure, which may resolve later in childhood.[3,4] However, adults with a long-standing patent ductus arteriosus have also been shown to develop associated calcifications (readily assessed with ECG-gated multidetector CT), which, along with ductal morphology, may affect therapeutic options.[5]

2. MRI with phase-contrast flow analysis can be very helpful for quantification of Qp/Qs (ratio of pulmonary to systemic flow, normally 1:1, but increased with left to right shunts) and assessment of ventricular size and function.

3. Injuries to the recurrent laryngeal nerve, phrenic nerve, and thoracic duct.

REFERENCES

1. Goitein O, Fuhrman CR, Lacomis JM. Incidental finding on MDCT of patent ductus arteriosus: Use of CT and MRI to assess clinical importance. *AJR Am J Roentgenol.* 2005;184(6):1924–1931.
2. Slovis TL, Shankaran S. Patent ductus arteriosus in hyaline membrane disease: Chest radiography. *AJR Am J Roentgenol.* 1980;135(2):307–309.
3. Currarino G, Jackson JH. Calcification of the ductus arteriosus and ligamentum botalli. *Radiology.* 1970;94(1):139–142.
4. Bisceglia M, Donaldson JS. Calcification of the ligamentum arteriosum in children: A normal finding on CT. *AJR Am J Roentgenol.* 1991;156(2):351–352.
5. Morgan-Hughes GJ, Marshall, AJ, Roobottom C. Morphologic assessment of patent ductus arteriosus in adults using retrospectively ECG-gated multidetector CT. *AJR Am J Roentgenol.* 2003;181(3):749–754.

Randolph K. Otto

CLINICAL HISTORY *A 5-year-old boy who presents with hypertension*

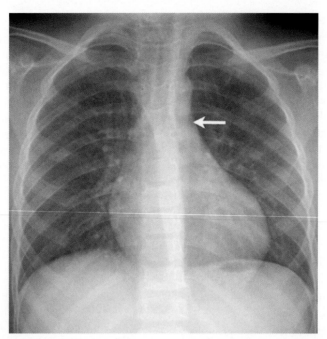

FIGURE **5.31A**

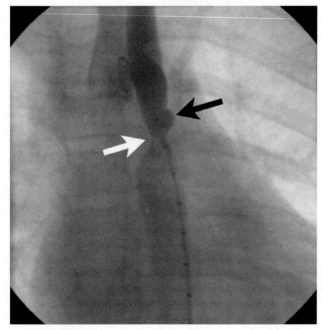

FIGURE **5.31B**

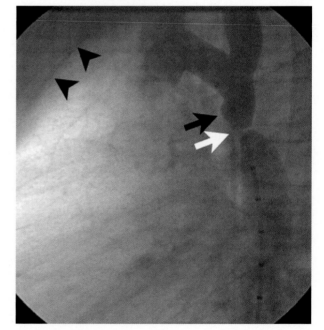

FIGURE **5.31C**

FINDINGS Frontal chest radiograph (**A**) demonstrates a focal indentation of the proximal descending aorta (*white arrow,* "three sign"). Frontal (**B**) and lateral (**C**) projections from a thoracic aortogram demonstrate a severe focal narrowing of the proximal descending aorta (*white arrow*) immediately distal to a normal ductus bump (*black arrow*). An enlarged internal mammary artery is identified on the lateral projection (*black arrowheads*).

DIFFERENTIAL DIAGNOSIS Aortic coarctation, pseudocoarctation

DIAGNOSIS Aortic coarctation

DISCUSSION Coarctation of the aorta is a congenital focal narrowing of the aorta, typically just distal to the origin of the left subclavian artery (juxtaductal), although stenosis may extend to involve the arch and isthmic regions. Aortic coarctation represents approximately 7% of all congenital heart disease, with a male predominance.[1]

The exact pathogenesis is unknown, but migration of ductal tissue into the aortic wall is perhaps the most widely accepted theory. Another theory suggests that abnormalities in preductal aortic flow, such as with HLH syndrome, bicuspid aortic valve, or a large VSD, produce hemodynamic alterations leading to the coarctation.[2]

Aortic coarctation is frequently an isolated finding, but multiple associated conditions are known, including Turner syndrome (occurring in 35%), bicuspid aortic valve (22% to 42%), intracranial aneurysms (10%), aortic aneurysm, VSD, ASD, and Shone complex. Coarctation is often associated with tubular hypoplasia, which is defined as a combination of a small diameter (for the distal arch, less than 50% of the ascending aorta) and increased length between arch segments.[2]

Classic radiographic findings of aortic coarctation include rib notching relating to collateral blood flow, the "three sign" (indented contour of the proximal descending aorta corresponding to the site of coarctation), and post-stenotic dilation. However, aortic coarctation is now most often first identified on echocardiography in the neonatal period and early childhood, prior to development of radiographic signs. Aortic coarctation may currently be managed surgically or via transcatheter interventional techniques (balloon angioplasty without or with stent placement).

Questions for Further Thought

1. What are the complications of untreated aortic coarctation?
2. What are potential complications of treated aortic coarctation?
3. What are other etiologies of aortic narrowing/stenosis, and how do they differ from typical coarctation?

Reporting Responsibilities

- Precise description of primary coarctation morphology.
- Any associated conditions, including location, shape, and length of associated hypoplastic segments.
- Presence of collateral arterial supply.
- Hemodynamic assessment (MRI).

What the Treating Physician Needs to Know

- MRI with phase-contrast analysis can be quite helpful in determining the presence of any hemodynamically significant stenosis or collateral blood supply to the distal aorta.[3]
- Any morphologic abnormalities which may guide therapeutic options (aneurysm, extensive stenosis or associated hypoplasia, involvement of brachiocephalic vessels, etc.).

Answers

1. Congestive heart failure may occur in the neonatal period as well as later in adulthood. Long-term complications of hypertension include aortic rupture, dissection, valvular insufficiency, infectious endocarditis, coronary artery disease, and intracranial hemorrhage from associated intracranial aneurysms.

2. Recurrent stenosis, dissection, aneurysm formation, and rupture.[4]

3. Other etiologies of aortic narrowing/stenosis include Williams syndrome, Takayasu arteritis, neurofibromatosis, and middle aortic syndrome, but these generally have differing anatomic distribution (ascending, abdominal, generalized, or multifocal) and morphologic appearances (long segment, mural thickening). Pseudocoarctation refers to an elongated redundant aorta with buckling in a similar juxtaductal location, but patients are asymptomatic without hemodynamic changes.

REFERENCES

1. Brickner ME, Hillis LD, Lange RA. Congenital heart disease in adults. First of two parts. *N Engl J Med.* 2000;342(4):256–263.
2. Kimura-Hayama ET, Meléndez G, Mendizábal AL, et al. Uncommon congenital and acquired aortic diseases: Role of multidetector CT angiography. *Radiographics.* 2010;30(1):79–98.
3. Konen E, Merchant N, Provost Y, et al. Coarctation of the aorta before and after correction: The role of cardiovascular MRI. *AJR Am J Roentgenol.* 2004;182(5):1333–1339.
4. Shih MC, Tholpady A, Kramer CM, et al. Surgical and endovascular repair of aortic coarctation: normal findings and appearance of complications on CT angiography and MR angiography. *AJR Am J Roentgenol.* 2006;187(3):W302–W312.

Paritosh C. Khanna

CASE 5.32

CLINICAL HISTORY *A 5-year-old female who presents with a tender right postauricular mass (Figs. 5.32A and B)*

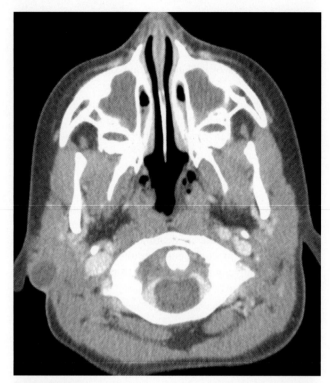

FIGURE 5.32A

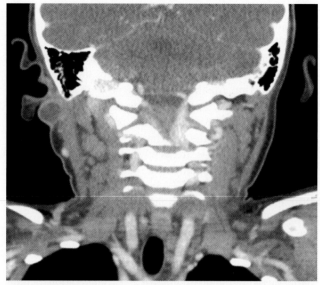

FIGURE 5.32B

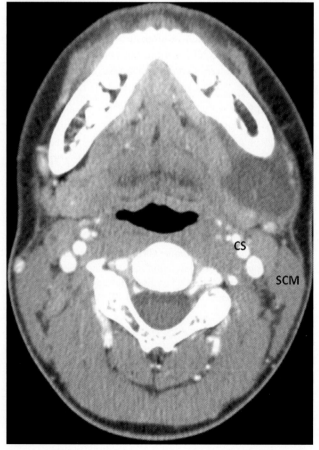

FIGURE 5.32C

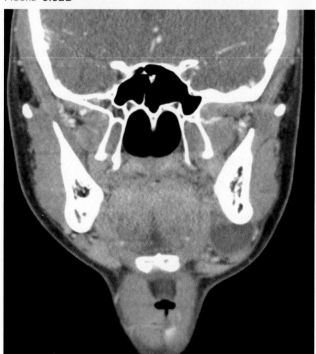

FIGURE 5.32D

FINDINGS Axial (**A**) and coronal (**B**) contrast-enhanced CT images demonstrate a well-circumscribed, rim-enhancing lesion within the posterior aspect of the parotid gland on the right, at the level of the mastoid tip. There is minimal surrounding fat stranding. In a different 16-year-old male who presented with focal swelling near the angle of the mandible on the left side, axial (**C**) and coronal (**D**) contrast-enhanced CT images demonstrate a well-circumscribed, hypodense lesion anterior to the sternocleidomastoid (SCM) muscle and anterolateral to the carotid space (CS).

DIFFERENTIAL DIAGNOSIS Branchial cleft cyst that is likely infected, soft-tissue abscess/parotid abscess, infected lymphangioma, necrotic infected lymph node(s), lymphoepithelial cysts

DIAGNOSIS Branchial cleft cyst that is likely infected

DISCUSSION Branchial cleft cysts (also known as branchial apparatus anomalies or branchial apparatus cysts) are remnants of the branchial apparatus due to incomplete involution during embryonic development. Although typically appearing as cysts, sinus tracts and fistulae may also occur. Branchial cleft cysts are often asymptomatic unless they become infected.

Four types of branchial cleft cysts have been described[1,2]:

First branchial cleft cysts (~5%) may be located around the pinna and the external auditory canal, adjacent to the mandibular angle, or in or around the parotid gland.

Second branchial cleft cysts represent the vast majority (~90%). These are further subdivided into four types. Type I: Superficial and anterior to SCM muscle; type II: most common, classically anterior to SCM, lateral to CS and posterior to submandibular gland; type III: between internal and external carotid arteries; and type IV: pharyngeal mucosal space.

Third branchial cleft cysts (rare) may be found anywhere along the following course: Starting at the pyriform sinus, posterior to common or internal carotid arteries, extending through the thyrohyoid membrane and into the superior mediastinum. The larynx may be involved.

Fourth branchial cleft cysts (rare) typically follow the course of the recurrent laryngeal nerve and may be found extending along left pyriform sinus, thyrohyoid membrane, and left lobe of the thyroid gland.

Branchial cleft cysts are generally unilocular, hypoattenuating on CT, and well circumscribed with walls that typically do not enhance with contrast unless infected, in which case walls may be thick and irregular with surrounding fat stranding. Previously infected cysts may have isodense contents from residual proteinaceous material. On MRI, branchial cleft cysts are typically hypointense on T1-weighted, and hyperintense on T2-weighted, short-tau inversion recovery (STIR) and fluid-attenuated inversion recovery (FLAIR) sequences. However, there may be variable signal intensity if previously or currently infected. On T2-weighted imaging, a sinus tract may be visualized. Ultrasound has also been found useful for imaging these lesions; probe-tenderness, internal echoes, and surrounding hyperemia confirm clinical suspicion of superimposed infection.[3,4]

DIFFERENTIAL DIAGNOSTIC CONSIDERATIONS

Soft-tissue abscess/parotid abscess: Can be indistinguishable from an infected branchial cleft cyst; may be multilocular and irregular with a lot of surrounding fat stranding.

Infected lymphangioma: Usually multilocular, insinuating along fascial planes within the soft tissues of the neck.

Necrotic, infected lymph node(s): Usually preceded by lymphadenopathy.

Lymphoepithelial cysts: Seen in patients with HIV; rare in children; often multiple and bilateral; hypertrophied lymphoid follicles may be associated.

Questions for Further Thought

1. How do patients with branchial cleft cyst?
2. What types of branchial cleft cyst do the above examples most likely represent?

Reporting Responsibilities

Lesion location, likely type, and whether the branchial cleft cyst appears infected by imaging.

What the Treating Physician Needs to Know

Location of branchial cleft cyst and whether it may be infected.

Answers

1. Palpable neck mass, tenderness, and erythema when infected.
2. Index case: First branchial cleft cyst. Additional case: Second branchial cleft cyst, type II.

REFERENCES

1. Benson MT, Dalen K, Mancuso AA, et al. Congenital anomalies of the branchial apparatus: Embryology and pathologic anatomy. *Radiographics.* 1992;12(5):943–960.
2. Koeller KK, Alamo L, Adair CF, et al. Congenital cystic masses of the neck: Radiologic-pathologic correlation. *Radiographics.* 1999;19(1):121–146.
3. Koch BL. Cystic malformations of the neck in children. *Pediatr Radiol.* 2005;35(5):463–477.
4. Rosa PA, Hirsch DL, Dierks EJ. Congenital neck masses. *Oral Maxillofac Surg Clin North Am.* 2008;20(3):339–352.

CASE 5.33

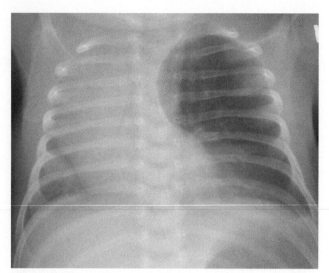

FIGURE **5.33A**

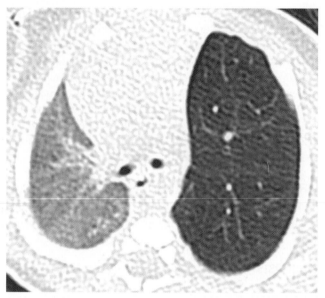

FIGURE **5.33B**

FINDINGS Frontal radiograph (**A**) and axial CT (**B**) images show hyperinflation of the left upper lobe with mass effect.

DIFFERENTIAL DIAGNOSIS Congenital lobar emphysema, congenital pulmonary airway malformation (CPAM), pulmonary artery hypoplasia, pulmonary hypoplasia, pulmonary interstitial emphysema (PIE)

DIAGNOSIS Congenital lobar emphysema

DISCUSSION Congenital lobar emphysema (also known as congenital lobar overinflation) usually involves a single lobe (most commonly the left upper lobe) and presents with respiratory distress in the neonate. It is thought to result from a check-valve mechanism at the bronchial level that causes progressive hyperinflation by allowing more air to enter the involved lobe on inspiration than what leaves on expiration. Classically, progression from a radiodense pulmonary lobe (due to retention of fetal lung fluid) to a progressively hyperlucent and hyperexpanded lobe is usually seen. Diagnosis is typically made by chest radiography. CT shows an expanded lobe with attenuated vascular structures, air trap-ping with lobar hyperinflation, and contralateral mediastinal shift with compression of the lung.[1] CT helps to confirm the diagnosis and to exclude other causes of hyperinflation.[2]

DIFFERENTIAL DIAGNOSTIC CONSIDERATIONS

In most cases of CPAM, air is contained in abnormal cystic spaces of varying sizes. In both pulmonary artery hypoplasia and pulmonary aplasia the affected lung is small and there is no air-trapping. Rarely, PIE can persist and present as an expanding hyperlucent mass. The pulmonary vessels and bronchi may be seen to be surrounded by air.[3]

Questions for Further Thought

1. In what percentage of cases can a cause for congenital lobar emphysema be found?

2. What is the incidence of associated abnormalities?

Reporting Responsibilities

• Describe the lobe involved and the extent of involvement.

• Exclude other causes of hyperlucent neonatal lung lesions.

What the Treating Physician Needs to Know

- The majority of cases of congenital lobar emphysema present in the neonatal period and infancy with respiratory distress. Diagnosis is typically made with chest radiography.
- Surgical lobectomy may need to be performed on an emergency basis if progressive hyperinflation occurs. Conservative treatment may be adopted for those with minimal symptoms or if found as an incidental finding. Over time, the involved lobe typically becomes atrophic.

Answers

1. A cause can be found in approximately 50% of cases, such as abnormality of bronchial wall, mucosal web, and extrinsic compression.

2. Congenital heart disease is associated in 14% to 50% of patients.

REFERENCES

1. Daltro P, Fricke BL, Kuroki I, et al. CT of congenital lung lesions in pediatric patients. *AJR Am J Roentgenol.* 2004;183(5): 1497–1506.

2. Berrocal T, Madrid C, Novo S, et al. Congenital anomalies of the tracheobronchial tree, lung, and mediastinum: Embryology, radiology, and pathology. *Radiographics.* 2004;24(1):e17.

3. Larson D. Congenital lobar emphysema. In: Donnelly LF, ed. *Diagnostic Imaging: Pediatrics.* 2nd ed. Salt Lake City, Utah: Amirsys; 2012;2:20–23.

CASE 5.34

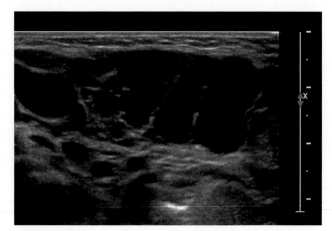

FIGURE **5.34A**

FINDINGS Ultrasound (**A**) and axial contrast-enhanced CT (**B**) at the level of the neck show a large cystic mass with multiple septations which are better appreciated by ultrasound.

DIFFERENTIAL DIAGNOSIS Lymphatic malformation, venous-lymphatic malformation, branchial cleft cyst, soft-tissue sarcoma

DIAGNOSIS Lymphatic malformation of the head and neck

DISCUSSION Lymphatic malformation of the head and neck (also know as cystic hygroma) represents abnormal dilation of endothelial lined lymphatic spaces that are thought to result from either an early sequestration of embryonic lymphatic channels or failure of lymphatics to drain adequately into adjacent veins. Most lymphatic malformations are detected by 2 years of age, with many identified in infancy. A typical presentation is that of an infant with a compressible soft-tissue neck mass. Rapid enlargement related to hemorrhage or infection may also lead to patient presentation. Patients are often asymptomatic but a large mass can cause symptoms due to extrinsic pressure such as feeding difficulties or symptoms related to airway compromise.[1,2]

Lymphatic malformations of the head and neck are usually multilocular, occasionally unilocular, thin-walled lymph-containing cystic spaces most commonly involving the posterior cervical space as well as the submandibular, parotid, and masticator spaces. These lesions are characteristically infiltrative with a propensity for local extension across multiple neck spaces, as well as inferiorly into the axilla and superior mediastinum or superiorly into the floor of the mouth and tongue.

On ultrasound, lymphatic malformations are typically seen as a multilocular cystic mass with septations of

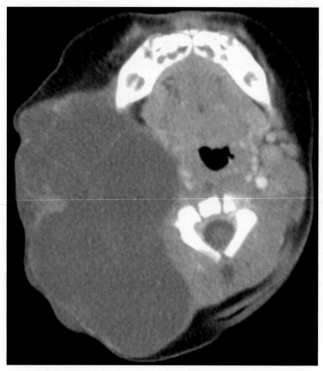

FIGURE **5.34B**

variable thickness. Fluid–fluid levels may be seen if there is internal hemorrhage. On CT, they are imaged as poorly circumscribed, multiloculated hypodense masses with fluid attenuation values. On MRI, the most common pattern is that of a mass or masses with intermediate to low T1 and hyperintense T2 signal intensity. Thin, almost imperceptible walls may be seen on both CT and MRI. Internal debris or fluid–fluid levels resulting from hemorrhage or less commonly infection may also be seen. An added venous component, if present, may show presence of phleboliths as well as dilated, variably enhancing vascular spaces following contrast administration. Treatment of lymphatic malformation may involve sclerotherapy or surgical resection. Venous-lymphatic malformations may also be treated in a similar manner.[3]

DIFFERENTIAL DIAGNOSTIC CONSIDERATIONS

Venous-lymphatic malformations also have a vascular component that enhances and may have phleboliths.

Branchial cleft cysts are generally unilocular and well circumscribed with walls that typically do not enhance with contrast unless infected.

Soft-tissue sarcoma should be suspected in the presence of associated soft tissue and lack of MR features which suggest a vascular/lymphatic malformation.

Questions for Further Thought

1. What imaging study is recommended for a posterior cervical space lymphatic malformation?
2. What complication may be seen due to a viral infection in a patient with lymphatic malformation?

Reporting Responsibilities

- Describe the location and extent of the lymphatic malformation, especially extension into the mediastinum and axilla.
- Evaluate for areas of internal hemorrhage and local mass effect.

What the Treating Physician Needs to Know

- Extent of the lymphatic malformation, including possible extension into the upper mediastinum and axilla.
- Although these masses usually grow slowly, they may suddenly increase in size secondary to hemorrhage, trauma, or viral infection. Mass effect may produce facial nerve paralysis and dysphagia.

Answers

1. Although ultrasound is usually sufficient for the diagnosis of posterior cervical space lymphatic malformation, MRI or CT scan is often required to evaluate for possible extension into the mediastinum and axilla.
2. Viral infections may cause a sudden increase in size of a lymphatic malformation, thought due to production of a large amount of lymphatic fluid from the lymphoid follicles located in the cyst wall.

REFERENCES

1. Koeller KK, Alamo L, Adair CF, et al. Congenital cystic masses of the neck: radiologic-pathologic correlation. *Radiographics.* 1999;19(1);121–146.
2. Koch BL. Lymphatic Malformation. In: Harnsberger HR, ed. *Diagnostic Imaging: Head and Neck.* 2nd ed. Salt Lake City, Utah: Amirsys; 2011;III:1:6–9.
3. Giguère CM, Bauman NM, Smith RJ. New treatment options for lymphangioma in infants and children. *Ann Otol Rhinol Laryngol.* 2002;111(12 Pt 1):1066–1075.

Randolph K. Otto

CASE 5.35

CLINICAL HISTORY *A 19-month-old female with cyanosis and harsh 5/6 holosystolic murmur.*

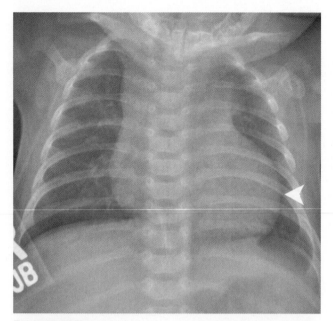

FIGURE **5.35A**

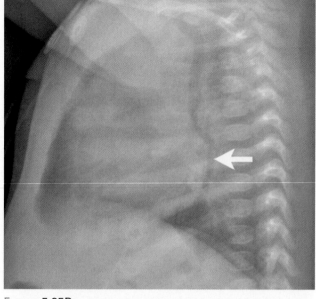

FIGURE **5.35B**

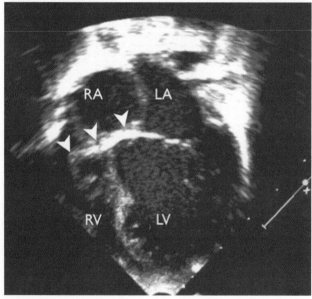

FIGURE **5.35C**

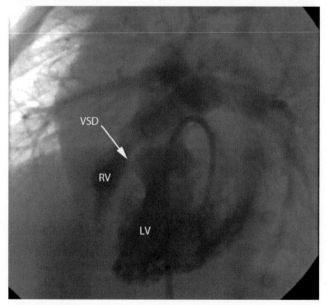

FIGURE **5.35D**

FINDINGS Frontal (**A**) and lateral (**B**) chest radiographs reveal a prominent left ventricular contour (*arrowhead*) and left atrium (*arrow*), with normal to decreased pulmonary vascularity. Horizontal long-axis echocardiographic image (**C**) demonstrates a solid echogenic tissue plate in the expected location of the tricuspid valve (*white arrowheads*), hypoplastic RV, and enlarged LV (LA, left atrium; RA, right atrium). LAO image from left ventriculography (**D**) demonstrates a VSD (*white arrow*) with opacification of the hypoplastic RV and enlarged LV.

DIFFERENTIAL DIAGNOSIS Tricuspid atresia or stenosis

DIAGNOSIS Tricuspid atresia with small VSD and normally related great arteries

DISCUSSION The radiographic differential diagnosis for a patient with cyanosis and decreased pulmonary vasculature includes tricuspid atresia/stenosis, TOF, pulmonary atresia, d-TGA with pulmonary stenosis, as well as Ebstein anomaly.

In the presented patient with tricuspid atresia, the diagnosis was initially made by prenatal sonography, confirmed postnatally, and the patient was referred for surgical consultation at the time of this evaluation.

Tricuspid atresia represents approximately 1.4% to 2.9% (clinical versus autopsy series) of all congenital heart disease and is the third most common form of cyanotic congenital heart disease, after TOF and TGA.[1] About 50% of patients with tricuspid atresia develop symptoms within the first day of life, and 80% present by 1 month. Most patients with tricuspid atresia present with cyanosis, but those with d-TGA have congestive heart failure and manifest with failure to thrive, recurrent respiratory tract infections, and perspiration. Late development of cyanosis, cardiac murmur, and exercise intolerance are also reported.

Classification of tricuspid atresia is based on position of the great arteries (types I to IV) as well as degree of pulmonary artery atresia/stenosis (a, b, or c):

Type I: Normally related great arteries, 70% to 80%.

Type II: d-TGA, 12% to 25%.

Type III: Great artery positional abnormalities other than d-TGA, 3% to 6%.

Type IV: Persistent truncus arteriosus.

a. Pulmonary artery atresia.

b. Pulmonary artery stenosis or hypoplasia.

c. No pulmonary artery stenosis.

Tricuspid atresia can also be classified according to the valvular morphology, with the muscular form accounting for 89%.

All instances of tricuspid atresia require the presence of an ASD to allow systemic venous return. Most (95%) also have a VSD of variable size, which dictates the resulting degree of right ventricular and pulmonary arterial hypoplasia. Generally, those patients with normally related great arteries (type I) present with cyanosis and decreased pulmonary vascularity on radiographs. In approximately 20% of cases of tricuspid atresia, the great arteries are transposed (d-TGA, type II), leading to pulmonary overcirculation from the LV. There is frequently associated subaortic stenosis, aortic coarctation, or interruption of the aortic arch, with failure to thrive, thought related to the decreased proximal aortic flow.

Diagnosis of tricuspid atresia is generally made during the prenatal[2] or early postnatal period with echocardiography. Radiographs can demonstrate left atrial enlargement (50%), left ventricular enlargement (frequently simulating right ventricular enlargement), and concavity in the region of the MPA. Decreased pulmonary vascularity is seen in 80%, and right aortic arch in 8%. Cardiac catheterization is often performed before surgical palliation for further anatomic definition, and MRI can be helpful in long-term assessment of ventricular function.

Questions for Further Thought

1. Can patients with tricuspid atresia survive without intervention?

2. What are the usual methods of surgical palliation for tricuspid atresia?

Reporting Responsibilities

- Include tricuspid atresia in the differential diagnosis of cyanotic congenital heart disease and normal to decreased pulmonary vasculature.

- Remember that for those patients with tricuspid atresia and d-TGA, the clinical presentation and radiographs are quite different, with increased pulmonary vasculature.

- Document the presence and size of the associated atrial and VSDs when identified with the use of advanced imaging modalities.

What the Treating Physician Needs to Know

- Currently, radiologists are most often asked to assist in the long-term care of patients with tricuspid atresia by measuring ventricular function and Qp/Qs (ratio of pulmonary to systemic flow). MRI can also be helpful in classification of the morphology of the atretic valve.[3]

- The coexistence of subaortic stenosis or arterial hypoplasia (pulmonary or aortic) is important, as it influences the surgical management of tricuspid atresia.[4]

Answers

1. If the ASD is unrestrictive with an adequately sized VSD, there may be sufficient pulmonary blood flow to allow survival without palliation.

2. Generally, those patients with normally related great arteries are initially managed with a systemic to pulmonary shunt, and ASD or VSD enlargement. Those patients with transposed arteries and pulmonary overcirculation receive pulmonary artery banding. Subsequent management includes staged creation of a bidirectional cavopulmonary shunt (Glenn) and modified Fontan procedure (IVC-pulmonary conduit).

REFERENCES

1. Rao PS. Demographic features of tricuspid atresia. In: Rao PS, ed. *Tricuspid Atresia*. 2nd ed. Mount Kisco, NY: Futura; 1992: 23–37.

2. Tongsong T, Sittiwangkul R, Wanapirak C, et al. Prenatal diagnosis of isolated tricuspid valve atresia: Report of 4 cases and review of the literature. *J Ultrasound Med.* 2004;23(7):945–950.

3. Fletcher BD, Jacobstein MD, Abramowski CR, et al. Right atrioventricular valve atresia: Anatomic evaluation with MR imaging. *AJR Am J Roentgenol.* 1987;148(4):671–674.

4. Sittiwangkul R, Azakie A, Van Arsdell GS, et al. Outcomes of tricuspid atresia in the Fontan era. *Ann Thorac Surg.* 2004; 77(3):889–894.

Sandra L. Wootton-Gorges

CLINICAL HISTORY *A 14-year-old boy with chest wall deformity*

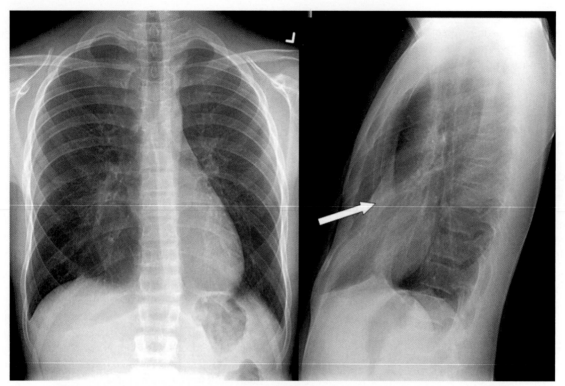

FIGURE 5.36A

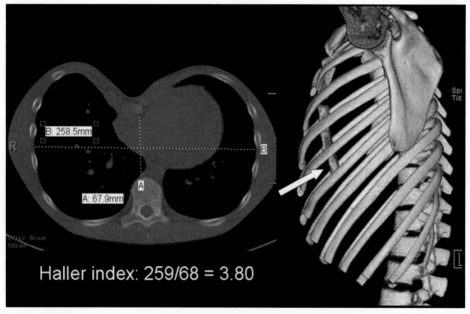

Haller index: 259/68 = 3.80

FIGURE 5.36B

FINDINGS Frontal and lateral views of the chest (**A**) show a blurred right heart border and vertically oriented anterior ribs and a depressed sternum (*arrow*). The patient does not have scoliosis. Non-contrast CT of the chest (**B**) shows a pectus (Haller) index of 3.8. The three-dimensional (3D) reconstruction nicely demonstrates the sternal depression (*arrow*) and deformity. The pectus or Haller index is calculated on this non-contrast CT chest image by dividing the lateral chest diameter by the A–P diameter. The postoperative images (**C**) after Nuss procedure show less depression of the lower sternum (*arrow*). There is postoperative pneumomediastinum, subcutaneous emphysema, and bilateral pleural effusions, as well as left basilar atelectasis.

DIAGNOSIS Pectus excavatum, or funnel chest

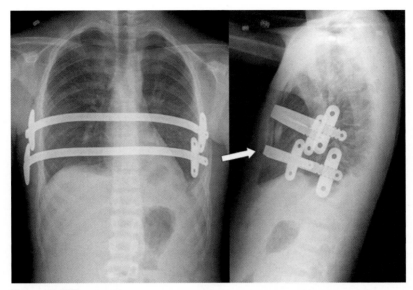

FIGURE **5.36C**

DISCUSSION Pectus excavatum is a common chest wall deformity in children, and is seen in up to 1/400.[1] It usually involves the lower sternum near the xiphoid, and is thought to develop from rapid and misdirected growth of coastal cartilages.[2] Most patients present during their pubertal growth spurt with deformity.[3] Some also have exercise intolerance. Eighty percent are boys, and up to 45% of cases are familial. Connective tissue disorders such as Marfan syndrome may be seen in about 20%. Twenty to thirty percent may have associated scoliosis. Workup includes physical examination, pulmonary function testing, and cardiac evaluation.[3] Chest radiography is used to define the deformity (**A**). Noncontrast CT is often obtained to calculate the Haller, or pectus, index. This is obtained by dividing the greatest width of the chest by the narrowest A–P diameter. The normal pectus index is 2.56 (standard deviation 0.35).[2] Three-dimensional reconstruction may further define the chest wall deformity. Recent studies have suggested the Haller index calculated from the chest radiograph (greatest width from the frontal radiograph, and A–P diameter from the lateral) is as useful as from CT, with much less radiation exposure.[1]

Pectus excavatum is treated with minimally invasive surgery, or the Nuss procedure (Fig. 5.36C). Indications for surgery, besides cosmetic issues, may include a Haller or pectus index of 3.25 or greater, restrictive or obstructive lung disease, cardiac compression (seen by echocardiography), conduction abnormalities, mitral valve prolapse, or murmurs.[3]

Questions for Further Thought

1. Why is the right heart border blurred on the frontal radiograph in patients with pectus excavatum?
2. What are other associated abnormalities which may be seen in patients with pectus excavatum.

Reporting Responsibilities

- Describe the pectus excavatum deformity.
- Calculate the pectus index.
- Note if associated abnormalities including scoliosis or changes of Marfan syndrome (dilated ascending aorta, for example) are present. Give the degree of scoliosis if present.

What the Treating Physician Needs to Know

- The pectus index.
- If there are associated abnormalities, such as scoliosis.

Answers

1. The right side of the heart is compressed between the depressed sternum and the spine. This blurs the right heart border, which may be mistaken for right middle lobe pneumonia. The heart is also displaced to the left, mimicking cardiomegaly.

2. While most often an isolated abnormality, pectus excavatum may be associated with prematurity, connective tissue disorders (Marfan syndrome, Ehlers–Danlos syndrome), homocystinuria, and Noonan syndrome.

REFERENCES

1. Khanna G, Jaju A, Don S, et al. Comparison of Haller index values calculated with chest radiographs versus CT for pectus excavatum evaluation. *Pediatr Radiol.* 2010;40:1763–1767.
2. Restrepo CS, Martinez S, Lemos DF, et al. Imaging appearances of the sternum and sternoclavicular joints. *Radiographics.* 2009;29:839–859.
3. Nuss D, Kelly RE. Indications and technique of Nuss procedure for pectus excavatum. *Thorac Surg Clin.* 2010;20:583–597.

Marguerite T. Parisi

CASE 5.37

CLINICAL HISTORY *Two newborns (Figs. 5.37A and B), each presenting for technetium 99m pertechnetate scintigraphy (Tc-99m O₄), following abnormal neonatal thyroid screening testing*

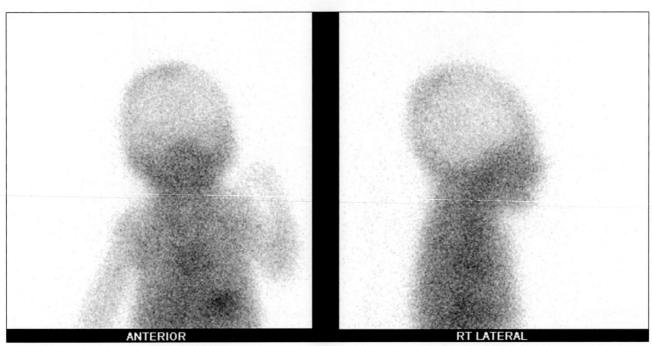

FIGURE 5.37A

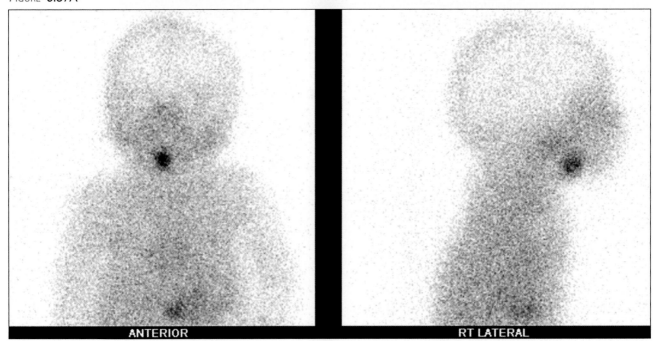

FIGURE 5.37B

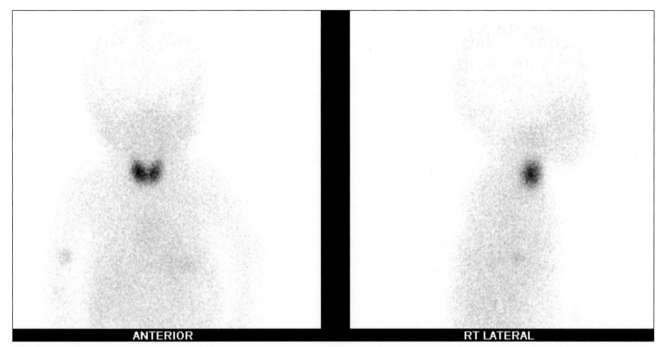

ANTERIOR　　RT LATERAL

FIGURE 5.37C

FINDINGS In the first child, anterior and lateral views from Tc-99m O$_4$ thyroid scan (**A**) reveal absence of radiotracer uptake in thyroidal tissue, in either an orthotopic or an ectopic location. In the second child, anterior and lateral views from Tc-99m O$_4$ scintigraphy (**B**) reveal absent uptake in the expected position of the thyroid gland. Rather, there is abnormal uptake in an ectopic, sublingual location. A normal Tc-99m O$_4$ thyroid scan (**C**) in a different newborn is presented for comparison.

DIFFERENTIAL DIAGNOSIS

- Absent radiotracer uptake (Fig. 5.37A): Primary hypothyroidism due to thyroid agenesis; secondary or central hypothyroidism (hypopituitarism, hypothalamic etiologies, others); transient hypothyroidism most commonly due to maternal thyrotropin receptor-blocking antibodies (TRB-Abs), among other causes.
- Ectopic radiotracer uptake (Fig. 5.37B): Ectopic thyroid gland; thyroid hemiagenesis (single-lobed gland typically in eutopic position).

DIAGNOSIS Both of the cases illustrated are due to primary congenital hypothyroidism (CH) caused by thyroid dysgenesis, that is, disordered thyroid gland development. Specific diagnoses are thyroid agenesis (**A**) and thyroid ectopia (**B**).

DISCUSSION CH, defined as thyroid hormone deficiency at birth, is one of the most common preventable causes of mental retardation. The overall incidence of CH is approximately 1 in 4000 with females affected twice as often as males.[1,2] The majority of cases of CH are sporadic (85%), due to thyroid dysgenesis, with an ectopic gland (66%) substantially more common than either thyroid agenesis or hypoplasia. The most common form of hereditary CH, occurring in 10% of patients, involves an inborn error of thyroxine (T4) synthesis (dyshormonogenesis), and is typically due to defects in thyroid peroxidase activity. A transient form of familial CH occurring in 5% of congenital hypothyroid patients is the result of transplacental passage of maternal TRB-Abs.

Physical examination detects only about 5% of infants with CH as most affected newborns lack the specific clinical features of hypothyroidism.[1] Rather, these patients first come to medical attention via newborn screening programs obtained from heel stick blood samples eluted from filter paper. Abnormal screening tests must be confirmed by serum thyroid function tests including free triiodothyronine (T3), T4, and thyroid stimulating hormone (TSH, thyrotropin) obtained from a venipuncture blood sample.

Once CH is confirmed, further diagnostic testing can be used to determine the underlying etiology.[1–5] Controversy exists as to whether or not supplemental testing should be performed as, in many cases, the results do not alter patient management.

Since thyroid dysgenesis is the most common form of CH, LaFranchi[1,2] and Sfakianaskis[3] consider thyroid scintigraphy using either Tc-99m O_4 or iodine-123 (I-123) to be the most informative supplemental test. Ultrasound is nearly as accurate as scintigraphy in detecting an enlarged or absent thyroid gland but occasionally misses an ectopic gland. Chang et al.[5] propose that the use of both scintigraphy and ultrasound results in a more complete depiction of neonatal CH than either test alone. As infants with thyroid agenesis have been shown to have a slightly worse intellectual prognosis than those with ectopic glands, the distinction is of prognostic significance.[2]

According to Sfakianakis,[3] there are four characteristic patterns of radiotracer uptake identified by Tc-99m O_4 scintigraphy: normal, nonvisualization, ectopic-hypoplastic, and dyshormonogenesis.

1. Normal study: There is radiotracer accumulation in a normal sized, bilobed gland in the normal/expected location of the thyroid bed (**C**).
2. Nonvisualization/absent radiotracer uptake (**A**) is due to primary (agenesis), secondary, or transient hypothyroidism due to maternal TRB-Abs. Ultrasound should be performed when there is absent radiotracer uptake to confirm thyroid agenesis.
3. Ectopic-hypoplasia:
   a. Ectopia: Abnormal radiotracer uptake in an ectopic location, typically sublingual (**B**); occasionally mediastinal; rarely pelvic. Hemiagenesis, a rare form of thyroid dysgenesis in which there is developmental failure of one lobe of the thyroid gland, results in the "hockey stick sign" on scintigraphy which can be confused with an ectopic gland on AP views. Lateral view demonstrates the hemiagenetic gland to be in normal position. While patients with hemiagenesis are clinically euthyroid, they may come to attention in the newborn period due to elevated TSH levels, which are the basis of newborn screening programs.
   b. Hypoplasia: Decreased radiotracer uptake in a small bilobed gland in the normal/expected location of the thyroid bed.
4. Dyshormonogenesis: Markedly increased radiotracer uptake in a bilobed gland in normal/expected location of

the thyroid bed is due either to a defect in T4 synthesis or transient hypothyroidism due to immaturity of the thyroid gland. Enlarged hyperactive glands can also be seen with maternal or neonatal Graves disease but in these cases, T4 should be elevated, not decreased as is present in those with primary CH.

Once CH is confirmed, treatment should be instituted immediately and not delayed until the exact etiology of the hypothyroidism is determined. This is because studies have demonstrated that neurocognitive outcome is worse in infants with CH in whom treatment commenced at a later age (after 30 days of age), in those treated with lower than recommended L-thyroxine doses and in those with more severe hypothyroidism.[2]

Questions for Further Thought

1. Why should one perform scintigraphy and/or ultrasound in the newborn diagnosed with CH rather than just instituting treatment?
2. Which are the preferred radiotracers for performing neonatal thyroid scintigraphy in those patients with presumed primary CH, and what are the advantages and disadvantages of each?

Reporting Responsibilities

The dose and specific radiotracer used should be reported. The report should include a description of the presence, the site, and the degree of radiotracer uptake, as well as the shape of the thyroid gland, if eutopic. If there is absence of radiotracer uptake, ultrasound should be suggested to confirm a presumed diagnosis of thyroid agenesis.

What the Treating Physician Needs to Know

Early diagnosis and treatment of CH are necessary for the prevention of severe mental retardation termed cretinism. Once CH is suggested either clinically or on newborn screening tests and confirmed by serum TSH and free T_4 tests, therapy should be instituted. Ancillary tests—including thyroid scintigraphy, ultrasound to confirm suspected thyroid agenesis, MRI in suspected secondary hypothyroidism, and other specific laboratory evaluations—are then performed at the discretion of an endocrinologist to determine the underlying etiology of the patient's CH.

Answers

1. Although the American Academy of Pediatrics Task Force Report on CH describes newborn thyroid imaging as optional, and while some clinicians believe that the presence, absence, or abnormal location of a thyroid gland does not alter the management of CH,[2] others[1-5] strongly believe that obtaining the maximal diagnostic data offers parents and clinicians the optimal opportunity for the most effective counseling and lifetime management of CH, beginning at birth.[4] Scintigraphy affords the maximal information on the anatomic status of the gland. If an absent (confirmed on thyroid ultrasound) or ectopic-hypoplastic gland is present, parents are informed about the lifelong need for thyroid replacement therapy. If a normal or enlarged eutopic gland is present, the parents are informed that their child will need reevaluation following controlled withdrawal of hormone replacement therapy at an older age (around 3 years) to determine if the neonatal hypothyroidism was a transient phenomenon.

2. Technetium-99m O_4 and I-123 are the preferred radiotracers for thyroid scintigraphy in neonates so as to minimize radioactivity exposure. I-131 should never be used in neonates as it delivers an unacceptably high radiation dose not only to the thyroid but to the whole body.

   Scanning with Tc-99m O_4 has the advantages of being inexpensive, readily available (often on-hand), quick and easy to perform, and nearly always diagnostic, while delivering the lowest radiation dose to the patient. Tc-99m O_4 scans are limited in that they may not be able to diagnose transient hypothyroidism[3] and may occasionally fail to demonstrate a small, poorly functioning eutopic gland.[4] Further, physiologic uptake of Tc-99m O_4 in adjacent salivary glands may confound scan interpretation.[4]

   I-123 is a more physiologic agent than Tc-99m O_4 in that it addresses the global function of the thyroid gland.[3] However, I-123 is more expensive and less readily available than Tc-99m O_4. The scan procedure takes 4 to 6 hours to complete, necessitating several hours of waiting in the clinic between oral administration and imaging. Dyshormonogenesis may not be promptly diagnosed with this technique as iodine uptake may be variable (absent or low), necessitating repeat imaging with perchlorate discharge technique to confirm the diagnosis.[3] While radiation exposure is within acceptable limits, it is higher than that imparted by Tc-99m O_4 scans.

REFERENCES

1. LaFranchi S. Congenital hypothyroidism: Etiologies, diagnosis, and management. *Thyroid.* 1999;9(7):735–740.

2. Rastogi MV, LaFranchi SH. Congenital hypothyroidism. *Orphanet J Rare Dis.* 2010;5:17.

3. Sfakianakis GN, Ezuddin SH, Sanchez JE, et al. Pertechnetate scintigraphy in primary congenital hypothyroidism. *J Nucl Med.* 1999;40(5):799–804.

4. Schoen EJ, Clapp W, To TT, et al. The key role of newborn thyroid scintigraphy with isotopic iodide (^{123}I) in defining and managing congenital hypothyroidism. *Pediatrics.* 2004;114(6): e683–e688.

5. Chang YW, Lee DH, Hong YH, et al. Congenital hypothyroidism: Analysis of discordant US and scintigraphic findings. *Radiology.* 2011;258(3):872–879.

CLINICAL HISTORY *A 14-year-old child with history of syncope (Figs 5.38A and B)*

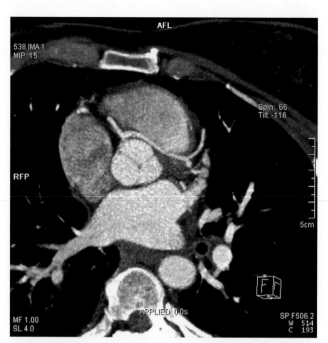

FIGURE 5.38A

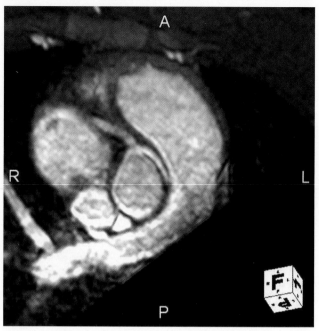

FIGURE 5.38B

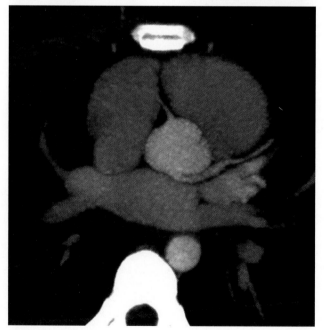

FIGURE 5.38C

FINDINGS Axial CT image and 3D steady-state free-precession (SSFP) MR sequence show anomalous origin of the left coronary artery (LCA) from the right coronary artery (RCA) and right aortic cusp, respectively, with interarterial course subsequently (**A** and **B**). For comparison, axial CT slice in a different patient (**C**) demonstrates normal coronary artery origins, with LCA arising from the left aortic cusp and the RCA arising from the right aortic cusp.

DIFFERENTIAL DIAGNOSIS None

DIAGNOSIS Anomalous left coronary artery origin

DISCUSSION Coronary anomalies are generally picked up incidentally in asymptomatic children; however, a small percentage present with syncope, chest pain, and even sudden cardiac arrest. Multidetector CT angiography (MDCTA) has fast acquisition time, volume imaging, high temporal and spatial resolution allowing better visualization of the origin and course of anomalous coronary artery. With SSFP MR sequence, which can be performed as a 3D acquisition, one can generate motion-free images using MRI as well. The classification for anomalous left coronary origin includes anomalous LCA from left main pulmonary artery (ALCAPA), LCA arising from the right aortic cusp or RCA, single coronary artery anomalies, and absent LCA with separate origins of the left anterior descending and circumflex arteries. The anomalous LCA can course between the aorta and MPA (interarterial), within the wall of the vessel (intra-arterial), or even have a segment which dives into the myocardium (bridge). This anomaly is not uncommonly symptomatic and is usually surgically repaired. ALCAPA presents very early in the neonatal age and may be associated with ASD, VSD, and coarctation.

Question for Further Thought

1. What is the most common form of ALCAPA?

Reporting Responsibilities

Anomaly of LCA origin, and anomalous course.

What the Treating Physician Needs to Know

- Type of coronary anomaly
- Interarterial course
- Associated congenital heart abnormalities

Answer

1. Bland–White–Garland syndrome where LCA arises from the MPA and the RCA from the aorta.

REFERENCE

1. Tariq R, Kureshi SB, Siddiqui UT, et al. Congenital anomalies of coronary arteries: Diagnosis with 64-slice multidetector CT. *Eur J Radiol.* 2011; July 11.

Prakash Masand

CLINICAL HISTORY *A 15-year-old girl with low-grade fever and recent weight loss*

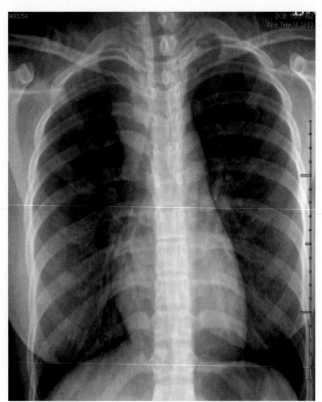

FIGURE **5.39A**

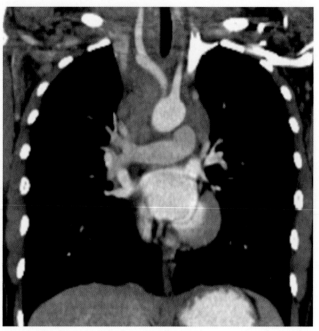

FIGURE **5.39B**

FINDINGS Frontal film of the chest (**A**) with abnormal right paratracheal density. CT chest (**B**) shows enlarged nonnecrotic mediastinal lymph nodes.

DIFFERENTIAL DIAGNOSIS Neoplasms such as lymphoma, metastases, infectious etiologies

DIAGNOSIS Hodgkin lymphoma

DISCUSSION Lymphomas account for 10% to 15% of childhood cancers and Hodgkin lymphoma has bimodal age distribution with a peak in second decade and after the age of 50. Hodgkin lymphoma is very rare under age 5. It presents with painless cervical, supraclavicular, or axillary adenopathy and at least two-third of children have mediastinal involvement. Plain radiographs show involvement of mediastinum and lungs. Contrast chest CT documents extent, allows staging, and shows parenchymal, pleural, or pericardial disease. Role of positron emission tomography (PET) CT is unclear and may be of benefit in follow-up of tumor burden and establishing the need for radiation.

Questions for Further Thought

1. What does Ann Arbor staging system take into account?
2. How often does one get lung involvement in Hodgkin lymphoma?

Reporting Responsibilities

Important to document extent of disease before therapy.

What the Treating Physician Needs to Know

Is the tumor volume bulky? (Defined as ratio of maximum tumor diameter to chest diameter at the level of diaphragm being more than one-third)

Answers

1. Infradiaphragmatic tumor burden/systemic symptoms.
2. 5% to 10% patients.

REFERENCES

1. Siegel M, ed. *Pediatric Body CT.* 2nd ed. Philadelphia, PA: Lippincott Williams & Wilkins; 2007.
2. Toma P, Granata C, Rossi A, et al. Multimodality imaging of Hodgkin disease and non-Hodgkin lymphomas in children. *Radiographics.* 2007;27:1335–1354.

CASE 5.40

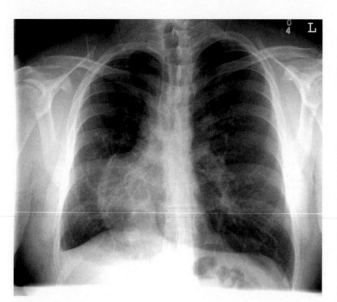

FIGURE **5.40A**

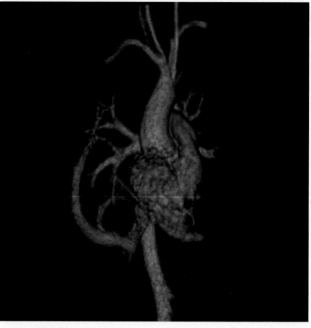

FIGURE **5.40B**

FINDINGS (**A**) Frontal radiograph of the chest demonstrates a small right hemithorax and a rightward mediastinal shift. The curvilinear density in the right lower lung represents an anomalous vein resembling a Turkish scimitar. (**B**) 3D volume-rendered image demonstrates the anomalous vein on the right draining into the IVC.

DIFFERENTIAL DIAGNOSIS Scimitar syndrome, lung hypoplasia, partial anomalous pulmonary venous connection (PAPVC).

DIAGNOSIS Scimitar syndrome (hypogenetic lung syndrome/venolobar syndrome)

DISCUSSION The first reported Cooper published case of Scimitar syndrome in 1836. There has a slight female preponderance with variable presentation ranging from respiratory insufficiency, cardiac failure, pulmonary hypertension, recurrent respiratory infections, and heart murmur. The syndrome typically consists of hypoplasia of the right lung, dextrorotation of the heart, hypoplasia of the right pulmonary artery, anomalous arterial supply to the lower lobe by the aorta or its branches below the level of the diaphragm, and anomalous venous drainage of all or part of the right lung to the IVC. The descending anomalous pulmonary vein is visible as a curvilinear density along the right heart, reminding a Turkish sword on the chest radiograph. Other associations include hemivertebrae, abnormal bronchial anatomy, ASD and VSD, coarctation of the aorta, dextrocardia, and genitourinary tract anomalies. Two different types of the syndrome are identified, an infantile form that presents with congestive heart failure due to right ventricular volume overload from a left to right shunt and an adult form, detected after the first year of life and often mildly symptomatic.

Question for Further Thought

1. Where does the anomalous venous drainage occur?

Reporting Responsibilities

Diagnose-associated anomalies

What the Treating Physician Needs to Know

- Anatomic depiction of anomalous arterial supply and venous drainage pattern
- Degree of left to right shunting, quantified with cardiac MR in conjunction with 2D echocardiography
- Presence of associated anomalies

Answer

1. IVC, azygous vein, coronary sinus, right atrium, hepatic veins or portal vein.

REFERENCE

1. Berrocal T, Madrid C, Novo S, et al. Congenital anomalies of the tracheobronchial tree, lung, and mediastinum: Embryology, radiology, and pathology. *Radiographics.* 2004;24(1):e17.

Prakash Masand

CLINICAL HISTORY *A 16-year-old child with bilateral lung masses and known testicular primary*

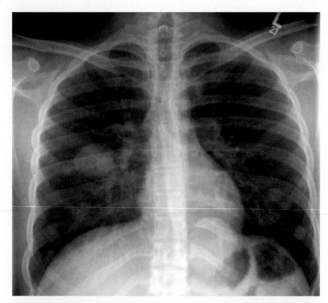

FIGURE **5.41A**

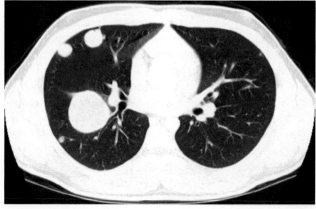

FIGURE **5.41B**

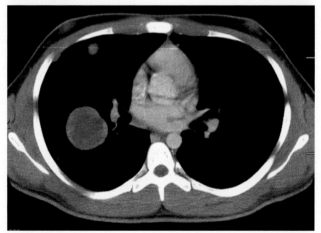

FIGURE **5.41C**

FINDINGS Frontal chest film shows bilateral round opacities concerning for metastases (**A**). Lung and mediastinal soft-tissue windows from a chest CT demonstrate non-calcific, discrete mass lesions suggesting metastases (**B** and **C**).

DIFFERENTIAL DIAGNOSIS Pulmonary metastases, Wegener granulomatosis, septic emboli, rheumatoid nodules, juvenile respiratory papillomatosis

DIAGNOSIS Pulmonary metastases

DISCUSSION Pulmonary metastases account for approximately 80% of all lung tumors in children and more than 95% of malignant tumors. The common tumors known to metastasize to lungs include Wilms tumor, testicular germ cell tumors, hepatoblastoma, and sarcomas such as osteogenic sarcoma, rhabdomyosarcoma, and rarely neuroblastoma. Wilms tumor and osteogenic sarcoma are the most frequently implicated malignancies. Lung metastases appear as single or multiple well-circumscribed nodules, variable in size, often peripheral, and preferentially involving the lower lobes in those with a hematogenous spread. A reticular or miliary pattern may occur with those demonstrating lymphangitic spread. Cavitation and pneumothorax are rare but are most often associated with Wilms tumor, Hodgkin lymphoma, and osteosarcoma. Osteosarcoma metastases can show calcification. While some metastatic lung nodules are excised for diagnosis and staging, others are removed as part of oncologic management to achieve long-term survival and effect cure.

Question for Further Thought

1. Lung metastases from which primary carry a poor prognosis?

Reporting Responsibilities

Location of metastases, presence of calcification or cavitation.

What the Treating Physician Needs to Know

• Number of lesions
• Associated pneumothorax, pleural and chest wall involvement
• Change on follow-up imaging

Answer

1. Rhabdomyosarcoma.

REFERENCE

1. Dishop MK, Kuruvilla S. Primary and metastatic lung tumors in the pediatric population: A review and 25-year experience at a large children's hospital. *Arch Pathol Lab Med.* 2008;132(7): 1079–1103.

CLINICAL HISTORY *A 3-year-old boy with fever and cough*

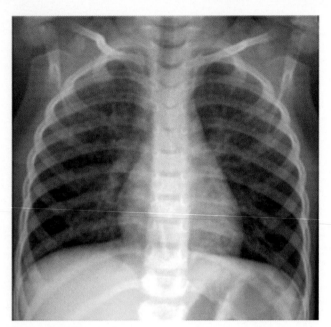

Figure **5.42A**

FINDINGS Frontal and lateral chest radiographs (**A** and **B**) show hyperinflated lungs with perihilar opacities.

DIFFERENTIAL DIAGNOSIS Bacterial versus viral pneumonia

DIAGNOSIS Viral pneumonia

DISCUSSION Pneumonia in children can be bacterial or viral and respiratory syncitial virus (RSV) being the common viral agent in children <5 years of age. RSV pneumo-

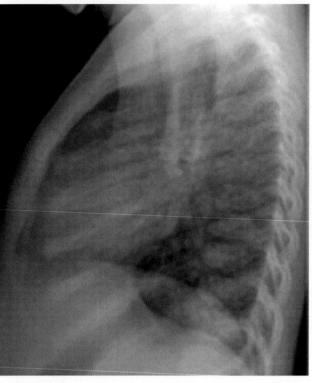

Figure **5.42B**

nia is highly contagious, spreading via droplet and fomite exposure. The infection is more common during the winter months, and presents as outbreaks in hospitals and long-term care facilities. Immunocompromised children are at a greater risk. The plain radiographic findings are nonspecific and diagnosis of viral pneumonia is suggested when the following are visualized: symmetrically hyperaerated lungs (lungs seen up to the level of the 10th rib posteriorly), interstitial process seen as bronchial wall thickening (peribronchitis) radiating from the hila centrally, and linear subsegmental atelectasis. The presence of a more focal alveolar infiltrate (airspace consolidation with air bronchograms) is suspicious for superimposed bacterial pneumonia. Viral pneumonia cannot be reliably differentiated from bacterial pneumonia by radiography; however, a more focal area of consolidation leans more toward a bacterial etiology, and justifies the subsequent use of antibiotics.

Question for Further Thought

1. What are some common causative agents of viral pneumonia?

Reporting Responsibilities

Presence of focal alveolar pneumonic infiltrate on chest film.

What the Treating Physician Needs to Know

• Presence of a focal airspace opacity to suggest bacterial etiology.
• Other pathologic processes such as pleural effusion, associated mass, and so on.

Answer

1. Respiratory syncitial, adenovirus, parainfluenza, and rhinovirus.

REFERENCES

1. Donnelly LF. Maximizing the usefulness of imaging in children with community acquired pneumonia. *AJR Am J Roentgenol.* 1999;172(2):505–512.
2. Virkki R, Juven T, Rikalainen H, et al. Differentiation of bacterial and viral pneumonia in children. *Thorax.* 2002;57(5): 438–441.

CASE 5.43

CLINICAL HISTORY *A 4-year-old male with incidental finding*

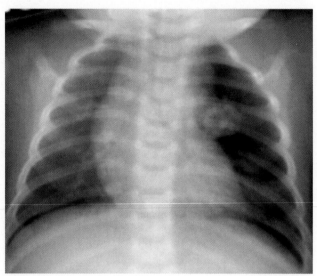

FIGURE **5.43A**

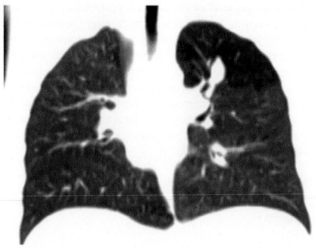

FIGURE **5.43B**

FINDINGS (**A**) Frontal radiograph demonstrates a hyperlucent left upper lobe with ill-defined density radiating from the left hilar region. (**B**) CT lung window image demonstrates a tubular dense structure near the left hilum (bronchocele) with hyperlucent left upper lobe.

DIFFERENTIAL DIAGNOSIS Bronchial atresia, congenital lobar emphysema (CLE), CPAM, bronchogenic cyst, pulmonary sequestration.

DIAGNOSIS Bronchial atresia

DISCUSSION Bronchial atresia was first described by Ramsay and Byron in 1953. It is a rare anomaly that occurs due to atresia of a proximal bronchus that lacks communication to central airways. The terminal airways beyond the obliterated bronchus are normal. In fact, the portion of the lung distal to this abnormal bronchus demonstrates air trapping resulting in hyperinflation. The air trapping is secondary to air supply from the adjacent lung segments via collateral pathways. The apicoposterior segmental bronchus of the left upper lobe is most commonly involved, followed by the right upper lobe, left lower lobe, right middle lobe, and right lower lobe in that order. The etiology may be related to an in utero traumatic or ischemic insult to the bronchial wall, or separation of distal bronchial cells from the proximal bronchial bud. The classic chest radiographic appearance is a branching tubular opacity near the hilum, which represents mucus plugging of a dilated subsegmental bronchus distal to the atretic portion, also called bronchocele. There is associated hyperlucency of the lung around this bronchocele. This entity is usually found incidentally on chest radiographs or CT scans in the second or third decade; however, occasionally, there is a history of asthma, pneumonia, chest pain, or dyspnea. In children, it may be rarely associated with respiratory distress. Usually no further treatment is required.

Question for Further Thought

1. Can bronchial atresia coexist with type 2 CPAM/sequestration?

What the Treating Physician Needs to Know

- Is it congenital bronchial atresia
- Which bronchus and corresponding lobes/segments are involved
- Coexisting lesions, if any

Answer

1. Yes, and these are then referred to as hybrid lesions.

REFERENCES

1. Berrocal T, Madrid C, Novo S, et al. Congenital anomalies of the tracheobronchial tree, lung and mediastinum: Embryology, radiology, and pathology. *Radiographics.* 2004;24(1):e17.
2. Desir A, Ghaye B. Congenital abnormalities of intrathoracic airways. *Radiol Clin North Am.* 2009;47(2):203–225.

Prakash Masand

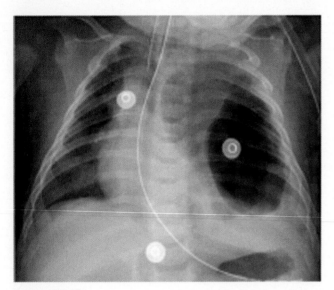

FIGURE **5.44A**

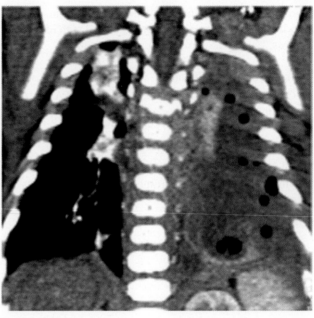

FIGURE **5.44B**

FINDINGS Frontal chest radiograph showing a left pleural effusion and mediastinal deviation to the right (Fig. 5.44**A**). Coronal soft-tissue window from a CT shows a left pleural collection with air and enhancing pleural margin, compatible with an empyema (Fig. 5.44**B**).

DIFFERENTIAL DIAGNOSIS Empyema, pleural effusion, necrotizing pneumonia

DIAGNOSIS Left-sided empyema

DISCUSSION A parapneumonic effusion containing pus is termed as an empyema. The American Thoracic Society (ATS) divides the empyema process into three stages: (1) exudative where pleural fluid has low cell content, (2) fibrinopurulent in which frank pus is present, and (3) organizing phase where there is a thick peel formed by fibroblasts. On plain radiography, there is partial or complete opacification of the hemithorax, with or without a mediastinal shift. On ultrasound, there is a septated fluid collection, with consolidation of the underlying lung. CT demonstrates fluid collection, pleural enhancement, and thickening (split pleura sign), increased density in the extrapleural fat, loculation, foci of air, and underlying parenchymal changes. Septations are not visible on CT and may not be able to differentiate simple effusion from an empyema. Hence, ultrasound is better at differentiating transudative from exudative pleural fluid collection, and is used to guide treatment as well. Drainage of a pleural collection depends upon whether it is enlarging in size or compromising respiratory function.

Questions for Further Thought

1. Is empyema frequently associated with pneumonia?
2. What are the management options for empyema?

Reporting Responsibilities

Suggest the diagnosis based on CT criteria, ultrasound finding of loculations and septations leans toward empyema formation.

What the Treating Physician Needs to Know

- Is the fluid loculated
- Are there septations within the collection
- Are there underlying abnormality, such as necrotizing pneumonia, and bronchopleural fistula

Answers

1. Yes.
2. Insertion of a drain with or without fibrinolytics, limited open decortication, and video-assisted thoracoscopic surgery (VATS).

REFERENCES

1. Jaffe A, Calder AD, Owens CM, et al. Role of routine computed tomography in paediatric pleural empyema. *Thorax.* 2008;63:897–902.
2. Calder A, Owens CM. Imaging of parapneumonic pleural effusions and empyema in children. *Pediatr Radiol.* 2009;39:527–537.

CASE 5.45

CLINICAL HISTORY *Premature infant with respiratory distress*

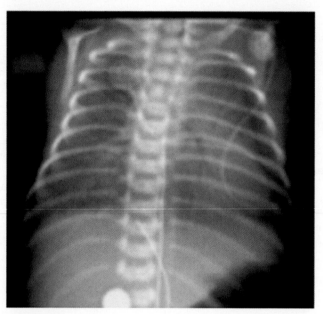

FIGURE **5.45**

FINDINGS Frontal chest film shows a diffuse granular pattern in a 2-day-old neonate (Fig. 5.45).

DIFFERENTIAL DIAGNOSIS Surfactant deficiency, pneumonia, pulmonary edema, meconium aspiration

DIAGNOSIS Surfactant deficiency

DISCUSSION Surfactant deficiency or hyaline membrane disease (HMD) affects premature infants and infants of diabetic mothers. The problem is lack of surfactant lipoprotein superimposed on lung immaturity. Clinically, they have tachypnea, cyanosis, and retractions in a few minutes after birth. The early radiographic findings include underaeration of lungs with diffuse bilateral reticular and granular opacities. Later, a more generalized opacification or complete whiteout pattern is seen. This may be due to edema, pneumonia, hemorrhage, or atelectasis. Clinical use of artificial surfactant has been an important therapeutic advance. It is given at birth with more frequent doses in the first 24 to 48 hours after birth. This has reduced the need for long-term high-pressure ventilation and high oxygen concentration. Barotrauma from high-frequency ventilation is a problem and causes complications such as PIE and pneumothorax.

Question for Further Thought

1. What is the associated problem in patients with surfactant deficiency that contributes to the lung disease?

Reporting Responsibilities

Recognize the reticulonodular pattern in premature neonates to suggest surfactant deficiency

What the Treating Physician Needs to Know

- Degree of lung inflation and presence of atelectasis

- Signs of barotrauma in the form of a PIE, pneumothorax, or pneumomediastinum
- Position of the endotracheal tube

Answer

1. Patent ductus arteriosus.

REFERENCE

1. Baert AL, Knauth M, Sartor K. Radiological Imaging of the Neonatal Chest. 2nd revised ed. Springer, New York; 67–70.

CLINICAL HISTORY *A 6-month-old male with respiratory distress*

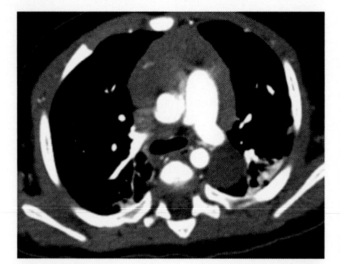

FIGURE **5.46A**

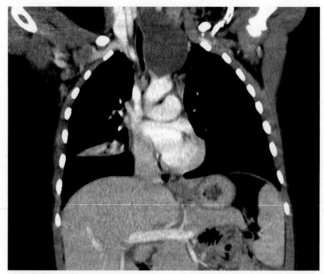

FIGURE **5.46B**

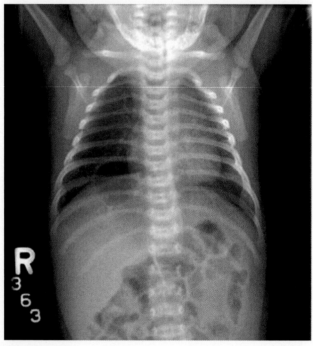

FIGURE **5.46C**

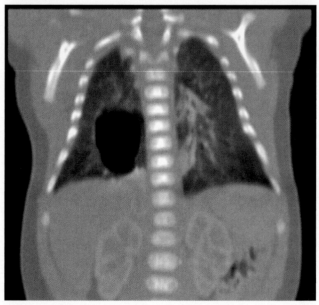

FIGURE **5.46D**

FINDINGS (**A**) Discrete nonenhancing low-density mass arising in the mediastinum at the carinal level. (**B**) Low attenuation mass in the lower neck and mediastinum, causing airway compression, pathologically proven bronchogenic cyst. (**C**) Frontal chest radiograph showing right lower lobe parenchymal cyst lesion. (**D**) Intrapulmonary bronchogenic cyst on CT.

DIFFERENTIAL DIAGNOSIS Bronchogenic cyst, other bronchopulmonary foregut malformation such as duplication cyst, round pneumonia, neurenteric cyst, CPAM

DIAGNOSIS Bronchogenic cyst (bronchopulmonary foregut malformation)

DISCUSSION Bronchogenic cysts arise due to abnormal budding of primitive ventral foregut and the airway, are lined by respiratory epithelium, and contain proteinaceous or serous fluid. Almost 70% are located in the middle or posterior mediastinum, with intraparenchymal (lung) and lower neck being other sites. Within the mediastinum, they may be hilar, carinal, or paratracheal with carinal being the most frequent location. These cysts typically do not communicate with the airway but if they do, can contain air and have air/fluid levels secondary to infection. Bronchogenic cysts are found incidentally or with history of cough, wheezing, stridor, and pneumonia from airway compression. On non-contrast-enhanced CT and T1-weighted MRI sequences, they can have slightly higher attenuation than water or bright signal, respectively, due to proteinaceous fluid within. The cyst contents do not enhance. Thick enhancing wall and air/fluid levels can be seen if infected. These lesions are resected due to potential for hemorrhage, infection, and rupture.

Question for Further Thought

1. Do bronchogenic cysts occur in sites such as the retroperitoneum and base of the tongue?

Reporting Responsibilities
Correct diagnosis (age and location are fairly typical)

What the Treating Physician Needs to Know

- Location and internal characteristics of mass lesion
- Is the mass responsible for airway compression

Answer

1. Yes, rarely.

REFERENCE

1. Kocaoğlu M, Frush DP, Uğurel MS, et al. Bronchopulmonary foregut malformations presenting as mass lesions in children: Spectrum of imaging. *Diagn Interv Radiol.* 2010;16:153–161.

CASE 5.47

CLINICAL HISTORY *A 1-day-old infant with tachypnea and grunting*

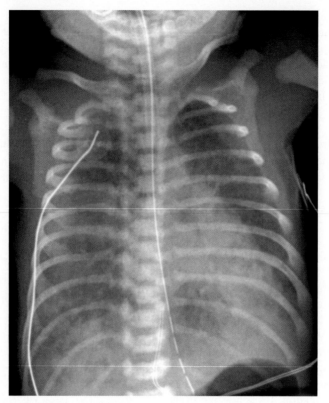

FIGURE **5.47**

FINDINGS Hyperaerated lungs with diffuse reticulonodular opacities scattered throughout both lungs. No pleural effusion.

DIFFERENTIAL DIAGNOSIS Neonatal pneumonia, meconium aspiration, respiratory distress syndrome, TTN, pulmonary edema

DIAGNOSIS Neonatal pneumonia

DISCUSSION Neonatal pneumonia is not very common and underlying risk factors include maternal chorioamnionitis and prematurity. The routes of infection include hematogenous and ascending infection via infected amniotic fluid while passage through the birth canal. It will present in the first 24 hours with severe respiratory problems. Plain radiography shows diffuse homogeneous opacities within both lungs and it may be difficult to differentiate from HMD in a premature child. Also reticulonodular pattern can be seen, with symmetrically hyperaerated lungs. There may be an associated pleural effusion. More focal airspace consolidation is unusual this early on. If the infection is systemic, other organ systems maybe involved. Evaluation includes cultures of blood and tracheal aspirate, chest x-ray, and full evaluation for sepsis, including a lumbar puncture.

Question for Further Thought

1. What is the most common cause of early onset pneumonia occurring right after birth?

Reporting Responsibilities

Include neonatal pneumonia in differential with mentioned radiographic features in the right clinical setting.

What the Treating Physician Needs to Know

- Abnormality on the chest radiograph
- Associated pleural effusion
- Involvement of other sites

Answer

1. Generalized sepsis with implicated organism being gram-positive cocci such as *Staphylococcus aureus* or gram-negative bacilli such as *Escherichia coli.*

REFERENCES

1. Slovis TL. *Caffey's Pediatric Diagnostic Imaging.* 11th ed. Philadelphia, PA:Mosby Elsevier; 2008;1:120–122.
2. Haney PJ, Bohlman M, Sun CC. Radiographic findings in neonatal pneumonia. *AJR Am J Roentgenol.* 1984;143(1):23–26.

CLINICAL HISTORY *A 10-year-old child with chronic cough (Fig. 5.48A)*

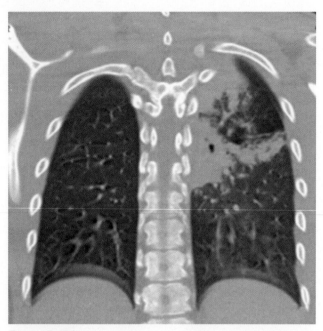

FIGURE **5.48A**

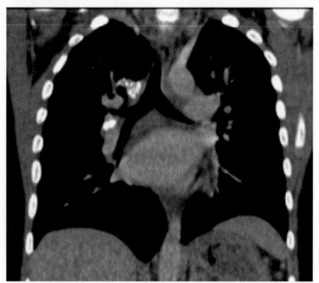

FIGURE **5.48C**

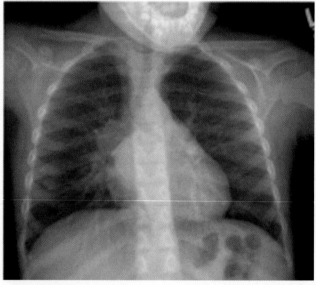

FIGURE **5.48B**

FINDINGS Lung windows from a chest CT show patchy left upper lung alveolar infiltrates with centrilobular nodularity (**A**). Frontal chest radiograph shows right hilar adenopathy in a different child with H/O tuberculosis (TB) (**B**). Coronal CT images show right hilar calcific nodes in a third patient with old pulmonary TB (**C**).

DIFFERENTIAL DIAGNOSIS Infectious etiologies such as TB, fungal disease, and atypical mycobacteria. Histoplasmosis and postradiation change if calcific nodes in mediastinum

DIAGNOSIS Pulmonary TB

DISCUSSION Pulmonary TB is not common in the US. Immunocompromised children are a greater risk, and clinical presentation is variable with low-grade fever, cough, malaise, and loss of weight being common. The causative organism is *Mycobacterium tuberculosis* and caseation necrosis is typical within lesions, particularly with nodal disease. About 20% to 30% develop extrapulmonary TB with lymph nodal disease and meningitis as the usual presentations. The primary complex develops after inhalation of the bacillus, which multiplies and spreads via lymphatics (local adenopathy and contiguous parenchymal disease) or hematogenously (extrapulmonary spread). The plain films in active TB show lymph node enlargement, consolidation, nodules, and miliary pattern. Cavitation within nodular infiltrates is common. Bronchiectasis and tracheobronchial stenosis are other findings. Complicating features include empyema, pneumothorax, pericarditis, and fibrosing mediastinitis.

Question for Further Thought

1. What is Pott disease?

Reporting Responsibilities

Include TB in differential if involvement of nodes and multifocal upper lobe predominant lung infiltrates, nodules, cavitary lesions.

What the Treating Physician Needs to Know

- Presence of necrotic nodes and parenchymal changes
- Pleural, pericardial, and chest wall complications
- Extrapulmonary spread

Answer

1. TB spondylitis caused by hematogenous spread, usually affecting the lower thoracic spine.

REFERENCE

1. Fonseca-Santos J. Tuberculosis in children. *Eur. J Radiol.* 2005; 55:202–208.

Prakash Masand

CLINICAL HISTORY *A 15-year-old child with hepatomegaly and abnormality on chest radiograph*

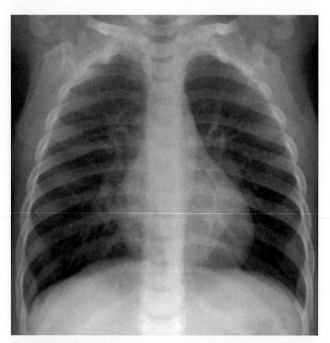

FIGURE 5.49A

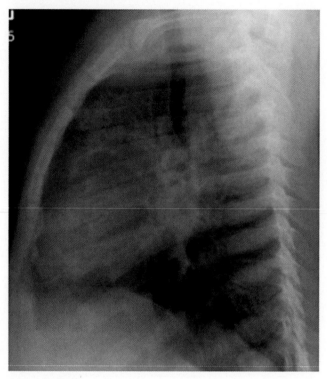

FIGURE 5.49B

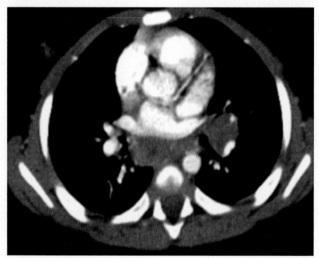

FIGURE 5.49C

FINDINGS (**A** and **B**) Frontal and lateral chest film with hilar enlargement. (**C**) Axial CT image showing hilar and mediastinal lymphadenopathy.

DIFFERENTIAL DIAGNOSIS Sarcoidoisis, postinfectious cat-scratch disease, lymphoma, leukemia

DIAGNOSIS Childhood sarcoidosis

DISCUSSION Sarcoidosis in children is a rare multisystem disorder, with slightly higher incidence in African Americans, and mean age at presentation being 14 years even though the range is wider. The etiology is unknown and diagnosis is based on clinical findings and pathologic evidence of noncaseating granulomas in the affected organ. Like in adults, the radiographic features include hilar and mediastinal lymphadenopathy. Lung parenchymal involvement is common and high-resolution chest CT shows septal line thickening, perilymphatic distribution of nodules, and even fibrosis. Pleural effusion may be seen. Cutaneous lesions, hepatosplenomegaly, and peripheral lymphadenopathy are other features. Early onset childhood sarcoidosis is typically seen before 1 year of age, and presents with ocular problems such as uveitis. Liver, spleen, and lymph nodes are also involved. The overall prognosis is good with mainstay of treatment being oral corticosteroids.

Question for Further Thought

1. What is the definitive diagnostic test for childhood sarcoidosis?

Reporting Responsibilities

Multisystem involvement with characteristic hilar lymphadenopathy should raise the concern for sarcoidosis.

What the Treating Physician Needs to Know

- Distribution of lymphadenopathy within the chest
- Other sites of involvement in the body
- Easiest site for tissue biopsy

Answer

1. Tissue sampling from an involved organ generally provides an answer.

REFERENCES

1. Shetty AK, Gedalia A. Childhood sarcoidosis: A rare but fascinating disorder. *Pediatr Rheumatol Online J.* 2008;6:16.
2. Milman N, Hoffmann AL. Childhood sarcoidosis: Long term follow-up. *Eur Respir J.* 2008;31(3):592–598.

CLINICAL HISTORY *A 12-year-old boy with fever and cervical lymphadenopathy*

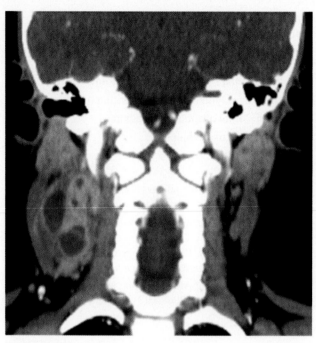

FIGURE **5.50A**

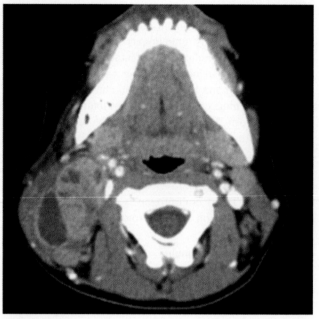

FIGURE **5.50B**

FINDINGS Coronal and axial contrast-enhanced CT neck images (**A** and **B**) show enlarged necrotic cervical nodes.

DIFFERENTIAL DIAGNOSIS Cat-scratch disease, infection including TB, neoplasms such as lymphoma, metastatic lesions.

DIAGNOSIS Cat-scratch disease

DISCUSSION Cat-scratch disease is characterized by regional adenopathy, often painful, commonly involving cervical and axillary nodes with spontaneous resolution within 3 months. Young adults are affected with recent exposure to a cat/kit-

ten, and causative agent is *Bartonella henselae.* About 10% to 35% nodes progress to suppuration and imaging shows central hypodensity on CT or heterogeneity on ultrasound. Multiple hypodense lesions representing granulomas develop in the liver/spleen with or without hepatosplenomegaly. Serologic tests and PCR from nodal biopsy are confirmatory. Antibiotics are not indicated unless immunocompromised.

Questions for Further Thought
1. What does systemic infection with *B. henselae* cause?
2. What is typical about the lymphadenopathy in cat-scratch disease?

Reporting Responsibilities

Include cat-scratch disease as one of the differentials with the imaging findings of necrotic appearing enlarged lymph nodes, especially in a young adult or child.

What the Treating Physician Needs to Know

With high index of suspicion for this disease, ask about history of exposure to a cat/kitten and perform appropriate serologic tests

Answers

1. Systemic infection causes cutaneous vascular lesions (bacillary angiomatosis), subcutaneous nodules, and osteolytic lesions.

2. The enlarged nodes proximal to site of inoculation have necrosis and surrounding edema.

REFERENCES

1. Wang CW, Chang WC, Chao TK, et al. Computed tomography and magnetic resonance imaging of cat-scratch disease: A report of two cases. *Clin Imaging.* 2009;33:318–321.

2. Hopkins KL, Simoneaux SF, Patrick LE, et al. Imaging manifestations of cat-scratch disease. *AJR Am J Roentgenol.* 1996; 166:435–438.

Note: Page number followed by f denotes figure.